RURAL NURSING

CONCEPTS, THEORY, AND PRACTICE

2nd Edition

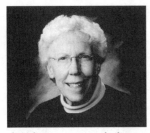

Helen J. Lee, PhD, RN, is a Professor Emeritus in the College of Nursing, Montana State University-Bozeman, Missoula Campus. She holds a BSN and Masters of Nursing from Montana State College, Bozeman and a PhD in nursing from The University of Texas at Austin. Her research interests are in rural, gerontological, and end-of-life issues, rural nursing theory development, and the variables of hardiness, perception of health, and mobility. Her memberships include the American Nurses' Association, Oncology Nursing Society, National Rural Health Association, Rural Nurse Organization, Western Institute of Nursing, Zeta Upsilon Chapter of Sigma Theta Tau International, and charter member of the International Council of Nursing—Rural and Remote Nurses Network.

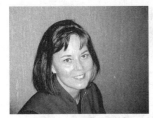

Charlene A. Winters, DNSc, APRN, BC, is an Associate Professor in the College of Nursing at Montana State University-Bozeman, Missoula Campus. She is Interim Coordinator of the Clinical Nurse Specialist Programs and Associate Director of the Center for Research on Chronic Health Conditions in Rural Dwellers (CRCHC). Dr. Winters' research interests are illness uncertainty, chronic illness self-management, and rural nursing theory development. She is an active member of the American Association of Critical Care Nurses, the Western Institute of Nursing, the Montana Association of Clinical Nurse Specialists, Sigma Theta Tau International, and charter member of the International Council of Nursing—Rural and Remote Nurses Network. Dr. Winters holds a doctorate degree in Nursing Science from Rush University, Chicago, Illinois, and a bachelor and a master's degree of science in nursing from California State University, Long Beach.

RURAL NURSING

CONCEPTS, THEORY, AND PRACTICE

2nd Edition

Helen J. Lee, PhD, RN
Charlene A. Winters, DNSc, APRN, BC
Editors

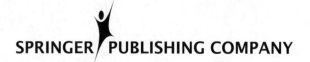

SPRINGER PUBLISHING COMPANY

Springer Publishing Company, Inc.
11 West 42nd Street
New York, NY 10036

Acquisitions Editor: Ruth Chasek
Production Editor: Sara Yoo
Cover design by Mimi Flow
Cover photo by Kay Rosenthal
Typeset by Straight Creek Bookmakers, Boulder, CO

06 07 08 09 10 / 5 4 3 2

Library of Congress Cataloging-in-Publication-Data

Rural nursing : concepts, theory, and practice/edited by Helen J. Lee &
   Charlene A. Winters.—2nd ed.
      p. ; cm.
   Rev. ed. of : Conceptual basis for rural nursing. c1998.
   Includes bibliographical references and index.
   ISBN 0-8261-6955-4
   1. Rural nursing.   I. Lee, Helen J., PhD.   II. Winters, Charlene A.
   III. Conceptual basis for rural nursing.
   [DNLM: 1. Nursing.   2. Rural Health Services.   WY 101 R9485
   2006]
   RT120.R87C66 2006
   610.73'43—dc22
                                                              2005021589

Printed in the United States of America by Bang Printing.

This book is dedicated to Meg K. McDonagh and Elizabeth H. (Betty) Thomlinson (deceased 2004), her mentor, from the University of Calgary, Alberta, Canada, who inspired the continuation of the rural nursing theory development activity that began at Montana State University-Bozeman College of Nursing nearly three decades ago.

by 1/ 22

by 1/22 yd   9.14.22.
221-12.

Contents

Editorial Board   x

Contributors   xi

Preface   xix

Acknowledgments   xxiii

Part I. The Rural Nursing Theory Base

1   Rural Nursing: Developing the Theory Base   3
    Kathleen Ann Long and Clarann Weinert

2   Examining the Rural Nursing Theory Base   17
    Helen J. Lee and Meg K. McDonagh

3   Exploring Rural Nursing Theory Across Borders   27
    *Charlene A. Winters, Elizabeth H. Thomlinson, Chad
    O'Lynn, Helen J. Lee, Meg K. McDonagh, Dana S. Edge, and
    Marlene A. Reimer*

Part II. Perspectives of Rural Persons

4   Old-Timers   43
    Robin L. Boland and Helen J. Lee

5   Health Needs and Perceptions of Rural Persons   53
    Ronda L. Bales, Charlene A. Winters, and Helen J. Lee

6   Health Perceptions, Needs, and Behaviors of Remote Rural
    Women of Childbearing and Childrearing Age   66
    Ronda L. Bales

7   Rural and Remote Women Developing Resilience to Manage
    Vulnerability   79
    Beverly D. Leipert

8   Strategizing Safety: Perinatal Experiences of Rural Women   96
    Katharine S. West

9   Rural Family Health: Enduring Acts of Balancing   110
    Sonja J. Meiers, Sandra K. Eggenberger, Norma K. Krumwiede,
    Mary M. Bliesmer, and Patricia A. Earle

Part III. The Rural Dweller and Response to Illness

10 Patterns of Responses to Symptoms in Rural Residents:
    The Symptom-Action-Time-Line Process   129
    Janice A. Buehler, Maureen Malone, and
    Janis M. Majerus-Wegerhoff

11 Updating the Symptom-Action-Time-Line Process   138
    Chad O'Lynn

12 The Chronic Illness Experience of Isolated Rural Women:
    Use of an Online Support Group Intervention   153
    Charlene A. Winters and Therese Sullivan

13 Acceptability: One Component in Choice of
    Health Care Provider   166
    Jean Shreffler-Grant

Part IV. Rural Nursing Practice

14 The Distinctive Nature and Scope of Rural Nursing Practice:
    Philosophical Bases   179
    Jane Ellis Scharff

15 Rural Health Professionals' Perceptions of Lack of Anonymity   197
    Susan J. Raph and Janice A. Buehler

16 The Rural Nursing Generalist in Community Health   205
    Linda E. Troyer and Helen J. Lee

17 The Rural Nursing Generalist in the Acute Care Setting:
    Flowing Like a River   218
    Kathryn (Kay) Ayres Rosenthal

18 Men Working as Rural Nurses: Land of Opportunity   232
    Chad O'Lynn

19 Continuing Education and Rural Nurses   248
    Lori Hendrickx

Part V. Rural Public Health

20 Public Health Emergency Preparedness in Rural or
Frontier Areas 259
Sandra K. Kuntz, Jane Smilie, and Melanie Reynolds

21 Environmental Risk Reduction for Rural Children 270
Wade G. Hill and Patricia Butterfield

22 Rural School Health: Who Covers for the Rural School Nurse
When There is None? 282
Laurie Bernhardt Glover

23 Improving the Health Literacy of Rural Elders:
An Interdisciplinary Approach 291
*M. Susan Jones, Marilyn M. Gardner, Janelle A. Peeler, Serena
Merry Britt, and Marilyn Lewis Graves*

24 The Culture of Rural Communities: An Examination of Rural
Nursing Concepts at the Community Level 301
Nancy Findholt

Part VI. Looking Ahead

25 Further Development of the Rural Nursing Theory Base 313
Helen J. Lee and Meg K. McDonagh

26 Implications for Education, Practice, and Policy 322
Jean Shreffler-Grant and Marlene A. Reimer

APPENDIX

An Analysis of Key Concepts for Rural Nursing 331
Helen J. Lee and Charlene A. Winters

Index 343

Editorial Board

Contributors

Ronda L. Bales, MN, RN, is an Adjunct Assistant Professor, Montana State University-Bozeman, College of Nursing, Billings Campus. Her baccalaureate and master's degrees are from Montana State University-Bozeman. Her research interests are women's health, cardiovascular care, and rural health issues. She teaches undergraduate students in medical-surgical nursing.

Mary M. Bliesmer, DNSc, MPH, RN, Interim Associate Dean and Professor, has taught at Minnesota State University, Mankato for 25 years. Focus areas for teaching include foundations of nursing, gerontological nursing and health policy. Dr. Bliesmer is a certified Gerontological Nurse Practitioner and received a BS from Mankato State University, a master's degree in public health from the University of Minnesota, Minneapolis, and a doctorate of nursing science from Rush University in Chicago.

Robin L. Boland, MN, RN, FNP-C, earned her BSN from Montana State University-Bozeman in 1976. She worked in critical care nursing for 20 years in central Montana before obtaining her MN in the Rural Family Nurse Practitioner Master of Nursing program from Montana State University-Bozeman in 2000. She currently works as a Family Nurse Practitioner in Great Falls, Montana.

Serena Merry Britt is a full-time graduate student in the Master's of Social Work Program at Western Kentucky University in Bowling Green. Her baccalaureate degree is from Transylvania University, Lexington, Kentucky. Her social work interests include child welfare, elder, and rural issues. Because of her experiences with her graduate assistantship with the Health Enhancement for the Rural Elderly project, she has research interests in rural elders and their unique health concerns.

Janice A. Buehler, PhD, RN, is a retired Associate Professor, College of Nursing, Montana State University-Bozeman, Billings Campus. She earned her BSN from Oregon Health Sciences Center, her MS in psychiatric-mental health nursing from the University of Colorado, Denver, and her PhD from the University of California, San Francisco. Her research interests are in Native American and rural issues and in developing substantive grounded theory.

Patricia Butterfield, PhD, RN, FAAN, is the Director of the Occupational and Environmental Health Nursing Program at the University of Washington, Seattle. She also serves as the Interim Assistant Chair for the Department of Psychosocial and Community Health Nursing. Her research interests include household environmental risk reduction with low income families, environmental justice, environmental risk perception, and occupational health issues faced by small businesses.

Patricia A. Earle, PhD, RN, is an Associate Professor, School of Nursing, Minnesota State University, Mankato. She completed her BS at Mankato State University, and an MS and a PhD in educational administration at University of Minnesota, Minneapolis. She is currently teaching communication courses in the undergraduate program. Dr. Earle has participated in a variety of community and legislative activities to promote the health of women and families in the rural setting. Her research interests are families and chronic illness.

Dana S. Edge, PhD, RN, is an Associate Professor, University of Calgary Faculty of Nursing, Alberta, Canada. She received her BSN from the University of Iowa and her MSN from the University of North Carolina, Chapel Hill; her PhD in epidemiology is from the University of Toronto, Ontario, Canada. Her research interests include rural health, occupational epidemiology, cancer etiology, and population health.

Sandra K. Eggenberger, PhD, RN, is an Associate Professor, School of Nursing, Minnesota State University, Mankato. She holds degrees from Minnesota State University, Mankato (baccalaureate), the University of California, San Francisco (MS), and Texas Woman's University, Denton (PhD). Her research expertise is in the area of family research using phenomenology and grounded theory methodology.

Nancy Findholt, PhD, RN, is an Assistant Professor, Oregon Health & Science University School of Nursing, La Grande Campus. She has a baccalaureate degree from the University of Wisconsin, Eau Claire, a master's degree from the University of Washington, Seattle, and a PhD in nursing from Oregon Health & Science University. Her research interests are rural health, school health, community-based health promotion, and community-based participatory research. She teaches community health and leadership and management in nursing to undergraduate students.

Marilyn M. Gardner, PhD, MS, is an Assistant Professor for the Department of Public Health, Western Kentucky University, Bowling Green. Her doctoral degree is in health behavior from the University of Alabama, Birmingham. Her areas of expertise are in behavioral theory and health program evaluation. Teaching responsibilities include evaluation, epidemiology, biomedical ethics, and applied interdisciplinary research.

Laurie Bernhardt Glover, MN, APRN, FNP, is an Adjunct Assistant Professor, Montana State University-Bozeman College of Nursing, Great Falls Campus. Her baccalaureate and master's degrees are from Montana State University-Bozeman; she is a board-certified Family Nurse Practitioner. Her practice interests are community health, including school nursing, and underserved populations. She teaches undergraduate students in community health, psychosocial concepts, care management, and pathophysiology.

Marilyn Lewis Graves, MSN, RN, is adjunct faculty at Belmont University in Nashville, Tennessee. Her baccalaureate is from Mississippi College, Clinton, and her master's degree is from Western Kentucky University, Bowling Green. Her research interests are rural, elder, and end-of-life issues, cultural competency, and international immersion experiences. She teaches community health to undergraduate students and works part-time for Alive Hospice in Nashville.

Lori Hendrickx, EdD, RN, CCRN, is Associate Professor of Nursing, South Dakota State University, Brookings. Her BSN is from the University of North Dakota, Grand Forks, her MSN is from the University of Wisconsin-Eau Claire, and her EdD is from the University of Montana, Missoula. She has practiced in critical care and rural hospitals, has served on the American Association of Critical Care Nurses' Board of Directors, and is a member of the National Rural Health Association. Her research interests are issues facing rural nurses.

Wade G. Hill, PhD, RN, is an Assistant Professor, Montana State University-Bozeman College of Nursing, Bozeman Campus. His baccalaureate and master's degrees in nursing are from the University of Wyoming, Laramie; his PhD in Public Health is from Oregon State University, Corvallis. His research interests include children's environmental health, health behavior change, and psychosocial determinants of health. Dr. Hill teaches graduate students in epidemiology and research methods.

M. Susan Jones, PhD, RN, is an Associate Professor of Nursing, Western Kentucky University, Bowling Green. Her baccalaureate degree is from the University of Tennessee, Memphis, her master's degree is from Vanderbilt University, Nashville, Tennessee, and her PhD in Nursing is from the University of Cincinnati, Ohio. Her research interests are rural, elder, and agricultural health and safety issues. Teaching responsibilities include community health nursing, pharmacology, and an interdisciplinary rural health and safety course.

Norma K. Krumwiede, EdD, RN, is an Associate Professor, in the School of Nursing, Minnesota State University, Mankato. She holds degrees from Augustana College (baccalaureate) Sioux Falls, South Dakota, Montana State University-Bozeman (Minnesota), St. Scholastica College (MEd), Duluth, Minnesota and the University of South Dakota (EdD). Her problem-based research agenda has focused on rural, family, oncology, orthopedic, and cultural diversity issues.

Sandra K. Kuntz, PhD, RN, is an Assistant Professor, Montana State University-Bozeman College of Nursing, Missoula Campus. She holds a baccalaureate degree in nursing from California State University, Long Beach; an MS in community health nursing from Texas Woman's University, Dallas, and a PhD in community health services from Walden University, Minneapolis, Minnesota. Her research interests include rural public health infrastructure related to collaboration and preparedness and environmental health issues including risk reduction and prevention.

Beverly D. Leipert, PhD, RN, is Chair in Rural Women's Health Research and Associate Professor, University of Western Ontario Faculty of Health Sciences and Faculty of Medicine and Dentistry, London, Ontario. Her baccalaureate degrees, BA and BSc in Nursing, are from the University of Saskatchewan, Saskatoon; her master's degree in nursing is from the University of British Columbia, Vancouver; and her PhD in nursing is from the University of Alberta Edmonton. Her research interests are rural women's health and empowerment and the development of rural women's health theory.

Kathleen Ann Long, PhD, APRN, FAAN, earned a BSN from Catholic University, Washington, District of Columbia, an MSN from Wayne State University, Detroit, Michigan, and a PhD in Behavioral Sciences from Johns Hopkins University, Baltimore, Maryland. She currently serves as Dean, University of Florida College of Nursing, Gainsville; previously she was Dean of Nursing at Montana State University, Bozeman. Dr. Long's clinical work, research and publications have focused on rural health, child and family mental health, and innovations in nursing education.

Janis M. Majerus-Wegerhoff, MN, RN, received her BSN and MN from Montana State University-Bozeman. She lives in Calgary, Alberta, Canada.

Maureen Malone, MN, RN, is a public health nurse with the Indian Health Service, Hardin, Montana. She earned a BSN from the University of Maryland, College Park, and an MN from Montana State University-Bozeman.

Sonja J. Meiers, PhD, RN, is Director of Graduate Programs and Associate Professor, School of Nursing, Minnesota State University, Mankato. She holds a PhD in nursing from the University of Minnesota, Minneapolis. Dr. Meiers teaches adult health in the undergraduate program and family nursing theory in the graduate program. Her research expertise is in the areas of family nursing, knowledge development, phenomenology, grounded theory, instrument development, and intervention design.

Meg K. McDonagh, RN, MN, ENC(C), is an Instructor in the Faculty of Nursing, University of Calgary, Alberta, Canada. Her baccalaureate degree is from the University of Alberta, Edmonton, and her master's of nursing degree is from the University of Calgary. Her research interests are health beliefs of rural Canadians, preceptorships in the education of rural health professionals, and the use of health research among rural and remote health practitioners. She teaches rural nursing to undergraduate nursing students and practices in a small rural Alberta hospital.

Chad O'Lynn, PhD, RN, CNRN, is an adjunct assistant professor, Montana State University-Bozeman, College of Nursing, Missoula Campus. He teaches undergraduate medical-surgical nursing and research courses and works part-time as a staff nurse at a local hospital. He earned his MSN at Oregon Health & Science University, Portland, and his PhD in Health Administration from Kennedy-Western University, Agoura Hills, California. He is currently working on his PhD in Nursing from Oregon Health & Science University, Portland. His research interest is caring from a masculine perspective.

Janelle A. Peeler, LCSW, CMSW, MSSW, is an Instructor in the Department of Social Work, Western Kentucky University, Bowling Green. Her baccalaureate degree is from Eastern Kentucky University, Greenville, North Carolina, and her master's degree is from the Kent School at the University of Louisville in Kentucky. Her social work interests include clinical practice. She is the baccalaureate Social Work Field Director and her teaching responsibilities include practice and introductory classes.

Susan J. Raph, MN, RN, CNAA, BC, is an Adjunct Assistant Professor and Campus Director, Montana State University-Bozeman College of Nursing, Great Falls Campus. Her baccalaureate and master's degrees are from Montana State University-Bozeman. Her research interests include rural nursing, nursing administration, and nursing education. She teaches fiscal issues in public health nursing to graduate students.

Marlene A. Reimer, RN, PhD, CNN(C), is a Professor, Faculty of Nursing, University of Calgary, Alberta, Canada. She received her diploma from the Calgary General Hospital School of Nursing, a post-diploma baccalaureate from the University of Manitoba, Winnipeg, and an MN and

PhD degrees from the University of Calgary. She is a founding member of the Canadian Association for Rural and Remote Nursing. Her research interests include quality of life and outcomes measurement with adults experiencing cognitive impairment.

Melanie Reynolds, MPH, is Supervisor of the Public Health System Improvement and Training Section at the Montana Department of Public Health and Human Services. She has worked for over 24 years in public health including workforce development, women's health, maternal child health, and public health improvement and emergency preparedness. She received her MPH from the University of Washington School of Public Health and Community Medicine, Seattle.

Kathryn (Kay) Ayres Rosenthal, PhD, RN, is the Director of Options for Health Living. Her BSN is from Creighton University, Omaha, Nebraska. Her MSN and PhD are from the University of Colorado Health Sciences Center, Denver. Options for Healthy Living programs include individual wellness appointments, community health education programs, therapeutic horseback riding for persons with disabilities, and parish nursing. Her interests include family, writing, nature photography, and speaking internationally.

Jane Ellis Scharff, MN, RN, is an Adjunct Assistant Professor, Montana State University-Bozeman College of Nursing, Billings Campus. Her baccalaureate and master's degrees are from Montana State University-Bozeman. She is a doctoral candidate in nursing at the University of Rochester in New York. Her research interests include phenomena related to rural nursing and health and historical research related to nursing's social contract. She teaches foundations, physical assessment, and nursing research.

Jean Shreffler-Grant, PhD, RN, is an Associate Professor and Campus Director at Montana State University-Bozeman, College of Nursing, Missoula Campus. She has taught at both the undergraduate and graduate levels in the areas of leadership and management. Her BSN and MSN are from the University of Cincinnati, College of Nursing and Health, Ohio, and her PhD from the University of Washington, Seattle. Her scholarly interests include rural health care, specifically focused on formal (traditional) and informal (complementary) health care services for residents.

Jane Smilie, MPH, is Chief of the Public Health System Improvement and Preparedness Bureau at the Montana Department of Public Health and Human Services. She has worked in public health for more than 15 years in chronic disease prevention, health promotion, public health system improvement and emergency preparedness. Her MPH is from the University of Washington School of Public Health, Seattle.

Therese Sullivan, PhD, RN, is a Research Associate Professor, College of Nursing, Montana State University-Bozeman, Bozeman Campus. She earned her undergraduate degree from Carroll College in Helena, Montana, her master's degree from Montana State University, Bozeman and her PhD at the University of Washington, Seattle. Her specialty area is gerontological nursing and her interest areas are chronic illness, concept development, and nursing history. She is a member of the American Nurses' Association and Sigma Theta Tau International.

Elizabeth H. Thomlinson, RN, PhD, (deceased March 31, 2004), was an Associate Professor and Associate Dean, Undergraduate Programs, Faculty of Nursing, University of Calgary, Alberta. Her baccalaureate and master's degrees were from the University of Manitoba, Winnipeg and her PhD in nursing was from the University of Minnesota, Minneapolis. Her research interests were family violence, failure to thrive, rural and remote health and nursing, and aboriginal health. She shared her knowledge and expertise with both undergraduates and graduate students.

Linda E. Troyer, MN, FNP, RN, is employed at a hospital emergency room and with Big Horn Hospice. Her baccalaureate degree is from the University of Washington, Seattle. Her MN is from Montana State University-Bozeman, College of Nursing. Her research interests are rural nursing and Native American and end-of-life issues.

Clarann Weinert, SC, PhD, RN, FAAN, is a Professor, College of Nursing, Bozeman Campus, Montana State University-Bozeman and Sister of Charity of Cincinnati, Ohio. Her BSN is from College of Mount St. Joseph Cincinnati, Ohio; her MS is from The Ohio State University, Columbus; and her MA/PhD in sociology is from the University of Washington, Seattle. Published widely in social support, rural health, and chronic illness, she is the Director of the Center for Research on Chronic Health Conditions in Rural Dwellers, Vice President of Sigma Theta Tau International, and a Fellow in the Western Academy of Nurses.

Katharine S. West, MPH, MSN, RN, CNS, is the Program Director of the South Eastern California Hearing Coordination Center, California Newborn Hearing Screening Program. She has a baccalaureate from Excelsior University, Albany, New York; a MPH in Population and Family Health from the University of California, Los Angeles; and an MSN from Azusa Pacific University in Azusa, California. Her research interests are rural maternal-child health, infant survival, breast-feeding, newborn hearing and language development, infant attachment, and spiritual care in nursing.

Preface

This book will provide nurses with a broad understanding of the characteristics of health care in rural settings and what is required for effective nursing practice in this context. The book had its genesis in a small working group at Montana State University, which has been developing a theoretical model of the practice of rural nursing for nearly 30 years. This expanded edition contains information of interest to all nurses whose practices are primarily in rural settings as well as those who are preparing nurses for this type of practice. The unique characteristics of this environment present issues for both recipients and givers of care that are explored in this text.

Several differences exist between the first edition of *Conceptual Basis for Rural Nursing* and this edition, now titled *Rural Nursing: Concepts, Theory, and Practice*. The first edition contained chapters written only by Montana State University College of Nursing faculty, graduate students, and former faculty. In this edition we demonstrate a branching out to our colleagues throughout the United States and Canada. Authors from California, Kentucky, Minnesota, Oregon, and South Dakota in the United States and from British Columbia, Alberta, and Manitoba in Canada have contributed to the text.

As with the first edition, we are reporting on the continuing quest to provide a theory structure, the "seeking of patterns which [are helping and those that] ultimately will help rural nurses provide better care for persons in rural communities" (Lee, 1998, p. xxi). Part I contains the seminal article on the rural nursing theory base, followed by two chapters in which the authors examine the rural theory base and report the exploration of rural nursing theory in a comparison research study discussed in chapter 3. Part II includes chapters about the perspectives of rural persons, and Part III focuses on rural dwellers and their response to illness. Part IV begins with the seminal article about rural nurse practice and follows with reports of studies conducted with nurses in differing rural nurse practice settings. Part V contains chapters devoted to rural public health. Part VI, the final section, contains two chapters: in the first the authors provide suggestions for further development of the rural nursing theory base, and in the second the authors outline implications for rural nursing education, practice, and policy. The Appendix contains a summary of the key concepts that we analyzed for the first edition.

The second edition of this text can be attributed to several events. The first was the visit made in 1998 by Meg K. McDonagh to the Missoula campus of Montana State University-Bozeman College of Nursing. Enrolled as a graduate nursing student at the University of Calgary, Meg elected to spend a portion of an independent study practicum in Montana, to learn about the rural theory development process and about emergency care in the United States. Her visit coincided with the reviewing of the galley proofs for the first edition of this text. Subsequent to Meg's visit, she and her colleagues, under the leadership of Elizabeth "Betty" H. Thomlinson, conducted a study of health perceptions and needs of rural Canadian dwellers. This research study forms part of the basis of the comparison study between Canadian and Montana rural residents reported in chapter 3.

The second event was our assignment to teach together a graduate course, Rural Health: Needs and Perceptions, at Montana State University-Bozeman. Nursing students enrolled in the course were to interview rural residents to determine their perceptions of and needs for health care. In earlier years, students enrolled in the course had collected data from specific groups of rural residents, particularly those engaged in extractive industry occupations—logging, farming, ranching; the compilation of that data led to the initial rural nursing theory development. In the intervening years, students selected groups of rural persons to interview who were of personal interest to better understand the rural health care environment. We decided it was time to refocus on rural nursing theory development, only this time from the perspective of those employed in service industries. We developed a proposal, obtained human subjects permission, obtained a small College of Nursing grant to offset associated expenses and asked the students to join our effort. This research study provided the Montana data for the Canadian-U.S. comparison study reported in chapter 3.

The third event was our attendance at the Third International Congress of Rural Nurses at the Decker School of Nursing, Binghamton University, State University of New York, in October 2002. We had the opportunity to present our findings of the aforementioned study and to network with others interested in rural nursing. At that conference we made arrangements to collaborate with Meg McDonagh and Betty Thomlinson in a study to compare health perceptions and needs between Canadian and

Montana residents. Also, at the conference we facilitated a round table discussion about rural nursing theory development and formed a listserv of persons interested in rural nursing theory.

Shortly following the third event, we were contacted by Springer Publishing Company regarding the possibility of a second edition of *Conceptual Basis for Rural Nursing*. Through the compilation of the outcomes of the previously mentioned three events, the review of the rural nursing theory work in which we were engaged, and the results of a solicitation of manuscripts from within and outside MSU College of Nursing, we developed the proposal for this book. We contacted Binghamton presenters regarding their interest in publishing their work in this text. Many responded positively and their articles comprise the contents of this text.

The experience of working with the many authors from the variety of rural settings and our editorial board members has been enjoyable. We hope our readers find the second edition thought provoking, and we look forward to the comments and critique from our rural nursing colleagues.

Helen J. Lee, PhD, RN
Charlene A. Winters, DNSc, APRN, BC

REFERENCE

Lee, H. J. (1998). Preface. In H. J. Lee (Ed.), *Conceptual basis for rural nursing*. New York: Springer Publishing.

Acknowledgments

We acknowledge the administrative support of Montana State University-Bozeman College of Nursing. We appreciate the support of supplies, communication access, and staff. We particularly want to acknowledge the assistance of Bev May, who assisted us with working through the glitches of Microsoft Word; Linda Gooley, who assisted with typing and mail-outs; and Ryan Wuellner, who assisted with computer access.

We express our appreciation to the members of the editorial board who gave their time and expertise, to the students who participated in our research endeavors, and to the participants who shared their perceptions in the studies reported within the contents of this text. Finally, we thank the contributors for their time and effort in preparing manuscripts.

PART I

The Rural Nursing Theory Base

The first part of this edition of *Rural Nursing: Concepts, Theory, and Practice* contains three chapters. The first is the seminal article first published in 1989 by Long and Weinert. It is a publication that made the rural nursing community aware of the theory development activity taking place at Montana State University-Bozeman. In the second chapter, Lee and McDonagh examine the rural nursing theory base through an extensive review of the relevant literature. It is followed by the chapter in which Winters, Thomlinson, O'Lynn, Lee, McDonagh, Edge, & Reimer report a study that examines rural nursing theory through a comparison of the health perceptions and needs between residents living in Montana in the United States and the Canadian provinces of Alberta and Manitoba.

CHAPTER ONE

Rural Nursing: Developing the Theory Base*

Kathleen Ann Long and Clarann Weinert

A logger suffering from "heart lock" does not have a cardiovascular abnormality. He is suffering from a work-related anxiety disorder and can be assisted by an emergency room nurse who accurately assesses his needs and responds with effective communication and a supportive interpersonal relationship. A farmer who has lost his finger in a grain thresher several hours earlier does not have time during the harvesting season for a discussion of occupational safety. He will cope with his injury assisted by a clinic nurse who can adjust the timing of his antibiotic doses to fit with his work schedule in the fields.

Many health care needs of rural dwellers cannot be adequately addressed by the application of nursing models developed in urban or suburban areas but require unique approaches emphasizing the special needs

Acknowledgments: Qualitative data collected and analyzed by Montana State University, College of Nursing graduate students and faculty, form the basis for a substantial portion of this paper. Ethnographic data collection and analysis was supported, in part, by a U.S. Department of Health and Human Services, Division of Nursing, Advanced Training Grant to the Montana State University, College of Nursing (#1816001649AI). The project that provided the survey data was funded by a Montana State University Faculty Research/ Creativity Grant. This article is based partially on a paper presented at the Western Society for Research in Nursing Conference, Tempe, AZ, May 1987.

of this population. While nurses are significant, and frequently the sole, health care providers for people living in rural areas, little has been written to guide the practice of rural nursing. The literature provides vignettes and individual descriptions, but there is a need for an integrated, theoretical approach to rural nursing.

Rural nursing is defined as the provision of health care by professional nurses to persons living in sparsely populated areas. Over the past 8 years, graduate students and faculty members at the Montana State University College of Nursing, have worked toward developing a theory base for rural nursing. Theory development has used primarily a retroductive approach, and data have been collected and refined using a combination of qualitative and quantitative methods. The experiences of rural residents and rural nurses have guided the identification of key concepts relevant to rural nursing. The goal of the theory building process has been to identify commonalities and differences in nursing practice across all rural areas and the common and unique elements of rural nursing in relation to nursing overall. The implications of developing a theory of rural nursing for practice have been examined as a part of the ongoing process.

The theory building process was initiated in the late 1970s. At that time, literature and research related to rural health care were limited and focused primarily on the problem of retaining physicians in rural areas and providing assessments of rural health care needs and prescriptions for rural health care services based on models and experiences from urban and suburban areas (Coward, 1977; Flax, Wagenfield, Ivens, & Weiss, 1979). The unique health problems and health care needs of extremely sparsely populated states, such as Montana, had not been addressed from the perspective of the rural consumer. No organized theoretical base for guiding rural health care practice in general, or rural nursing in particular, existed.

QUALITATIVE DATA

The target population for qualitative data collection was the people of Montana. Montana, the fourth largest state in the United States, is an extremely sparsely populated state, with nearly 800,000 people and an average population density of approximately five persons per square mile. One half of the counties in Montana have three or fewer persons per square mile, with six of those counties having less than one person per square mile. There is only one metropolitan center in the state; it is a city of nearly 70,000 people, with a surrounding area that constitutes a center of approximately 100,000 *(Population Profiles, 1985)*.

Qualitative data were collected through ethnographic study by Montana State University College of Nursing graduate students. These data provided the initial ideas about health and health care in Montana. Since general propositions about rural health and rural health care did not exist, the gathering of concrete data was the first step toward subsequent development of more general theoretical propositions.

Graduate students used ethnographic techniques as described by Spradley (1979) to gather information from individuals, families, and health service providers. Interview sites were selected by students on the basis of specific interest and convenience. During a 6–year period, data were gathered from approximately 25 locations. In general, each student worked in depth in one community, collecting data from 10 to 20 informants over a period of at least 1 year. Data were gathered primarily from persons in ranching and farming areas and from towns of less than 2,500 persons. In some instances, student interest led to extensive interviews with specific rural subgroups, such as men in the logging industry or elderly residents in a rural town (Weinert & Long, 1987). Open-ended interview questions were developed using Spradley's (1979) guidelines. The questions emphasized seeking the informants' views without superimposing the cultural biases of the interviewer. The opening question in the interview was, "What is health to you … from your viewpoint? … your definition?" Interviewers used standard probes and a standard format of questions regarding health beliefs and health care preferences.

Spradley (1979) indicated that the goal of ethnographic study is to "build a systematic understanding of all human cultures from the perspective of those who have learned them" (p. 10). The goal of data collection in Montana was to learn about the culture of rural Montanans from rural Montanans. Emphasis in the cultural learning process was on understanding health beliefs, values, and practices. Rigdon, Clayton, and Diamond (1987) have noted that understanding the meaning that persons attach to subjective experiences is an important aspect of nursing knowledge. The ethnographic approach captured the meanings that rural dwellers ascribe to the subjective states of health and illness and facilitated the development of a rich database.

As the database developed, the following definitions and assumptions were accepted as a foundation for theory development. Rural was defined as meaning sparsely populated. Within this context, states such as Montana, which are sparsely populated overall, are viewed as rural throughout, despite the existence of some population centers within them. Further, based on this definition, rural regions or areas can be identified within otherwise heavily populated states. The assumption is made that, to some degree, health care needs are different in rural areas from that of urban areas. Also, all rural areas are viewed as having some common health care needs. Finally, the assumption is made that urban models are not appropriate to, or adequate for, meeting health care needs in rural areas.

Retroductive Theory Generation

Faculty work groups were developed to examine and organize the qualitative data. The work groups involved three to five nursing faculty members, each with rural nursing experience, but with varied backgrounds and expertise. Thus, a work group included experts from various clinical areas, as well as persons with direct experience either in small rural hospitals or in larger, metropolitan centers within rural states. Standard ethnographic content analysis (Spradley, 1979) was used to sort and categorize the ethnographic data. Groups worked toward consensus about the meaning and organization of specific data. Recurring themes were identified, and these were viewed as having relevance and importance for the rural informants in relation to their views of health.

A retroductive approach, as originally described by Hanson (1958), was used to examine the initial ethnographic data and build the theory base. Specific concepts and relational statements were derived from the data, and more general propositions were induced from these statements. The new propositions were then used to develop additional specific statements which could be supported by existing data or which were categorized for later testing. The retroductive approach was literally a "back and forth" process that permitted persons familiar with the data to move between the data and beginning-level theoretical propositions. The process was orderly and consistent and required group consensus about data interpretation and the relevance of derived propositions. The retroductive process continued in work groups over several years as additional ethnographic data were gathered. Consultants participated at key points in the process, in order to raise questions, add insights, and critically evaluate the group's theory building approach. Walker and Avant (1983) have noted that the retroductive process "adds considerably to the body of theoretical knowledge. It is, in fact, the way theory develops in the 'real world'" (p. 176).

QUANTITATIVE DATA

Following several years of ethnographic study, the faculty members involved in theory development wished to enrich the qualitative database by collecting relevant quantitative data. Kleinman (1983) stated, "Qualitative description, taken together with various quantitative measures, can be a standardized research method for assessing validity. It is especially valuable in studying social and cultural significance, e.g. illness beliefs interaction norms, social gain, ethnic help seeking, and treatment responses" (p. 543). Hinds and Young (1987) noted, "The combination of different methodologies within a single study promotes the likelihood of uncovering multiple dimensions of a phenomenon's empirical reality" (p. 195).

A survey developed by Weinert in 1983 attempted to validate some of the rural health concepts that had emerged from the ethnographic data. These concepts were: health status and health beliefs, isolation and distance, self-reliance, and informal health care systems. Survey instruments with established psychometric properties were selected to measure the specific concepts of interest. A mail questionnaire completed by the respondents included the Beck Depression Inventory (Beck, 1967) and the Trait Anxiety Scale (Spielberger, Gorsuch, & Lushene, 1970) to tap mental health status, and the General Health Perception Scale (Davies & Ware, 1981) to measure physical health status and health beliefs. A background information form assessed demographic variables, including length of residence and geographic locale. The Personal Resource Questionnaire (Brandt & Weinert, 1981) assessed use of informal systems for support and health care.

The convenience sample of survey participants was located through the Agricultural Extension Service, social groups, and informal networks. All participants lived in Montana, completed the questionnaires in their homes, and returned them by mail to the researcher. The 62 survey participants were middle-class whites, with an average of 13.5 years of education and a mean age of 61.3 years, who had lived in Montana an average of 45.6 years. The survey sample consisted of 40 women and 22 men residing in one of 13 sparsely populated Montana counties. The most populated county has a population density of 5.9 persons per square mile and one town of nearly 6,000 people. In the most sparsely populated county, there is one town of 600 people and an average population density of 0.5 persons per square mile.

Findings from the quantitative study were used throughout the theory development process to support or refute concept descriptions and relational statements derived from the ethnographic data. Survey findings are discussed in the following section as they relate to key concepts and relational statements.

REFINING THE BUILDING BLOCKS OF THEORY

To order the data and foster the formation of relational statements, an organizational scheme for theory development was adopted. Using the paradigm first described by Yura and Torres (1975) and later by Fawcett (1984), ethnographic data were categorized under the four major dimensions of nursing theory: person, health, environment, and nursing. The data were then ordered from the more general to the more specific. This process led to the identification of constructs, concepts, variables, and indicators.

An example helps to illustrate this process. Ethnographic data had been gathered from "gypo" loggers. These men are independent logging

TABLE 1.1 Data Ordering Scheme

Component	Examples
Dimension	Person
Construct	Psychological/sociocultural
Concept	"Present time" orientation
	Crisis orientation to health
Variable	Definitions of time
	Definitions of crisis
Indicators	Hours, minutes, days
	Seasons, work seasons
	Number of injuries
	Number of illnesses

contractors from northwestern Montana who work in rugged isolated areas, usually living in trailers or tents while working. Examples of quotes from these loggers and their associates as found in the data are: A logger states, "We worry about the here and now;" a local physician says, "Loggers enter the health care system during times of crisis only;" the public health nurse in the area says, "Loggers don't want to hear about health care problems; they don't return until the next accident."

Table 1.1 shows the scheme used to organize these data. The concepts "present time" orientation and crisis orientation to health are identified. These are placed under the person dimension. In this example, the constructs are not fully developed, but are viewed as psychological and/or sociocultural. The important variables identified thus far are definitions of time and of crisis. Possible indicators are measures of time, such as hours or seasons, and measures of crisis, such as numbers of illnesses or injuries.

Key Concepts

In the process of data organization it was noted that some concepts appeared repeatedly in ethnographic data collected in several different areas of the state. In addition, aspects of several of these concepts were supported by the quantitative survey data (Weinert, 1983). Using Walker and Avant's (1983) model of concept synthesis, these concepts were identified as key concepts in relation to understanding rural health needs and rural nursing practice. These key concepts are as follows: work beliefs and health beliefs, isolation and distance, self reliance, lack of anonymity, outsider/insider, and old timer/newcomer.

As key concepts in this theory, work beliefs and health beliefs are viewed as different or rural dwellers as contrasted with urban or suburban residents. These two sets of beliefs appear to be closely interrelated among rural persons. Work, or the fulfilling of one's usual functions, is of primary importance. Health is assessed by rural people in relation to work role and work activities, and health needs are usually secondary to work needs.

The related concepts of isolation and distance are identified as important in understanding rural health and nursing. Specifically, they help in understanding health care-seeking behavior. Quantitative survey data indicated that rural informants who lived outside of towns traveled a distance of almost 23 miles, on average, for emergency health care and over 50 miles for routine health care. Despite these distances, ethnographic data indicated that rural dwellers tended to see health services as accessible and did not view themselves as isolated.

Self-reliance and independence of rural persons are also seen as key concepts. The desire to do for oneself and care for oneself was strong among the rural persons interviewed and has important ramifications in relation to the provision of health care.

Two key concept areas, lack of anonymity and outsider/insider, have particular relevance for the practice of rural nursing. Lack of anonymity, a hallmark of small towns and surrounding sparsely populated areas, implies a limited ability for rural persons to have private areas of their lives. Rural nurses almost always reported being known to their patients as neighbors, part of a given family, members of a certain church, and so on. Similarly, these nurses usually know their patients in several different social and personal relationships beyond the nurse-patient relationship. The old timer/newcomer concept, or the related concepts of outsider/insider, is relevant in terms of the acceptance of nurses and of all health care providers in rural communities. The ethnographic data indicated that these concepts were used by rural dwellers in organizing their view of the social environment and in guiding their interactions and relationships. Survey data revealed that those who had lived in Montana over 10 years, but less than 20, still considered themselves to be "newcomers" and expected to be viewed as such by those in their community (Weinert & Long, 1987).

Relational Statements

In an effort to move from a purely descriptive theory to a beginning level explanatory one, some initial relational statements were generated from the qualitative data and were supported by the quantitative data that had been collected thus far. The statements are in the early stages of testing.

The first statement is that rural dwellers define health primarily as the ability to work, to be productive, to do usual tasks. The ethnographic data indicate that rural persons place little emphasis on the comfort, cosmetic, and life-prolonging aspects of health. One is viewed as healthy when able to function and be productive in one's work role. Specifically, rural residents indicated that pain was tolerated, often for extended periods, so long as it did not interfere with the ability to function. The General Health Perception Scale indicated that rural survey participants reported experiencing less pain than an age-comparable urban sample (Weinert & Long, 1987). Further, scores on the Beck Depression Inventory and the Trait Anxiety Scale (Weinert, 1983) revealed that they experienced less anxiety and less depression.

The second statement is that rural dwellers are self-reliant and resist accepting help or services from those seen as "outsiders" or from agencies seen as national or regional "welfare" programs. A corollary to this statement is that help, including needed health care, is usually sought through an informal rather than a formal system. Ethnographic data supported both the second statement and its corollary. Numerous references were found showing, for example, a preference for "the 'old doc' who knows us" over the new specialist who was unfamiliar. Data from the Personal Resource Questionnaire (Weinert, 1983) indicated that rural dwellers relied primarily on family, relatives, and close friends for help and support. Further, the rural survey respondents reported using health care professionals and formal human service agencies much less frequently than did comparable urban respondents in previous studies.

A third statement is that health care providers in rural areas must deal with a lack of anonymity and much greater role diffusion than providers in urban or suburban settings. This statement has marked significance for rural nursing practice. Although limited ethnographic and survey data have been collected from rural nurses thus far, some emerging themes have been identified. In addition to identifying a sense of isolation from professional peers, rural nurses emphasize their lack of anonymity and a sense of role diffusion. There is an inability to keep separate the activities and behaviors of the individual nurse's various roles. In a small town, for example, the nurse's behavior as a wife, a mother, and a church attendee are all significantly related to her effectiveness as a health care professional in that community. Further, in their professional role, nurses reported experiencing role diffusion. Nurses are expected to perform a variety of diverse and unrelated tasks. On a single shift, a nurse may work in obstetrics delivering a baby, care for a dying patient on the medical-surgical unit, and initiate care of a trauma patient in the emergency room. Likewise, on evening shift or weekends, a nurse may be required to carry out tasks reserved for the pharmacist or dietitian on the day shift.

RELATIONSHIP OF CONCEPTS AND STATEMENTS TO THE LARGER BODY OF NURSING KNOWLEDGE

How people define health and illness has a direct impact on how they seek and use health care services and is a key concept in understanding client behavior and in planning intervention.

Definition of Health

The rural Montana dwellers primarily define health as the ability to work and to be productive. The work of other researchers supports the finding that residents of sparsely populated areas view health in terms of ability to work and remain productive. Ross (1982), a nurse anthropologist, studied the health perceptions of women living in the Lake District along the coast of Nova Scotia. She conducted in-depth interviews with 60 women of both British and French backgrounds in small coastal fishing communities. Similar to the rural dwellers in Montana, these women described good health as being "able to do what you want to do" and to "be able to work." Lee's (1987) recent work in Montana supports earlier findings on which the rural nursing theory was built. She found that work and health practices were closely related among farmers and ranchers; health is viewed as a functional state in relation to work. Scharff's (1987) interviews with nurses practicing in small rural hospitals in eastern Washington, northern Idaho, and western Montana indicated that they viewed the health needs of rural people as overlapping those of people living in urban situations in many instances. The nurse informants, however, noted that rural people equate health with the ability to work or function in their daily activities. Rural people were viewed as delaying health care until they were very ill, thus often needing hospitalization at the point of seeking care.

Self-Reliance

The statement derived from the Montana data that "rural dwellers resist accepting help from outsiders or strangers" has been supported in data from research in rural Maryland (Salisbury State College, 1986). People living in the rural eastern shore area were described as highly resistant to care from persons viewed as outsiders, and rural shore residents often refused to go "across the bridge" to Baltimore to seek health care, even though this was a trip of less than 100 miles and would allow access to sophisticated, specialized treatment. Like the rural people in Montana, these Maryland residents sought health care information and assistance from local, and often informal, sources. The self-reliance of rural persons and their resistance to outside help were also reported by Counts and Boil (1987) in relation to residents of the Appalachian area. Self-reliance was noted as a major feature that must be considered in planning nursing care services for this population.

The rural Nova Scotia women studied by Ross (1982) indicated informal personal networks of family, friends, and neighbors as important sources of health information who also provided the physical, financial, emotional and social support that contributes to well-being. When these women were asked what connection there was between health and the availability of hospitals, doctors, and other medical care, 42% indicated that it was the individual's responsibility for health knowledge and care; 25% thought professionals were useful to a certain point in providing advice and services such as routine physical exams; 19% indicated that these services were for sick persons, not healthy persons; and 9% felt the formal health care system had no relationship to health (Ross, 1982, p. 311). One woman commented, "Health is not a topic to discuss with doctors and nurses" (Ross, 1982, p. 309).

Rural Nursing

The Montana data and the theory derived from it indicate that nurses and other health care providers in rural areas must deal with a lack of anonymity. Nurses are known in a variety of roles to their patients, and in turn, know their patients in a variety of roles. Most of the nurses interviewed by Scharff (1987) felt that by knowing their patients personally they could give better care. Other nurses, however, noted that providing professional care for family or friends can be a frightening experience. Nurses indicated that there was no anonymity for them in the rural community, which, at times, was reassuring, and at other times, constricting (Scharff, 1987).

The concept of role diffusion in the rural hospital setting was very apparent in Scharff's (1987) work. She reported that a rural hospital nurse must be a jack-of-all-trades who often practices within the realm of numerous other health care disciplines, including respiratory therapy, laboratory technology, dietetics, pharmacy, social work, psychology, and medicine. Examples of the intersections between rural nursing and other disciplines include doing EKGs, performing arterial punctures, running blood gas machines, drawing blood, setting up cultures, going to the pharmacy to pour drugs, going to the local drugstore to get medications for patients, ordering x-rays and medications, delivering babies, directing the actions of physicians, and cooking meals when the cook gets snowed in. As Scharff (1987) noted, some of these functions are carried out by urban nurses practicing in particular settings such as a trauma center or intensive care unit. Rural nurses, however, are usually not circumscribed by assignment to a particular unit or department and are expected to function in multiple roles, even within one work shift.

This generalist work role and the lack of anonymity of rural nurses are substantiated by findings and descriptions from several other rural areas of the United States (Biegel, 1983; St. Clair, Pickard, & Harlow, 1986). A study of nurses in rural Texas noted, "Nurses play roles as nurse, friend, neighbor, citizen, and family member" within a community; further, rural nurses in their work roles were described as needing to be "all things to all people" (St. Clair et al., 1986, p. 28).

Generalizability

The issue of a situation or locale-specific theory and its relationship to the larger body of nursing knowledge needs serious consideration. The work of Scharff (1987) indicated that the core of rural nursing is not different from urban nursing. The intersections, however, those "meeting points at which nursing extends its practice into the domains of other professions;" the dimensions, that is, the "philosophy, responsibilities, functions, roles, and skills;" and the boundaries, which "respond to new and growing needs and demands from society" (American Nurses Association, 1980), appear to be very distinct for rural nursing practice.

Questions still remain as to how generalizable findings from Montana residents are to other rural populations. Clearly, there is a need for more organized and rigorous data collection in relation to rural nursing before these questions can be answered. A sound theory base for rural practice requires continued research, conducted across diverse rural settings.

IMPLICATIONS FOR NURSING PRACTICE

The findings from the Montana research about people living in sparsely populated areas have implications for nursing practice in rural areas. Since work is of major importance to rural people, health care must fit within work schedules. Health care programs or clinics which conflict with the rural economic cycle, such as haying or calving, will not be used. Since health is defined as the ability to work, health promotion must address the work issue. For example, health education related to cardiovascular disease should highlight strategies for preventing conditions that involve long-term disability, such as stroke. These aspects will be more meaningful to rural dwellers than preventive aspects that emphasize a longer, more comfortable life.

The self-reliance of rural dwellers has specific nursing implications. Rural people will often delay seeking health care until they are gravely ill or incapacitated. Nursing approaches need to address two distinct aspects: non-judgmental intervention for those who have delayed treatment and a strong emphasis on preventive health teaching. If the nurse can provide adequate health knowledge, the rural dweller's desire for self-reliance may lead to health-promotion behaviors. With a good information base, rural people can make appropriate decisions about self-care versus the need for professional intervention.

Health care services must be tailored to suit the preferences of rural persons for family and community help during periods of illness. Nurses can provide instruction, support, and relief to family members and neighbors, who are often the primary-care providers for sick and disabled persons.

The formal health care system needs to fit into the informal helping system in rural areas. A long-term community resident, such as the drugstore proprietor, can be assisted in providing accurate advice to residents through the provision of reference materials and a telephone back-up system. One can anticipate greater acceptance and use by rural residents of an updated but old and trusted health care resource, rather than a new, professional, but "outsider" service (Weinert & Long, 1987).

Nurses who enter rural communities must allow for extended periods prior to acceptance. Involvement in diverse community activities, such as civic organizations and recreational clubs, may assist the nurse in being known and accepted as a person. In rural communities acceptance as a health care professional is often tied to personal acceptance. Thus it appears that rural communities are not appropriate practice settings for nurses who prefer to maintain entirely separate professional and personal lives.

The stresses that appear to affect nurses in rural practice settings have particular importance. Rural nurses see themselves as cut off from the professional mainstream. They are often in situations where there is no collegial support to assist in defining an appropriate practice role and its boundaries. The educational preparation of those who wish to practice in rural settings needs to emphasize not only generalist skills, but also a strong base in change theory and leadership techniques. Nurses in rural practice need a sound orientation to techniques for accessing diverse sources of current information. If the closest library is several hundred miles away, for example, can all arrangement for interlibrary loan and access to material via telephone, bus, or mail be arranged? Networks that link together nurses practicing in distant rural sites are particularly useful, both for information exchange and for mutual support.

SUMMARY

It is becoming increasingly clear that rural dwellers have distinct definitions of health. Their health care needs require approaches that differ significantly from urban and suburban populations. Subcultural values, norms, and beliefs play a key role in how rural people define health and from whom they seek advice and care. These values and beliefs, combined with the realities of rural living—such as weather, distance, and isolation—markedly affect the practice of nursing in rural settings. Additional ethnographic and quantitative data are needed to further define both the common and the locale-specific conditions and characteristics of rural populations. Continued research can provide a more solid base for the nursing theory that is required to guide practice and the delivery of health care to rural populations.

REFERENCES

American Nurses Association. (1980). *Nursing. A social policy statement* (No. NP-63 20M 9/82R). Kansas City MO: Author.

Brandt, P., & Weinert, C. (1981). The PRQ: A social support measure. *Nursing Research, 30,* 277–280.

Beck, A. (1967). *Depression: Causes and treatment.* Philadelphia: University of Pennsylvania Press.

Biegel, A. (1983). Toward a definition of rural nursing. *Home Health Care Nursing, 1,* 45–46.

Counts, M., & Boyle, J. (1987). Nursing, health and policy winner a community context. *Advances in Nursing Science, 9,* 12–23.

Coward, R. (1977). Delivering social services in small towns and rural communities. In R. Coward *(Ed.), Rural families across the life span: Implications for community programming* (pp. 1–17). West Lafayette, IN: Indiana Cooperative Extension Services.

Davies, A., & Ware, J. (1981). *Measuring health perceptions in the health insurance experiment.* Santa Monica, CA: Rand.

Fawcett, J. (1984). *Analysis and evaluation of conceptual models of nursing.* Philadelphia: F. A. Davis.

Flax, J., Wagenfeld, M., Ivens, R., & Weiss, R. (1979). *Mental health and rural America: An overview, and annotated bibliography.* Rockville, MD: U.S. Government Printing Office.

Hanson, N. (1958). *Patterns of discovery.* Cambridge: Cambridge University Press.

Hinds, P., & Young, K. (1987). A triangulation of methods and paradigms to study nurse-given wellness care. *Nursing Research, 36,* 195–198.

Kleinman, A. (1983). The cultural meanings and social uses of illness: A role for medical anthropology and clinically oriented social science in the development of primary care theory and research. *Journal of Family Practice, 16,* 539–545.

Lee, H. (1987). *Relationship of hardiness and current life events to perceived health and rural adults.* Manuscript submitted for publication.

Population profiles of Montana counties: 1980. (1985). Bozeman, MT: Montana State University Center for Data Systems and Analysis.

Rigdon, I., Clayton, B., & Diamond, M. (1987). Toward a theory of helpfulness for the elderly bereaved: An invitation to a new life. *Advances in Nursing Science, 9,* 32–43.

Ross, H. (1982). Women and wellness: Defining, attaining, and maintaining health in Eastern Canada. *Dissertation Abstracts International, 42,* DEO 82–12624.

Salisbury State College. (1986, June). *Discussion of Salisbury Slate College rural health findings.* Presented at the Contemporary Issues in Rural Health Conference, Salisbury, MD.

Scharff, J. (1987). *The nature and scope of rural nursing: Distinctive characteristics.* Unpublished master's thesis, Montana State University, Bozeman, MT.

Spielberger, C., Gorsuch, R., & Lushene, R. (1970). *STAI manual for the State-Trait Anxiety Questionnaire.* Palo Alto, CA: Consulting Psychologist.

Spradley, J. (1979). *The ethnographic interview.* New York: Holt, Rinehart, and Winston.

St. Clair, C., Pickard, M., & Harlow, K. (1986). Continuing education for self actualization: Building a plan for rural nurses. *Journal of Continuing Education in Nursing, 17,* 27–31.

Walker, L., & Avant, K. (1983). *Strategies for theory construction in nursing.* Norwalk, CT: Appleton-Century-Crofts.

Weinert, C. (1983). [Social support: Rural people in their new middle years]. Unpublished raw data.

Weinert, C., & Long, K. (1987). Understanding the health care needs of rural families. *Journal of Family Relations, 36,* 450–455.

Yura, H., & Torres, G. (1975). *Today's conceptual frameworks with the baccalaureate nursing programs* (NLN Pub. No. 15–1558, pp. 17–75). New York: NLN.

CHAPTER TWO

Examining the Rural Nursing Theory Base

Helen J. Lee and Meg K. McDonagh

Our purposes in this chapter are threefold. First, we present a short historical perspective of the rural nursing theory development. A summary of the rural nursing theory structure explicated by Long and Weinert in 1989 follows. Then, we present a review of the literature supporting or refuting the viability of the theoretical statements and concepts.

HISTORICAL PERSPECTIVES

"Sparsely Populated Areas: Toward Nursing Theory" was the title of a Western Council on Higher Education for Nursing (now Western Institute of Nursing) symposium presented in 1982 by Montana State University-Bozeman. Organized by faculty member, Jacqueline Taylor (1982), the symposium was introduced to its audience by the Dean of the School of Nursing, Anna Shannon. In her introductory remarks, Dean Shannon (1982) stated that the presentation to the council members would demonstrate to its audience how a school could "maximize its resources, provide opportunities for faculty and student research and contribute ... to the development of an empirically based theory of rural nursing" (pp. 70–71). She noted the lack of literature and research about rural nursing plus the placement of little emphasis on the context of environment within nursing theories.

The symposium comprised five graduate students and faculty studies about (a) the beliefs and practices of Crow Indian women, Hmong refugees, and Hutterite colony members, (b) sodium in drinking water and adolescent blood pressure, and (c) the role of distance in home dialysis adjustment. Concluding remarks, given by faculty member Ruth Ludeman, included the information that a plan for theory construction and testing was in place using *retroduction,* a process involving both inductive and deductive reasoning. Theory development activity continued at Montana State University-Bozeman College of Nursing and resulted in the subsequent publication of an article titled, "Rural Nursing: Developing the Theory Base." (Long & Weinert, 1989) (see chapter 1.)

THE RURAL NURSING THEORY STRUCTURE

"Many disciplines exist to generate, test, and apply theories that will improve the quality of people's lives" (Fawcett, 1999, p. 1). The quality of the lives of rural persons and the lack of empiral studies about their health care was of concern to Montana State University-Bozeman nursing researchers. The middle-range theory that emerged came from a recognized need of rural nurses for a practice framework that acknowledges the unique perceptions of rural persons and the requirements of nurses who practice in rural settings. Prior to the development of the theory, it was assumed that nursing care of rural persons was similar to the care of persons living in urban environments.

The resulting descriptive theory is the "most basic type of middle range theory" (Fawcett, 1999, p. 15). The theory emerged from observations gathered through qualitative and quantitative descriptive studies conducted in the sparsely populated rural setting of Montana. It describes specific characteristics and observations made of rural persons seeking health care and their health care providers. The published theory contains several key concepts and three statements identified as "relational" (Long & Weinert, 1989). The first statement is descriptive and describes rural persons' definition of health. The first statement, a definition, states that "rural dwellers define health primarily as the ability to work, to be productive, to do usual tasks" (Long & Weinert, p.120). Key concepts associated with this statement are *work beliefs* and *health beliefs.*

The remaining two statements are relational as they describe relationships between key concepts. The second statement proposes that "rural dwellers are self-reliant and resist accepting help or services from those seen as 'outsiders' or from agencies seen as national or regional 'welfare' programs" (Long & Weinert, 1989, p. 120). Rural persons preferred to seek health care from *insiders,* persons with whom they were familiar.

Additional key concepts pertaining to this statement are *old-timer* and *newcomer*. A corollary to the second statement is "that help, including needed medical care, is usually sought through an informal rather than a formal system" (p. 120).

The third statement focuses on health care providers; it indicates that *lack of anonymity* and *role diffusion* is experienced more acutely among rural providers than among providers in urban or suburban settings. Lack of anonymity also applies to the recipients of health care in rural areas as all persons in that environment have a "limited ability ... to have private areas of their lives" (Long & Weinert, 1989, p. 119).

In addition to the above three statements, an understanding of the concepts "isolation" and "distance" is important in the health care-seeking behavior of rural residents. The concept of *isolation* refers to separation from or being placed alone (Lee, Hollis, & McClain, 1998). *Distance* is measurable time and physical distance from place to place. The qualitative data upon which the theoretical work was based indicated that rural residents did not feel isolated despite the fact that they averaged 23 miles of travel to their nearest emergency room and over 50 miles to their primary health care source (Long & Weinert, 1989, p. 119). It is important to note that both isolation and distance can be affected by perception. For example, Allison who lives a distance of 200 miles from the nearest health services does not perceive herself as isolated, while Barbara does. Both live the same distance from health services in terms of mileage and travel time. However, Allison used to live 350 miles from the nearest health services, and Barbara just moved from a city with a population of 40,000 that had a wide range of health services available 24 hr a day, the nearest facility being located three blocks away from her home. As this case illustrates by using a sociopsychological lens, some people would define isolation as decreased access to something perceived to be a valuable resource, in this case, health services.

RELATED NURSING LITERATURE

The contents of Long and Weinert's (1989) rural nursing theory article was and is widely quoted in nursing literature, community health and rural nursing texts, and presentations given about rural nursing. However, a rural nursing literature review that we conducted in the spring of 2003 contained few citations that specifically focused on health perceptions and needs of rural persons. We located three qualitative studies through conference proceedings (Bales, 2002a; Lee & Winters, 2002; Thomlinson, McDonagh, Reimer, Crooks, & Lees, 2002). A fourth source was a nursing master's thesis (Bales, 2002b). A fifth research source was a study that focused on the health care meanings, values, and practices of Anglo-American males in the rural Midwest (Sellers, Poduska, Propp, & White, 1999). We found other journal articles about rural research, mostly qualitative studies, that touched on the related rural concepts. In the following sections, each statement is followed by findings from the literature supporting or refuting the statement.

Theoretical Statement #1

> ... rural dwellers define health primarily as the ability to work, to be productive, to do usual tasks (Long & Weinert, 1989, p. 120)

The findings of three qualitative studies conducted in the United States (one with rural men aged 25–49 years and two with older rural persons aged 60–85), provided support for the above descriptive statement that defines health as being able to carry out important functions (Niemoller, Ide, & Nichols, 2000; Pierce, 2001; Sellers, Poduska, Propp & White, 1999). Another researcher (Averill, 2002) found that definitions of health varied across her sample that included older, more recent retirees, and Hispanic elders. The older retirees from mining and ranching communities viewed health in a similar manner to the original qualitative theory development samples while more recent retirees focused on strategies to remain healthy—proper diet, regular exercise, and regular health exams. The Hispanic elders in Averill's sample frequently mentioned incorporating home remedies and herbal preparations into their health maintenance practices.

Participants in the four health perceptions and needs studies (Bales, 2002a; Bales, 2002b; Lee & Winters, 2004; Thomlinson et al., 2002) conducted in the United States and Canada were more likely to define health holistically. Lee and Winters (2004) found that for rural persons working in service occupations, being able to function included being physically, mentally, and emotionally fit. Participants in a study conducted by Bales (2002b) thought that being healthy meant being mentally and physically active, eating well, and having an overall sense of well-being. Thomlinson and her colleagues (2002) interpreted their participants' responses by saying that health was a "holistic relationship between the physical, mental, social and spiritual aspects of their lives." This same view of health was echoed by Canadian middle-aged women in Thurston and Meadows' (2003) study and by Australian older women in de la Rue and Coulson's (2003) study of rural women's perspectives of health.

Summary. The literature both supports and refutes the first theoretical statement. Support appears in studies of rural male adults and of older persons and retirees from the extractive industries (mining, farming). Lack of support for the functional definition of health emerges from a variety of settings and from differing rural samples. It may be that age, the influence of the work ethic, and culture are factors in defining health (de la Rue & Coulson, 2003). Potentially, younger rural participants may be influenced by increased media exposure and its emphasis on health promotion and use of preventive health practices. In addition, health care providers may be expanding their view of health beyond the illness care model and sharing this with their patients.

Relational Statement #2

... rural dwellers are self-reliant and resist accepting help or services from those seen as "outsiders" or from agencies seen as national or regional welfare programs. (Long & Weinert, 1989, p. 120)

The characteristic of self-reliance runs through most of the literature about rural persons and their health-seeking behaviors (Davis & Magilvy, 2000; Jirojwong & MacLennan, 2002; Lee & Winters, 2004; Niemoller et al., 2000; Sellers et al. 1999; Thomlinson et al., 2002). Care was sought by rural residents after first "consulting books" (Jirojwong & MacLennan, p. 251) and trying "to deal with an illness themselves" (Thomlinson, McDonagh, Reimer, Crooks, & Lees, in press, p. 10). Because of the presence of chronic illnesses, older adults were knowledgeable about medical resources (physicians, physician's assistants, and nurse practitioners) in nearby areas (Niemoller et al., 2000; Pierce, 2001; Roberto & Reynolds, 2001), and if available, would use them "to achieve their desired level of independence" (Niemoller et al., p. 39). However, if the desired resources were not available, these same older adults would "manage" (p. 39).

Corollary to Relational Statement #2

... help, including needed health care, is usually sought through an informal rather than a formal system (Long & Weinert, 1989, p. 120).

The literature revealed a variety of findings related to the relational statement corollary. Bales (2002b) found that mothers living in frontier settings would seek advice from family, friends, and neighbors and would initiate self-care activities if the health care situation was not considered serious. However, if the illness or injury was gauged as serious, professional health care was accessed. Bypassing the informal for the formal system because of the seriousness of the illness or injury also was found in studies conducted by Buehler, Malone, and Majerus (1998) and Thomlinson et al. (2002).

Participants in a Canadian study (Thomlinson et al., 2002) indicated that family, friends, and neighbors were cited as a major source of support. Although older rural women in the U.S. study conducted by Pierce (2001) stated they were eager to help neighbors and the less fortunate, they also shared their reluctance to tell family and neighbors about their needs unless really necessary.

Help gained through accessing knowledge via the media, popular magazines, books, libraries, and the Internet was cited in two studies (Roberto & Reynolds, 2001; Thomlinson et al., 2002). A sample of older women living in the United States actively sought information about living with their osteoporosis (Roberto & Reynolds); members of a Canadian sample stated that they frequently made use of formal information sources through libraries, books, and computers (Thomlinson et al., 2002).

Summary. The second theoretical statement and its corollary is both sustained and refuted by the findings in the literature. Self-reliance remains a characteristic attribute of rural persons and influences the way they respond to illness or injury and their subsequent care-seeking behaviors. The informal system (family, friends, neighbors) is still frequently used as a resource. However, the rural cultural barrier to accessing care through formal resources appears to be changing. The accessibility of knowledge through a variety of sources and the need to have information about health and the chronic illnesses they are experiencing may be beginning to remove the cultural barrier of approaching "outsiders" for health and medical care. In part, this may be occurring because desired health information can now be obtained while maintaining anonymity. Prior to the current age of information technology, maintaining anonymity while seeking health information was not an option.

Relational Statement #3

> ... health care providers in rural areas must deal with a lack of anonymity and much greater role diffusion than providers in urban or suburban (Long & Weinert, 1989, p. 120).

The findings for the two elements forming this relational statement—lack of anonymity and role diffusion—are sustained in the literature about health care providers from Australia, New Zealand, and the United States. In relation to the lack of anonymity, authors state that "in close knit communities ... news travels fast" (Lau, Kumar, & Thomas, 2002, Results and Discussion, paragraph 7) and that "social life realities in small communities frequently blur professional boundaries" (Blue & Fitzgerald, 2002, p. 319–320). Social factors pertaining to practice in rural communities include privacy issues for both the professional and the clients for whom they give care (Lau et al., 2002). Health care practitioners in rural environments who are known by their clients may find that older women prefer receiving professional care from a familiar person (Courtney, Tong, & Walsh, 2000; Pierce, 2001) whereas middle-aged women will prefer to go elsewhere for care because of that familiarity (Brown, Young, & Byles, 1999; Lee & Winters, 2004). Lee and Winters found this particularly true for women's health care and mental health.

Role diffusion was found in studies conducted with psychiatrists in Australia (Lau et al., 2002) and by Rosenthal (1996) in her study of rural nursing in America. Hegney (1997) described role diffusion in her study of Australian rural nursing practice as the generalist and extended practice role. Role diffusion was evident in the practice of hospice nurses in New Zealand (McConigley, Kristjanson, & Morgan, 2000). The reality in sparsely populated areas is that with fewer persons to perform the multiple tasks, more tasks must be undertaken by the individuals who chose to practice in those areas.

Summary. The third theoretical statement about lack of anonymity and role diffusion is well supported in the available literature. The concept of familiarity, the antonym of lack of anonymity, can be a facilitator or a barrier to seeking health and illness care from local health care practitioners. It is a distinguishing feature of rural nursing that allows rural nurses a special knowledge of those for whom they provide care within their communities (Hegney, 1997).

Distance

Although distance was not part of any of the three theoretical statements making up the rural nursing theory base, the content of the rural literature we accessed for this review frequently touched on the concept. In the seminal article by Long and Weinert (1989), the participants included in the multiple studies tended to see health services as accessible and did not view themselves as isolated. The author of one article sustaining that perception stated that distance may not be a problem but said the concept exerts a strong influence in providing health care in rural areas (MacLeod, Browne, & Leipert, 1998). This view affirms Johnson, Ratner, and Bottorff's (1995) assertion that one's geographic location may influence or even determine the form of health-seeking behaviors rural residents demonstrate. In an article cited earlier, the older women described distance and geographical barriers with concern; yet, they seemed to take problems with accessibility "in stride" (Pierce, 2001, p. 52). However, the participants did express concern about the quality of available health services.

The remainder of the articles all refuted the initial findings about distance and access to health care in Long and Weinert's (1989) theory-based article. Fitzgerald, Pearson, and McCutcheon (2001) and Racher and Vollman (2002) stated that access to health care services is a major concern for residents across North America's rural and remote areas and the health professionals serving them. Access to care is particularly a concern for rural individuals with chronic illness; an expressed problem was finding the "best" doctor (Fitzgerald, Pearson, & McCutcheon, 2001). Buehler and Lee (1992) found the more rural the persons with cancer, the more limited were formal health care resources available to assist them and their families. Distances to emergency care was an expressed concern of service providers in rural areas (Lee & Winters, 2004) and of mothers of children living in frontier areas (Bales, 2002b). In a survey of middle-aged women, Brown and colleagues (1999) concluded that experiencing difficulties with accessing health care results in greater reliance on self-treatment and self-care, thereby leading to development of "attitudes of independence and self-reliance [sic]" (p. 151)

Summary. Distance and its part in the overriding construct of access to health care are of major concern to the majority of rural residents. This change may have resulted from fewer resources being available and increased consumer concerns about available resources particularly emergency and pharmaceutical services. In addition, the changing demographics mean an increase in older residents who experience illnesses, want quality care, and are seeking specialist care to obtain quality. Dealing with distance may be one of the major factors contributing to the resulting perception of self-reliance in rural and remote environments.

CONCLUSION

The review of the literature pertaining to the descriptive middle range rural nursing theory base reveals a variety of findings. The rural residents' definition of health in the first descriptive statement is changing from that of a functional nature to a more holistic view that includes physical, mental, social, and spiritual aspects. The self-reliance of rural residents in the second relational statement is broadly supported; however, the resistance to seeking help from those seen as "outsiders" is changing. The third relational statement pertaining to health care providers and their lack of anonymity and role diffusion is supported. The findings for the concept of distance in the original rural theory development work are not supported. This literature appraisal of the rural nursing theory base structure supports a need for change.

REFERENCES

Averill, J. B. (2002). Voices from the Gila: Health care issues for rural elders in south-western New Mexico. *Journal of Advanced Nursing, 40,* 654–662.

Bales, R. L. (2002a, April). *Health needs and perceptions: A study of six persons in Cooke City, MT.* Paper presented at the Proceedings of the 35th Annual Communicating Nursing Research Conference, Palm Springs, CA.

Bales, R. L. (2002b). *Health perceptions, needs, and behaviors of remote rural women of childbearing and childrearing age.* Bozeman, MT: Montana State University-Bozeman.

Blue, I., & Fitzgerald, M. (2002). Interprofessional relations: Care studies of working relationships between registered nurses and general practitioners in rural Australia. *Journal of Clinical Nursing, 11,* 314–321.

Brown, W. J., Young, A. F., & Byles, J. E. (1999). Tyranny of distance? The health of mid-age women living in five geographical areas of Australia. *Australian Journal of Rural Health, 7,* 148–154.

Buehler, J. A., & Lee, H. J. (1992). Exploration of home care resources for rural families with cancer. *Cancer Nursing, 15,* 299–308.

Buehler, J. A., Malone, M., & Majerus, J. M. (1998). Patterns of responses to symptoms in rural residents: The symptom-action-time-line process. In H. J. Lee (Ed.), *Conceptual basis for rural nursing* (pp. 318–328). New York: Springer Publishing.

Courtney, M., Tong, S., & Walsh, A. (2000). Older patients in the acute care setting: Rural and metropolitan nurses' knowledge, attitudes and practices. *Australian Journal of Rural Health, 8,* 94–102.

Davis, R., & Magilvy, J. K. (2000). Quiet pride: The experience of chronic illness by rural older adults. *Journal of Nursing Scholarship, 32,* 385–390.

de la Rue, M., & Coulson, I. (2003). The meaning of health and well-being: Voices from older rural women. *The International Electronic Journal of Rural and Remote Health Research, Education, Practice, and Policy, 3* (192) 1–10. Retrieved October 4, 2003 from http://rrh.deakin.edu.au,

Fawcett, J. (1999). *The relationship of theory and research* (3rd ed.). Philadelphia: Davis.

Fitzgerald, M., Pearson, A., & McCutcheon, H. (2001). Impact of rural living on the experience of chronic illness. *Australian Journal of Rural Health, 9,* 235–240.

Hegney, D. (1997). Rural nursing practice. In L. Siegloff (Ed.), *Rural nursing in the Australian context* (pp. 25–43). Deacon Act, Australia: Royal College of Nursing.

Jirojwong, S., & MacLennan, R. (2002). Management of episodes of incapacity by families in rural and remote Queensland. *Australian Journal of Rural Health, 10,* 249–255.

Johnson, J. L., Ratner, P. A., & Bottorff, J. L. (1995). Urban-rural differences in the health-promoting behaviours of Albertans. *Canadian Journal of Public Health, 86,* 103–108.

Lau, T., Kumar, S., & Thomas, D. (2002). Practicing psychiatry in New Zealand's rural areas: Incentives, problems and solutions. *Australian Psychiatry, 10*(1), 33–38.

Lee, H. J., Hollis, B. R., & McClain, K. A. (1998). Isolation. In H. J. Lee (Ed.), *Conceptual basis for rural nursing* (1st ed., pp. 61–75). New York: Springer Publishing.

Lee, H. J., & Winters, C. A. (2002, October). *Testing the theory base: Perceptions and needs of rural service providers.* Paper presented at the Third International Congress of Rural Nurses, Binghamton, NY.

Lee, H. J., & Winters, C. A. (2004). Testing rural nursing theory: Perceptions and needs of service providers. *Online Journal of Rural Nursing and Health Care, 4*(1). Retrieved September 16, 2004, from http://www.rno.org/journal/issues/vol-4/issue.1/Lee_article.htm

Long, K. A., & Weinert, C. (1989). Rural nursing: Developing the theory base. *Scholarly Inquiry for Nursing Practice: An International Journal, 3,* 113–127.

MacLeod, M., Browne, A. J., & Leipert, B. (1998). International perspective: Issues for nurses in rural and remote Canada. *Australian Journal of Rural Health, 6,* 72–78.

McConigley, R., Kristjanson, L., & Morgan, A. (2000). Palliative care nursing in rural Western Australia. *International Journal of Palliative Nursing, 6*(2), 80–90.

Niemoller, J. K., Ide, B. A., & Nichols, E. G. (2000). Issues in studying health-related hardiness and use of services among older rural adults. *Texas Journal of Rural Health, 18,* 35–43.

Pierce, C. (2001). The impact of culture of rural women's descriptions of health. *The Journal of Multicultural Nursing and Health, 7,* 50–53, 56.

Racher, F. E., & Vollman, A. R. (2002). Exploring the dimensions of access to health services: Implications for nursing research and practice. *Research and Theory for Nursing Practice: An International Journal, 16,* 77–90.

Roberto, K. A., & Reynolds, S. G. (2001). The meaning of osteoporosis in the lives of rural women. *Health Care for Women International, 22,* 599–611.

Rosenthal, K. A. (1996). *Rural nursing: An exploratory narrative description.* Unpublished Dissertation, University of Colorado, Denver.

Sellers, S. C., Poduska, M. D., Propp, L. H., & White, S. E. (1999). The health care meanings, values, and practices of Anglo-American males in the rural midwest. *Journal of Transcultural Nursing, 10,* 320–330.

Shannon, A. (1982). Introduction: Nursing in sparsely populated areas. In J. Taylor, Sparsely populated areas: Toward nursing theory. *Western Journal of Nursing Research, 4*(3)suppl, 70–71.

Taylor, J. (1982). Sparsely populated areas: Toward nursing theory. *Western Journal of Nursing Research, 4*(3)suppl, 69–77.

Thomlinson, E., McDonagh, M. K., Reimer, M., Crooks, K., & Lees, M. (2002). *Health beliefs of rural Canadians: Implications for practice.* Poster presented at the Third International Congress of Rural Nurses, Binghamton, NY.

Thomlinson, E., McDonagh, M. K., Reimer, M., Crooks, K., & Lees, M. (In press). Health beliefs of rural Canadians: Implications for practice. *Australian Journal of Rural Health.*

Thurston, W. E., & Meadows, L. M. (2003). Rurality and health: Perspectives of mid-life women. *The International Electronic Journal of Rural and Remote Health Research, Education, Practice, and Policy, 3* (219)), 1–12. Retrieved November 6, 2003, from http://rrh.deakin.edu.au

CHAPTER THREE

Exploring Rural Nursing Theory Across Borders

Charlene A. Winters, Elizabeth H. Thomlinson, Chad
O'Lynn, Helen J. Lee, Meg K. McDonagh, Dana S. Edge,
and Marlene A. Reimer

The descriptive rural nursing theory first published by Long and Weinert in 1989, and republished in 1999, is widely accepted and frequently quoted in presentations and articles. However, little testing of the theory has taken place. Recently, nurse scientists from the United States and Canada joined forces to validate the rural theory concepts. Lee and Winters (2004) conducted qualitative studies to explore rural persons' health perceptions and needs in the state of Montana and Thomlinson, McDonagh, Reimer, Crooks and Lee (2002) did the same in the Canadian provinces of Alberta and Manitoba. Then we compared the findings from these two studies. Our specific aim in the comparison were to (1) validate existing rural nursing theory concepts, (2) identify new emerging concepts, and (3) determine areas for further theoretical development and research.

BACKGROUND AND SIGNIFICANCE

Rural nursing is the provision of health care by professional nurses to persons living in sparsely populated areas (Long & Weinert, 1989). Rural

This research was funded by Montana State University-Bozeman College of Nursing Block Grant, Sigma Theta Tau International, Zeta Upsilon Chapter, and Visiting Scholar, University of Calgary, Alberta, Canada.

nursing theory evolved because of a recognized need for a framework for practice that considers the special needs of this population. The theory-building process began in the late 1970s with the collection of qualitative and quantitative data by Montana State University-Bozeman College of Nursing graduate students and faculty. A rich database resulted in the identification of several key concepts and the development of three theoretical statements related to understanding rural health needs and rural nursing practice. The first statement was that "rural dwellers define health primarily as the ability to work, to be productive, to do usual tasks" (Long & Weinert, 1989, p. 120). Two closely interrelated concepts associated with this statement pertain to work beliefs and health beliefs. Health is defined in relation to work and health needs are secondary to work needs.

The second theoretical statement was that "rural dwellers are self-reliant and resist accepting help or services from those seen as 'outsiders' or from agencies seen as national or regional 'welfare' programs" (Long & Weinert, 1989, p.120). Closely associated to this statement is the tendency of rural dwellers to rely on informal social networks for health care. Key concepts pertaining to this statement are "self-reliance," "outsider," "insider," "old-timer," and "newcomer." Rural dwellers tend to engage in self-care and prefer the familiarity of the people and professionals who know them in contrast with the newcomer, or specialist, who is unfamiliar. Other concepts identified as important in understanding the health care-seeking behavior of rural residents are distance, isolation, and lack of anonymity, which are descriptive of the rural context in which these people live and work. The qualitative data from Montana, upon which the theoretical work was based, indicated that rural residents accepted distance as a normal part of living in a rural area. The degree of distance involved, whether actual or perceived, led some rural dwellers to experience a sense of isolation. Lastly, a lack of anonymity implies a limited ability for rural persons to have private areas in their lives, a phenomenon common to small towns and sparsely populated areas.

The third theoretical statement was that health care providers in rural areas "must deal with a lack of anonymity and much greater role diffusion than providers in urban or suburban settings" (Long & Weinert, 1989, p. 120). In a small community, everyone knows who the nurse is and this knowledge affects the nurse's effectiveness as a health care professional in that community. Furthermore, nurses are expected to function as expert generalists. For example, on a given day, a nurse working the day shift in a rural hospital may care for a laboring woman, recover an elderly man following surgery, triage in the emergency room, and prepare a pediatric trauma patient for transport to a regional medical center.

When the theory-building process began, literature and research related to rural health care were limited and focused primarily on rural health care delivery and access to service issues (Long & Weinert, 1989). A theoretical base for guiding rural health care did not exist. This prompted the faculty and students of Montana State University-Bozeman College of Nursing to begin the development of a theory base for rural nursing practice. Although rural nursing theory concepts are now widely accepted, a limited number of researchers have reported their efforts to test these initial findings. Our recent search of the literature resulted in only two citations for work that specifically related to rural nursing theory (Nichols, 1989, 1999). Both were response articles to Long and Weinert's theory-based article. Much of the published rural literature and research continues to focus on issues related to health care delivery and access. Given the paucity of research, we designed a study to test the rural nursing concepts described nearly 20 years ago.

METHODS AND PROCEDURES

The Montana study and the Canadian study were similar in design and purpose but the researchers (Lee & Winters, 2004; Thomlinson, Mc-Donagh, Reimer, Crooks, & Lees, 2002) planned and carried them out separately. In both studies, they used an ethnographic approach (Miles & Huberman, 1994; Morse & Field, 1995; Rossman & Rallis, 2003). In an ethnographic study, researchers describe and interpret phenomenon of interest in a cultural or social group or system (Creswell, 1998). Consistent with this approach, they collected data through open-ended interviews of rural persons and observational field notes (Rossman & Rallis) that documented their insights, their interactions with participants, and the physical and cultural context of the communities in which the participants lived. Through these activities, Lee and Winters, and Thomlinson et al. were able to identify the perceptions of the rural persons and learn what they understood about their health and how they managed their day-to-day health care situations. Using this open-ended approach, Lee and Winters, and Thomlinson et al. found that themes emerged from the interview narratives (Miles & Huberman), allowing us to make comparisons with the concepts and statements contained in the rural nursing theory proposed by Long and Weinert (1989).

Montana Study

Montana is the fourth largest state in the United States covering 147,042 square miles and stretching 700 miles from east to west. The state is sparsely populated with a density of 6.2 persons per square mile (*Census 2000 data for the state of Montana, n.d.*). According to the 2000 Census,

90.6% of the state's residents are Caucasian; the principle minority population is Native American (6.2%). Farming, fishing, and forestry occupations occupy 2.2% of the population whereas 42.4% of the population is employed in service, sales, and office occupations (*Census 2000 data for the state of Montana*, n.d.). The Rocky Mountains run north and south through the western part of the state, whereas eastern Montana is characterized by its rolling plains.

Lee and Winters (2004) conducted the Montana study according to the guidelines set forth by the Montana State University-Bozeman Human Subject Committee. They recruited participants through word of mouth (snowball sampling). Each participant signed a consent form that emphasized that only aggregate data would be reported. Lee and Winters maintained confidentiality of participants by removing names and identifiers. All participants were older than 18 years of age, employed in service occupations, and had lived in their respective communities for at least 5 years (Table 3.1).

Table 3.1 Demographics

	Montana Sample	Canadian Sample
Men	14	13
Women	24	42
Ethnicity		
Caucasian	35	52
Native American	3	
Aboriginal		3
Age range, years	22–85 ($m = 49$)	18–84*
Education	7–18 ($m = 13$)	8–16*
Marital status		
Married	26	37
Divorced	5	5
Single	7	9 (5 widow/widower)
Unknown		4
Occupation		
Grocery store clerks	4	
Secretaries	3	
Hospital workers	3	
Restaurant workers	3	
Beauty shop workers	2	
Animal care workers	2	
Museum operators	2	
County employees	2	

(continued)

Table 3.1 (*continued*)

	Montana Sample	Canadian Sample
Window treatment	2	
Post office workers	2	
Retirees		9
Ranchers		7
Education		19
Health care		3
Accountant		1
Bookkeeper		1
Other	13	15
Time in rural community, years	5–84 (*m* = 34)	3+*
Size of community, persons	70–1728	50–5,000
County density, persons per square mile	0.8–29.8	Not calculated
Distance to nearest large town, miles	12–250 (*m* = 60)	Not asked
Distance to nearest emergency care, miles	0.1–110 (*m* = 30)	3–90*
Self-reported health status		Not asked
Excellent	5	
Very good	3	
Good	17	
Fair	8	
Poor	1	
Did not respond	4	
Health insurance		
Yes	29	All have health care
No	8	insurance
No response	1	

*Means not available

Graduate nursing students enrolled in a rural nursing course conducted 38 interviews in the fall semesters of 2000 and 2001 with individuals living in rural towns with populations of 1,500 persons or less. Using open-ended questions, they asked participants about their perceptions of health and how they responded to illness and injury. Interviews lasted between 30–60 minutes and were audiotaped. Once transcribed, the students analyzed the interview narratives for themes. Students recorded observational field notes to document their activities, interactions, and insights. They wrote individual papers addressing the themes emerging from their interviews and field observations. Working separately, Lee and

Winters (2004) coded the transcripts and field notes identifying common themes. They then met to compare their findings with those identified by the students. They continually compared data supporting the emerging themes until they arrived at a consensus on the findings. Four major themes emerged from the analysis: (a) definition of health, (b) distance and access to resources, (c) symptom-action-time-line process (SATL), and (d) choice (see Table 3.2).

Canadian Study

The provinces of Alberta and Manitoba are approximately equal in size, with each province covering 250,000 square miles or roughly one and three-quarters the size of the state of Montana. The geography of Alberta closely parallels Montana, with rolling prairie and the Rocky Mountains bordering the western edge of the province. The terrain in Manitoba varies from flat farmland in the south to the Cambrian Shield, an area of granite rock with thin soil, in the north. In the north are large tracts of land covered with muskeg and forest. A major geographic difference between the two provinces is that 17% of Manitoba is covered with water compared with 3% of Alberta (*Statistics Canada,* 2004). The geographic diversity was a major reason for selecting these two distinct sites for the study.

In Alberta, the industries of farming, logging, ranching, and oil production employ 7% of the population, with sales, service, business, and finance employing 41% of Albertans. Similarly, in Manitoba farming, logging, mining, and fishing employ 7% of the population, whereas sales, service, business, and finance employ 41.6% of Manitobans (*Statistics Canada,* 2004).

Following ethical approval by the Conjoint Health Research Ethics Board at the University of Calgary, Thomlinson et al. (2002) sought par-

Table 3.2 Common Themes and Sub-themes

Theme	Sub-theme
Definitions of Health	a. Sickness
	b. Illness
Health-Seeking Behaviors	a. Symptom-Action-Time-Line (SATL)
	b. Resources
	c. Self-reliance
Choices	a. Residence
	b. Health care provider
Distance	a. Rural
	b. Northern

ticipants through newspaper advertisements and through word of mouth from other participants. In the first stage of the study, they selected 29 participants from municipal districts and small towns within 300 kilometers of Calgary. In the second stage, they sought 26 participants living in central and northern Manitoba for interviews (Table 3.1). As with the Montana study, all participants were over 18 years of age and signed consent forms that emphasized that only aggregate data would be reported. Thomlinson et al. maintained confidentiality of participants through the removal of names and identifiers. Thomlinson et al. and nursing student research assistants conducted face-to-face, semistructured interviews lasting between 45–60 minutes. Participants selected the locations for interviews, which were usually held in their homes.

Initially, four researchers (E. Thomlinson, M. McDonagh, K. Crooks, and M. Lees) coded five interview transcripts separately then compared findings. Two of the researchers (E. Thomlinson and M. McDonagh) completed the analysis of the remainder of the transcripts. The major themes that emerged from the transcripts included definitions of health, health-seeking behaviors, resources that were accessed, and definitions of rural and northern.

DATA ANALYSIS

In June 2003, we met at the University of Calgary, Alberta. We developed agreements regarding steps in the process of data comparison, responsibilities of team membership, dissemination of findings, and authorship. We conducted subsequent meetings via teleconference.

We began the process by viewing and comparing the demographic characteristics of the two samples. We compared the concepts, themes, salient characteristics, and relevant qualitative data excerpts from both studies and then displayed them using a concept-ordered matrix (Miles & Huberman, 1994). We collapsed concepts and themes having the same or very similar defining attributes into a common theme. We further evaluated concepts and themes that differed for differences in sample and methods and then added them to the matrix resulting in a combined dataset. We then compared findings with rural nursing theory concepts and theoretical statements. In this manner, we maintained methodological rigor of consistency, neutrality, truth-value, and applicability (Morse & Field, 1995).

FINDINGS

After much analysis and discussion, we identified by consensus four common themes and nine subthemes (Table 3.2) and summarized them below.

Common Themes

Definition of health. We identified the theme *definition of health* in both studies. In the Montana study, health was described primarily as the absence of conditions that would interrupt work or play and included physical, mental, and emotional fitness. In the Canadian study, the definition of health was similar but included the importance of spiritual and environmental considerations. Participants from both studies spoke of health as a concept that was to some degree related to age and the absence of chronic illness with comments such as, "I'm healthy for my age." Following further examination of the transcripts and discussion, we agreed upon the common theme definition of health as a holistic perspective in which optimal ability to function at work or play and to pursue desired activities is maintained. Optimal ability is obtained through health-seeking and health-promoting behaviors to achieve holistic balance, resolution of short-term disruptions, and adaptation to long-term health challenges.

In addition, Canadian participants differentiated between *sickness* and *illness,* noting that sickness is short in duration and is curable; whereas illness is either chronic in nature or serious and life threatening. We then determined that sickness and illness were subthemes of definition of health.

Health-seeking behaviors. The theme *Symptom-Action-Time–Line (SATL)* emerged from the Montana data and was used to describe the social process of identifying symptoms and seeking self, lay, or professional health care for illness and injuries (Buehler, Malone, & Majerus, 1998). SATL was similar to the theme health-seeking behaviors, which emerged from the Canadian data. We discussed the similarities and differences between these two themes noting that SATL focused on obtaining health resources once a health disruption is noted. Furthermore, the theme health-seeking behaviors incorporated SATL as well as behaviors designed to promote health and prevent health disruptions. We determined that health-seeking behaviors was a common theme and SATL was a subtheme of health-seeking behaviors. Health-seeking behaviors is defined as conscious behaviors designed to promote healthy relationships among physical, mental, social, and spiritual aspects of one's life so that life balance is maintained.

Resources was a theme identified in the Canadian data and defined as people and other sources of information and assistance one uses in health-seeking behaviors. Examples of resources that were provided by Canadian participants included community elders, trusted traditional healers, libraries, the Internet, and health care professionals who really listen. The Montana researchers also noted resources as a component of SATL. As a result, we determined resources to be an additional subtheme of health-seeking behaviors.

In reviewing the data, we noted a number of excerpts that described the self-reliance of rural dwellers. Participants engaged in self-care when managing illness and injury and when needed, chose to seek care first from friends and family members prior to seeing a health care professional. Participants commented that they kept their "medicine cabinets stocked" and when injured, they would pull the edges of the wound together if only a "couple of inches long." They would see a health care provider for injuries they didn't think they "could put a Band-Aid on" or handle themselves. Because of its prevalence in the data and the context in which the term appeared, we determined that *self-reliance* was a subtheme under health-seeking behaviors.

Choices. The conscious life choices one makes in terms of residence and accessing health services was a theme we identified as choices. The theme emerged from the Montana data based on participants' comments regarding their choice to live in rural areas and their decision-making processes regarding when and which health resources they access when ill or injured. Generally, participants expressed satisfaction with living in rural areas and commented on the benefits of rural living. The Canadian researchers did not initially identify choices as a theme. However, they did find that the participants exhibited a "taking charge" attitude, which we believed to be equated with making choices. And because the Canadian participants made comments similar to Montana participants regarding the benefits of rural living and how living in sparsely populated areas shaped their health care decision making, we reached a consensus in identifying choices as a theme.

Distance. Thomlinson et al. (2002) classified participants in their study as either rural or northern, and asked the participants to describe what these terms meant to them. They noted that the Canadian government has six definitions of rural and defines northern as the region north of a north and south line determined by 16 combined social, biotic, economic, and climatic aspects of geography (McNiven, 1999). Distance was the factor that differentiated rural from northern for Canadian participants, in that northern residents are more isolated and distances to all services, not just health services, are much farther than those for rural residents. Distance, was also described by the Montana participants, with comments focusing on distance to services, lack of service availability, and travel times to services. Thus, we determined that *distance* was a theme and rural and northern were subthemes of distance. Distance was defined as separation (space, time, and behavior) between the rural population and health care resources.

DISCUSSION

The definition of health we identified in this study, although more holistic than the original definition, continues to support the interrelatedness of work and health and provides partial support for the first theoretical statement identified by Long and Weinert (1989). Furthermore, the new definition of health adds to the original definition by including "ability to play," identifying the importance of mental and emotional fitness, and including the notion that health is qualified by age and the presence of illness. In addition, we determined health-seeking and health-promoting behaviors to be foundational to the maintenance of health.

Although variations existed within groups, health-seeking behaviors were demonstrated by participants from both countries. Therefore, we identified health-seeking behaviors, as a common theme and described the processes participants' used to promote healthy relationships among physical, mental, social and spiritual aspects of their life. Underlying the overall theme of health-seeking behavior, were three subthemes: (a) SATL, (b) resources, and (c) self-reliance.

The acronym SATL described previously by Buehler et al. (1998) is the social process of identifying symptoms and seeking self, lay, or professional health care for illness and injuries. With this process, participants choose the resources that they believe will be effective in promoting their health status or managing their health concern. We defined resources as people, other sources of information, and assistance one uses in health-seeking behaviors.

Self-reliance is described by Chafey, Sullivan, and Shannon (1998) as behaviors of accomplishing tasks without the help of others, stemming from values (such as autonomy) or contextual variables (such as barriers to resource access). Accordingly, we identified self-reliance in this collaborative study. Findings indicate that participants preferred to engage in self-care for illness and injuries and sought assistance from informal resources prior to seeking the services of health care professionals. The findings support the second theoretical statement (Long & Weinert, 1989), and the addition of three subthemes to health-seeking behaviors contributes to the expansion of the rural nursing theory base.

The theme choices refers to the participants'conscious decision-making processes regarding their place of residence and patterns of accessing health services. During data analysis, we realized that participants were constantly making choices, and these decisions affected their lifestyle, their personal health and health practices and that of their families, and their livelihood. Examples of such choices include decisions regarding when, where, and from whom to seek care for an injury, where they should reside (stay on the farm or move into town), and what kind of foods they should be eating to maintain health and yet stay within their allotted budget. Long and Weinert (1989) did not previously identify choices as part of rural nursing theory.

Distance was an important concept that Long and Weinert (1989) identified in their original descriptive theory and we also found it important in the comparison study. We defined it as separation (space, time, and behavior) between the rural population and health care resources, and then further broke it down on the basis of the degree of remoteness recognizing that distances to *all* services, not just health services, are much greater for isolated rural residents. Expanding the concept of distance to include definitions of rural and northern is one way that *degrees of remoteness* can be used to extend rural nursing theory. The identification and explication of the themes definition of health, health-seeking-behaviors, choices, and distance have implications for furthering health care providers' understanding of the health care-seeking behaviors, practices, and preferred resources of rural dwellers.

Implications for Rural Nursing Theory and Practice

The findings of this comparison study validate and expand upon existing rural nursing theory concepts and provide partial support for the first and second theoretical statements identified by Long and Weinert (1989). As the focus of this study was on the health perceptions and needs of rural persons, it is beyond the scope of this project to address the rural nursing theory concepts germane to the third theoretical statement regarding the role of rural health care providers.

Through the expansion of the previous understanding of health, educators and practitioners are provided the opportunity to view their specific rural population's health needs in a broader context. The data also reveal that a variety of health-seeking and health-promoting behaviors is important to rural dwellers. The information gained from this study about SATL, resources, and choices has significant implications for further rural nursing theory development and practice. By increasing the amount of information gathered and the breadth of the rural population sampled, the theory base solidifies its applicability to rural nurses and thus has the potential to positively impact the health care delivery to rural dwellers in North America. Understanding the health-care decision-making processes used by rural dwellers will assist nurses to provide care appropriate to their client's needs and rural lifestyle.

Although distance is not a new concept in the rural nursing theory base, our understanding of distance and what it means to specific rural groups has been expanded in this study. The data support the notion that distance is not constant, it is variable among specific populations and their contexts. This has implications for how the context of rural dwellers is understood by rural nurses and has the potential to affect future programs for health education and health program delivery.

Although each of the four themes and nine subthemes require further examination, the aforementioned findings suggest that major tenets of rural nursing theory can be applied across the western United States-Canadian border. This finding provides contextual information important to the further development of rural nursing theory. Additional research that compares and contrasts the health perceptions and needs of persons living in differing rural environments is necessary to further build upon the theory base. In addition, replication of this study is needed internationally as well as in other North American rural and remote areas to provide the necessary rigor and applicability of rural nursing theory. Finally, studies are needed that address the third theoretical statement, which focuses on the issues facing nurses practicing in rural and remote areas. A more solid base for rural nursing theory is required to guide the delivery of nursing care to rural and remote populations.

REFERENCES

Buehler, J., Malone, M., & Majerus, J. (1998). Patterns of response to symptoms in rural residents: The symptom-action-time-line process. In H. Lee (Ed.), *Conceptual basis for rural nursing* (pp. 318–328). New York: Springer Publishing.

Census 2000 data for the state of Montana. (n.d.). Retrieved December 15, 2002, from http://www.census.gov/census2000/states/mt.html

Chafey, K., Sullivan, T., & Shannon, A. (1998). Self-reliance: Characterization of their own autonomy by elderly rural women. In H. J. Lee (Ed.), *Conceptual basis for rural nursing* (pp. 156–177). New York: Springer Publishing.

Creswell, J. (1998). *Qualitative inquiry and research design: Choosing among five traditions*. Thousand Oaks, CA: Sage.

Lee, H. J., & Winters, C.A. (2004). Testing rural nursing theory: Perceptions and needs of service providers. *Online Journal of Rural Nursing and Health Care*, 4. Retrieved July 5, 2004, from http://www.rno.org/journal/issues/Vol-4/issue-1/Lee_article.htm.

Long, K. A., & Weinert, C. (1989). Rural nursing: Developing the theory base. *Scholarly Inquiry for Nursing Practice, 3*(2), 113–127.

Long, K. A., & Weinert, C. (1999). Rural nursing: Developing the theory base. 1989. *Scholarly Inquiry for Nursing Practice, 13*(3), 257–269.

McNiven, C. (1999). North is that direction. Canadian Social Trends, pp. 8–11. *Statistics Canada—Catalogue* No. 11–008. Retrieved July 23, 2004, from http://estat.statcan.ca/content/english/articles/pop-a.shtml

Miles, M. B., & Huberman, A. M. (1994). *Qualitative data analysis* (2nd ed.). Thousand Oaks, CA: Sage.

Morse, J. M., & Field, P. A. (1995). *Qualitative research methods for health professions* (2nd ed.). Thousand Oaks, CA: Sage.

Nichols, E. (1989). Response to "Rural nursing: Developing the theory base." *Scholarly Inquiry for Nursing Practice, 3,* 129–132.

Nichols, E. (1999). Response to "Rural nursing, Developing the theory base." 1989. *Scholarly Inquiry for Nursing Practice, 13,* 271–274.

Rossman, G. B., & Rallis, S. F. (2003). *Learning in the field* (2nd ed.). Thousand Oaks, CA: Sage.

Statistics Canada. (2004). Retrieved May 27, 2004, from http://www.statcan.ca/start.html

Thomlinson, E., McDonagh, M. K., Reimer, M., Crooks, K., & Lees, M. (2002). Health beliefs of rural Canadians: Implications for practice [Abstract]. *Charting the course for rural health in the 21st century,* 18.

PART II

Perspectives of Rural Persons

In this part we present current research findings about the perspectives of persons in a variety of rural settings. First, one of the key concepts (see Appendix) relevant to the rural nursing theory base is explored. Boland and Lee report on a qualitative study of the meaning of *old-timer* for older persons living in north central Montana. It is followed by a chapter by Bales, Winters, and Lee that reports on the health needs and perceptions of persons living in an isolated town in south central Montana where access in many of the winter months is limited to snowmobile or snowshoe.

The next three chapters contain studies of rural women. Bales reports on the health perceptions, needs and behaviors of remote rural women of childbearing and childrearing age. Leipert proposes a model explaining the development of resilience to manage vulnerability in rural women. Using grounded theory methods, West recommends a model for strategizing safety to manage the perinatal experience of rural women.

The last chapter in this part focuses on rural families. Meiers, Eggenberger, Krumwiede, Bliesmer, and Earle propose a model titled, "Enduring Acts of Balancing" as an explanation for how rural families respond to the expectations of the modern health care system.

CHAPTER FOUR

Old-Timers

Robin L. Boland and Helen J. Lee

Acceptance into a rural community as a health provider can be influenced by many variables. One such variable is the concept of *old-timer*. In 1987, Weinert and Long wrote "Rural dwellers used the concepts of 'old-timer' and 'newcomer' as a framework to organize their social interactions, their relationships within the community and were important to their 'view of the social environment'" (p. 453). In 1998, Caniparoli clarified the meaning of the term *old-timer* through a concept analysis; she concluded further clarification was needed. The purpose of this chapter is to explore the concept of old-timer and its relationship to the social function of a rural community. A discussion of the social order of rural communities is followed by a brief description of rural nursing theory development. A literature review and the recommendations regarding further work on the concept old-timer are explicated.

BACKGROUND

Rural Communities

The rural environment is characterized by low-density settlement (Rosenblatt & Moscovice, 1982). Rural communities consist of few people who are often related; their day-to-day interactions are face-to-face, occurring in local settings (Bushy, 2000). In contrast to urban populations, the support network that forms within rural families is more likely to rely on close relatives (those who share the household or live locally) or is locally integrated, consisting of local family, friends, and neighbors (Wenger, 1989). Family members look to members of their network, creating informal systems to interact within their communities. They look to the older, more experienced individuals for guidance and leadership in establishing a community's social order.

The presence of few persons is accompanied by a sparseness of social services, including health care (Rosenblatt & Moscovice, 1982). As a part of their culture, rural dwellers experience greater control in their daily lives, becoming independent and self-reliant. In adapting to their environment, they rely first on themselves and then on others within their informal network systems before tapping into formal resource systems. According to Long and Weinert (1989), the concepts of old-timer and newcomer were important to the rural community members' interactions and "relevant in terms of acceptance of nurses and all health providers in rural communities" (p. 125).

Rural Nursing Theory Development

In the late 1970s, limited information was available about the health needs of the rural population. Existing nursing models were applicable toward urban and suburban areas; however, because of the unique health problems and health needs of the rural population, they were inadequate in addressing rural health care concerns. "No organized theoretical base for guiding rural health care practice in general, or rural nursing in particular, existed" (Long & Weinert, 1989, p. 114). Long and Weinert reported the results of combined quantitative and qualitative studies conducted by faculty and graduate students that explored the health beliefs, values, and practice of rural dwellers. They identified key concepts, including health status and health beliefs, work beliefs, isolation and distance, self-reliance, informal health care systems, lack of anonymity, outsider, insider, old-timer, and newcomer.

Oldtimer

The term old-timer or descriptions of old-timers have been used extensively in Western and historical literature to describe older, adventurous, colorful, yet knowledgeable individuals. Folklore and Western movies have portrayed old-timers in this capacity. The majority of old-timers were men, as women were not considered part of the frontier experience (Malone, 1983).

Many times authors described old-timers according to their occupations, such as cowboys, miners, loggers, ranchers, and trappers. Their work was implied to be dangerous and usually involved working alone (El

Comancho, 1929). More recently in Western literature, McCumber (1999) used the term old-timer as a marker for respect and experience when he wrote "Yesterday's greenhorn is tomorrow's old-timer" (p. 93).

The popular media and health care organizations are similar in their views of old-timers as older, tenured, respected, and experienced. Chafetz, Childress, Glazer, Holmes, and Lande (1998) studied the preferences for nouns and adjectives that might be used in news stories to refer to older adults. They cited old-timer as one of the most disliked terms in referring to people aged older than 65 years. In newspaper articles published in the *Great Falls Tribune, Missoulian,* and Helena's *Independent Record,* writers reported survey results describing the attitudes of long-time Montana residents toward quality of life, jobs, and importation of new ideas and innovations caused by newcomers to the state (Johnson, 1996). *Long-time residents,* those identified as living in the same state longer than 10 years, were more likely to criticize the impact of newcomers and agreed that the number of newcomers moving into the state would negatively affect the environment of the state.

Caniparoli (1998) identified defining attributes of the term old-timer, which were "age, length of time in a community, and establishment of a relationship within the community" (p. 108). Because of the many differing interpretations of the use of the term old-timer, she concluded further clarification was needed. She suggested the following clarifying questions to guide further exploration of the concept of old-timer: (a)To what degree do communities of today use the concept of old-timer as it was understood in Western folklore? (b) How are old-timers identified in a community and how do they view themselves? (c) What roles do old-timers serve in a community organization and social order? and (d)Are the attributes of old-timer the same today as they were in the past? (p. 111).

METHODS

I (R. Boland) chose a qualitative descriptive design based on the grounded theory approach (Burns & Grove, 1997; Chinn & Kramer, 1995; LaBiondo-Wood & Haber, 1994) to clarify the concept of old-timer and explore the influence these individuals have on a community. I chose for the study the communities of Sand Coulee, Stockett, Tracy, and Centerville in Montana. The communities lie in close proximity to each other and are 10-15 miles south of the larger city of Great Falls. These communities have a rich agricultural and mining history. Many families emigrated into these communities in the early 1900s, and have maintained homesteads, family farms or ranches, as well as small businesses. Together these communities form what is commonly known as The Gulch. The study was conducted with the approval of the Montana State University-Bozeman College of Nursing Human Subject Committee.

Sample

The convenience sample comprised nine participants aged 72–92 years: three single women, two single men, and two married couples. All participants were Caucasian and native Montanans. Six participants had lived in the community since birth, two arrived in the community in early adulthood to teach school and married residents of the community, and one participant moved into the community at the age of 5 years. Eight participants had children or extended family living in the community, whereas the ninth participant was single and the last of her family to live in the community. The participants' occupations consisted of ranching and teaching. Four of the nine participants were retired; the remaining five were semiretired ranchers.

Data Collection

I conducted informal face-to-face interviews using open-ended questions in the participants' homes. Initially I contacted two participants known to me. I solicited additional names of potential participants from these interviewees, creating a snowball effect of gathering participants. I used the original questions and slight variations, dependent upon the responses, to elicit information from the remaining participants. I also gathered demographic data from the participants.

Data Analysis

I analyzed the data using a grounded theory method of comparative analysis (Chinn & Kramer, 1995). The data analyzed for this study consisted of transcribed interviews and field notes. Analysis of data involved coding, examining the units of analysis for patterns, and categorizing the data. I then analyzed the patterns for new categories and concepts and their relationships.

FINDINGS

From the comparative analysis of the data, four central themes emerged: (a) name descriptors of older residents, (b) characteristics of old-timers, (c) community functions of old-timers, and (d) old-timers' perceptions of their influence in the community. I further broke down the four central themes into subcategories. Old-timer stories interfaced each theme and provided insight and rich descriptions of the old-timers from The Gulch. Their stories painted a picture of earlier individuals who were knowledgeable, hardworking, fun loving, and committed to their neighbors and the rural way of life they shared.

Name Descriptors of Older Residents

Old-timer was the most common name identified by the participants, and all agreed the term was considered respectful in reference to older residents who had lived in the community a long time. Some participants delighted in reaching the status of old-timer. As indicated by one old-timer rancher, as old-timers from the previous generation passed away, his generation then became the old-timers. The participants viewed the status of old-timer as a rite of passage, "being part of the history."

Characteristics of old-timers

I identified age, long-time residency, and land ownership as common characteristics of old-timers. The participants were less clear about a specific age to identify old-timers. All participants shared stories of individuals they considered old-timers. These old-timers had "age on their side," usually aged 80 years or older, with a few aged as old as 98–100 years. It was a common belief that many of the old-timers were "gone," "passing away," or "there aren't that many left."

Age and long-time residency in the community were woven together to form the basis for "being born and raised here." "Living here all your life" was often quoted as a prerequisite to inclusion as an old-timer. In reference to one old-timer, "he grew up at No. 7 [a mine]" and continues to live in the community to this day. One participant offered this insight when asked to clarify between age and long-time residency in determining old-timer status: "I would say how long they have lived here. We haven't had anybody move in here that is an old-timer."

One exception to long time residency was land ownership. Many of the participants, as well as others identified as old-timers, had land holdings going back two and three generations. The land ownership was the tie to the community; land established a relationship with the community. One participant stated the relationship between land ownership and old-timer status this way:

> The ranch has been in our name 100 years. The neighbors down here, they came about the same time our Dad did, but the old people are both dead now. Their kids sold part of the ranch to me. So them old-timers are gone. Now we are the old-timers or old-duffers.

Another old-timer, also a rancher, offered this explanation regarding the discrepancy between old-time miners and old-time ranchers from his boyhood. "The miners would drink," with the implication the miners were less respectable than the ranchers. In his mind, the ranchers were the old-timers.

Many of the participants used stories to describe the old-timers they had known in the past and the old-timers of the present. Their stories reflected colorful, adventuresome, experienced, independent characters, sometimes with a peculiar quality that served to describe their physical appearance or habits. One old-timer participant recalled the story of a hired hand working for his father. The hired hand had been hauling manure and was injured when he fell off a wagon being driven by another hired hand. Angry, the injured ranch hand left for Stockett on foot. The participant continued:

> He went to Dr. [name] and got sauced up and he came back that night and the other kid was eating his supper and there was a gunshot, he shot him through the window. Didn't hit the guy. They had him arrested and he had ten dollars coming. The ten dollars he had coming, he spent for snooze. They called him Snooze [name]. He didn't chew it; he stuffed it up his nose.

The participants in the study were also risk takers at some point in their lives. The young women took teaching positions in unfamiliar rural one-room schoolhouses and the hardworking young men risked all during the depression years to keep the family ranch. These old-timer participants emerged from these experiences to form the backbone of the community, the glue holding the tight-knit community together.

Community Functions of Old-Timers

I identified work as an activity, sociability, keepers of the traditions, and historians as functions old-timers contributed to the community. Old-timers were described as hardworking. The times, the conditions, the elements necessitated they be so. Hard times helped to forge a common bond between the old-timers. The old-timers worked together out of necessity for survival, their personal survival and that of their livelihood or business.

> As far as getting together, the old-timers had to rely on one another, more so than today. We still work together. You have to. We ship [cattle] together. Otherwise, you just can't get help. When I grew up, there were about six of us that had a branding crew and working crew together, but I am the last one left.

The participant continued to explain that quite often working together was also a social event.

> The real old-timers, if you look way over there you see the roof of that big barn? That was Pete's place. That was a real old-timer. This is how they got together and worked. He called the neighbors and said I have a bunch of three-year-old steers to dehorn. You come next Sunday and we will do them. I will get a keg of beer. They made one mistake. They opened the keg of beer first. By the time they got to work the big steers, because they had to rope them and throw them, 1,500 pounds apiece, those guys were so looped they couldn't handle them. Pete said we can't do it, you come back next Sunday and we will do it again. They did the same darn thing. They opened the keg of beer again. Two Sundays in a row and they never got one animal done. The third Sunday, they did them [steers] before they opened the keg of beer.

All the participants agreed that old-timers of yesterday were more sociable than the old-timers of today. Activities of yesterday included dances, card parties, meetings, baseball, and, of course, just plain visiting. Community dances were especially important. Barns were built to hold dances and people would come from all over. One participant, a fiddle and saxophone player, explained "every ranch house had one or two fiddlers," and "I took my sax, tied it down [on the saddle], and away I would go."

One old-timer reflected:

> It was a close community because that is all there was. It was a long way from Great Falls and other entertainment and you didn't go to Great Falls until it was necessary, so they depended on one another for anything that was going on. You would leave notes on the board down at the store if there was anything going on or a shower or whatever, home demonstration meeting.

Today the old-timers continue to serve the community by sharing traditions from previous generations. Their community is steeped full of traditions from their ethnic forefathers. A female participant, very active in the Senior Citizen organization and Holy Trinity Parish, shared her philosophy regarding the passing on of traditions: "If it wasn't for them [old-timers], a lot of things wouldn't be done. See, the kids will see what they do and then they [kids] keep right on doing the same thing."

Old-timers also act as historians, passing down stories from generation to generation. These stories richly described the lives and characteristics of old-timers. Some participants served as informants for local history books or had written their own books. The pages of history written about The

Gulch owe their existence to the tales and trivia recorded or retold by old-timers. Old-timers hold the past knowledge of the community's rich mining history, the secrets of the abandoned homesteads scattered on the hillsides, and the stories of many persons who had come and gone from the community. The participants were eager to share their own stories, which spoke well of their knowledge of the history of the community. Yet, many participants said even though their stories were often sought, their influence had waned.

Old-Timers' Perceptions of Their Influence on a Community

The participants expressed that changing times had altered the influence old-timers have on a community. The community was not as tightly knit as it once was. Today there were fewer farms and ranches on the landscape. Even within the small communities, long-time residents did not know the "newcomer" neighbor living next door. The community's close approximation to the larger city of Great Falls had rendered The Gulch a bedroom community. Newcomers to the community reportedly showed little interest or actual involvement in community activities. Just as the characteristics of the community's population base had changed, so had the emphasis placed on community activities. The participants also noted less need to rely on one another, which they attributed to today's fast lifestyle, and technological advances, such as the telephone and automobile.

The loss of influence by old-timers was also linked to the loss of respect for elderly people in today's society. Participants thought the younger residents were less respectful and listened less to the advice the old-timers had to give. An old-timer shared in reference to the younger generations: "Oh, they like to listen and hear stories about the old times, but they don't want your advice." In some instances the identification of old-timers by family members did not mean they were necessarily influential. Unfortunately for some old-timers, the loss of influence had affected their self-esteem, and sadly enough, altered relationships with family or community members.

IMPLICATIONS

The implications and applications to the practice of nursing are numerous. Old-timer status and its relationship to a community's social order may still influence access and use of health care, but on a smaller scale than previously thought. Old-timers may influence individuals in a smaller social circle, such as organizations in which they are a member. Their sociability provides an avenue to share information directed toward accessing and using health care. For example, an elderly female patient who has learned the value of breast self-exam during a physical exam, in turn, may share this information with her Home Demonstration Group. If she is a respected member and her opinions valued, she may influence others in the group to either schedule a physical exam or to begin breast self-exam.

Another aspect to consider with regard to practice issues was the perceived lack of influence older long-time residents have on a community. Loss of respect for elderly people, decreased involvement in the community by newcomers, and less need to rely on ones' neighbors are credited for loss of influence older long-time residents have on a rural community. Health providers new to a rural area may be ill advised to target their advertising dollars only toward the elderly members of the community. To assume that utilization and acceptance by the older age group would ascertain utilization by the community as a whole could put the practitioners at financial risk.

This research indicates the need for further qualitative research to determine the context of old-timers' status and influence within organizations (Caniparoli, 1998). The study also could be replicated in other rural communities to determine the generalizability of the concept of old-timer and its relationship to the social function of a rural community.

REFERENCES

Burns, N., & Grove, S. K. (1997). *The practice of nursing research* (3rd ed.). Philadelphia: Saunders.

Bushy, A. (2000). *Orientation to nursing in the rural community.* Thousand Oaks, CA: Sage.

Caniparoli, C. (1998). Old-timer. In H. J. Lee (Ed.), *Conceptual basis for rural nursing* (pp. 102–112).New York: Springer Publishing.

Chafetz, P. K., Childress, E., Glazer, H. R., Holmes, H., & Lande, K. (1998). Older adults and the news media: Utilization, opinions, and preferred reference terms. *The Gerontologist,38,* 481–489.

Chinn, P. K., & Kramer, M. K. (1995). *Theory and nursing: A systematic approach* (4th ed.). St. Louis, MO: Mosby.

El Comancho. (1929). *The old timer's tale.* Chicago: Cantebury Press.

Johnson, P. (1996, February 5). Most Montanans see newcomers as threat to jobs. *The Great Falls Tribune,* 1B-2B.

LaBiondo-Wood, G., & Haber, J. (1994). *Nursing research: Methods, critical appraisal andutilization* (3rd ed.). St. Louis, MO: Mosby.

Long, K. A., & Weinert, C. (1989). Rural nursing: Developing the theory base. *Scholarly Inquiry for Nursing Practice, 3,* 113–127.

Malone, M. P. (1983). *Historians and the American West.* Lincoln: University of Nebraska Press.

McCumber, D. (1999). *The cowboy way: Seasons of a Montana ranch.* New York: Avon.

Rosenblatt, R. A., & Moscovice, I. S. (1982). *Rural health care.* New York: Wiley

Weinert, C., & Long, K. A., (1987). Understanding the health care needs of rural families. *Family Relations, 36,* 450–455.

Wenger, G. C. (1989). Support networks in old age—constructing a typology. In M. Jefferys (Ed.), *Growing old in the twentieth century.* London: Routledge. Cited in Community - a review of the theory. Retrieved October 13, 2004, from http://www.infed.org/community/community.htm

CHAPTER FIVE

Health Needs and Perceptions of Rural Persons

Ronda L. Bales, Charlene A. Winters, and Helen J. Lee

Health practices of rural dwellers are known to be influenced by their perceptions of health and illness. Long and Weinert (1998) remarked on the individuality of health perceptions among rural dwellers and noted that those assumptions regarding concepts of health cannot be generalized among rural populations. Understanding the health perceptions, needs, and behaviors of an individual, family, or community can be instrumental in health promotion planning. This chapter addresses the health needs, perceptions, and behaviors of six individuals living in one community in rural Montana.

INTRODUCTION TO THE COMMUNITY

With an elevation of 7,651 feet above sea level, the echoed phrase "closer to heaven than I may ever get" is a vivid reference to the vast and beautiful wilderness known as Montana City.* The community is nestled in the midst of mountain peaks and lies just east of the northeast entrance to a national park (Glidden, 1982). The location of Montana City is one of its unique attributes with access to and from the community varying from summer to winter. Although travel in and out of Montana City during the summer may be slow because of the winding mountain roads, it is not

*Names of communities have been changed for this chapter.

limited. The winter months, however, bring additional challenges beyond distance to the members of this community that other rural Montanans may not face. When the snow begins to fly in October, residents are faced with isolation in terms of travel outside their community. From October to May, when the snow typically melts, the only passable route by automobile is 55 miles on a narrow, winding highway through a national park with an additional 55 miles to expanded health care services (*National Geographic Road Atlas*, 2000). Passage via this route is dependent on snowplows to keep the roads passable. An alternative route out of Montana City is available. This route allows for travel to towns and cities in Montana and a neighboring state, about 100 and 120 miles respectively (Glidden; *National Geographic Road Atlas*). There is a catch, however; this route includes a stretch of road over a pass approximately 10 miles long that is left unplowed during the winter (Fahlberg, 1983). Therefore, access to and from Montana City via this route during the winter months is limited to those with snowmobiles. Thus, one can visualize that winter brings challenges to these rural dwellers that affect access not only to health care, but to all dimensions of life outside the community.

METHODS

My (R. Bales) purpose in this study was to explore the health needs and perceptions of rural persons living in Montana City, Montana. I chose descriptive qualitative research methods for this research project because they provide an opportunity "to try to understand how people make sense of their worlds" (Rossman & Rallis, 1998, p. 8). In this case, it allowed me an opportunity to understand how, when, where, and why the residents of Montana City seek health care and the factors that influence health care behaviors, access, and utilization.

After obtaining informed consent, I conducted semistructured interviews with members of the community. Initially, I identified participants through a key informant who owned a cabin located within the community. I approached the remaining participants directly and asked about their interest in participation in the study.

Sample

The convenience sample consisted of five women and one man, aged 37–76 years. The participants had lived in the community 3–30 years. Montana City met the definition of remote rural described by Koehler (1998): "a community with a population of 2,500 or less located forty miles or further from a city with a population of 50,000 or greater. Remote rural communities do not have a hospital or medical assistance facility" (pp. 238–239).

Data Collection and Analysis

I collected data by using a semistructured interview guide. Questions were open-ended and intended to elicit information regarding the individuals' health perceptions and needs. Interviews were audiotape recorded and transcribed. Field notes were kept to document observations and impressions about the community and persons interviewed. I analyzed the transcribed interviews and field notes for emergent themes

FINDINGS

Montana City

The population of this community varies drastically in accordance with the change of seasons. The participants of the study estimated the year-round population to be 70–100 persons and stated that it tripled during the summer. All participants identified themselves as "year-round" residents of the community.

I identified two main groups within the sample: (a) those who had lived in the community for a number of years and (b) those who had recently moved there. A comparison was provided by one participant who gave a description of the long-time members of the community.

> If you live here long enough, you can tell who lives here by how they dress, the snowmobiles they drive, the clothes they wear are patched up with duck tape. They have the old style stuff, but then maybe that's a sign of the culture too. I just think that some of that goes with it, that you choose to live that way because you want to. It is not important, material things are not important here. I am really speaking generally cause there are people moving in who have a lot more money to spend and they have the nicer homes. So you see, we are seeing a change in our culture here.

Health Care

Health care resources within the community of Montana City were limited. There was no clinic, hospital, or other formal health care. However, Emergency Medical Services (EMS) were available. The EMS network was composed of volunteers from the community who were mainly trained at the First Responder level, and one member who was available to practice at the Emergency Medical Technician (EMT) level at the time I conducted the interviews. There was a dedicated ambulance for the national park located at the entrance and the Park Ranger stationed there was an EMT. The EMS process was explained by a participant.

> If someone calls 911, they call me or someone on the roster. Then I go and appraise the situation and call for the ambulance if it is needed. See, we do have an ambulance available, but it is at the gate [to the national park]. But the park administration doesn't think the community should rely solely on the Park for its EMS services. So that is why they call someone on the list first, and then if we need it, we call for the ambulance.

The Park ambulance is equipped for advanced life support and can travel to a clinic located in Maryville, approximately 55 miles through the National Park. If transport to a hospital was necessary, a second ambulance from Littlewood had to meet the Park ambulance and transport the patient. Medical flight services are typically not available to Maryville community because the location presents a dangerous situation for helicopters.

All participants interviewed identified a retired doctor who lived in the community as a health care resource. Participants indicated they had accessed him at one time or another and that he had also helped them make judgments about whether or not it was necessary to obtain further or immediate care for a health-related issue. The identified retired physician had lived in Montana City for 5 years at the time I conducted the study. I contacted and interviewed this individual, not as a participant of the study, but rather to gain insight into the health care needs of the community in general. The retired physician indicated that he was available for emergencies and did what he could "on the spot," but that he did not encourage members of the community to use him as their regular health care provider. He also stated that he made decisions about what he would treat and how far he would go in treating a patient before sending them to a medical facility because he had very limited resources and equipment available to him in Montana City. He commented that he had very little besides his "five senses" with which to provide care.

Health Status

Two participants described themselves as having major medical illnesses. Several other participants made reference to the fact that there were a number of people in the community who had suffered major illnesses. According to the retired physician, the illnesses suffered by members of the community included heart failure, stroke, cancer, leukemia, pulmonary hypertension, and pheochromocytoma. Furthermore, he had the impression that the incidence of serious illness in the community was higher in comparison with other communities of similar size. Several interview participants also indicated that there appeared to be a high rate of smoking and alcohol consumption within the community. As one participant stated,

> There is a high rate of alcohol consumption and drugs too here, even for a small community. And that is a big factor in health issues here. And smoking, that is another issue, everybody smokes. I am sure for the percentage of smokers in a community, we are way off the top end.

Data such as average income, poverty rates, and unemployment percentages were not available for Montana City. Therefore, I could not draw any conclusions in regard to these data for the community.

Themes

Six major themes emerged from the analysis of the data. They included conscientious consumer, informed risk, self-reliance, hardiness, community support, and inadequate insurance. Two themes, (self-reliance and hardiness) were reported previously in rural nursing literature (Chafey, Sullivan, & Shannon, 1998; Wirtz, Lee, & Running, 1998). Four themes (conscientious consumer, informed risk, community support, and inadequate insurance) were new.

Self-Reliance. Self-reliance has been defined as "the capacity to provide for one's own need" (Agich, 1993, as cited in Chafey et al., 1998). Each participant expressed that they take care of themselves first. However, varying degrees of self-reliance were described. Two participants, a married couple who moved into the community to retire, expressed self-reliance but also stated they probably accessed formal health care more quickly than long-time residents of the community. Factors that may have influenced their self-reliance included good health insurance, easy access to health care prior to moving to Montana City, and one participant's diagnosis of pulmonary hypertension. They explained,

> We are a little different because we retired here from a very different background and there are several other couples like that. So you are seeing some different things in the rural areas than maybe before because our experience is to take advantage of good medical care where we were and so we sort of expect or do the same thing here, although it is a bit harder, but I think we would be much more apt to take advantage of it than people who have lived here for 50 years. They have had to do things on their own and are very resourceful and they take

care of things on their own. But we are spoiled the other way and so it
is a little [different].

Another participant who also moved into the community to retire
stated, "It has to be pretty bad [to seek health care]. I usually wait it out
or take care of it myself." Then he described a contrast between himself
and long-time residents of the community.

> I think that a lot of people here, because they have lived here all their
> life and haven't had access to immediate care, wait it out. The locals
> definitely try to treat themselves first and do wait it out when they prob-
> ably should leave right away and get there before it is too bad. So, in
> a way, I guess we are probably different from some of the people who
> have lived here a long time.

Another example of self-reliance was reported by a participant when
she described how she and her husband planned for surgery.

> We chose May because we knew we wanted to come after his surgery so
> he could recuperate up here. Since we live on Montana Pass and there
> was still snow, that meant we still had to get him to the house, and that
> had to be by snowmobile. The doctor said not to sit on the snowmobile,
> but that he could stand on our pull sled. So I drove the snowmobile and
> he stood up on the pull sled and I took him home.

Hardiness. The participants demonstrated several characteristics of
hardiness identified by Wirtz et al. (1998). Those included adaptability,
positive attitude, and endurance. The following excerpt from the interview
with the participant who was suffering from pulmonary hypertension
demonstrates adaptability and a positive attitude.

> I suppose I am concerned [about my health], but I happen to know this
> is a progressive disease and its just going to progress and so we will
> just deal with it as it comes. I think by nature I am an up person and
> so you just do it.

Another participant who suffered from a major medical condition
causing her severe pain demonstrated adaptability and endurance. She
commented, "I just worked ... I just go until I drop." "Our thing is we
go until I scream [because of pain] and if I scream, I go in."

An elderly participant recovering from surgery also demonstrated
endurance while caring for her terminally ill husband.

> I was in the hospital with my new shoulder when they called me at the
> hospital and told me that I had to either have him out of the hospital

by the tenth of June or come up with $118 a day. I can't afford $118 a day. They said I couldn't take him home with [my] shoulder and I said, 'well, I am going to. I don't have $118 a day.' My grandson came and stayed with me for four days and that really helped until I learned how to handle him, getting him in and out of bed and I had to lift. I felt more comfortable when I had him [my husband] at home, though I didn't sleep much, but I knew he was taken care of and that is where he wanted to be.

Conscientious consumer. The theme of conscientious consumer was a new theme identified in this study. Many participants made reference to making decisions about where to seek care depending on the type of illness or injury involved and the time of year. "In the summer you can go to Conway or Robertson or Littlewood, or Bowman or Lackwood. We have those options depending on how important it is." Another participant, a little over 8 months pregnant at the time of the interview, made a statement in regard to selecting a health care provider and making arrangements for the birth of her child.

I chose the Littlewood clinic but Conway would actually be a little closer but they have sometimes a little bit more weather concerns, while the road to Littlewood is always open. I chose it [Littlewood] after comparing it with Lackwood and other places.

Another participant demonstrated the concept of conscientious consumer by his explanation of his decisions about emergency care.

That [miles to emergency care] depends on what type of emergency. If right now if I cut my finger off working with the saw over there, I would head for Conway. If I was having chest pains, if I was able to make a conscious decision, I would be heading to Lackwood. Now they do have the clinic in Maryville and they are very good there. They have a really good doctor, but he is in the process of leaving. And it depends on who comes in there. If I like the doctor, I would go there for some things. If I don't like him, I wouldn't go back for anything. And in a few months if I cut my finger, I would be heading to the clinic in Maryville and then on to Lackwood because the road to Conway will be closing. And it really does depend on what is going on. I would base my decision on where to go on the situation and the problem.

Informed risk. Informed risk was a second new theme that emerged from the analysis. Informed risk was evidenced by the two participants with major health problems. One participant, who had pulmonary hypertension, explained that she was aware of the health risks associated with where she lived, but chose to remain in Montana City because of other benefits it provided that she valued. In other words, the risk was worth it to her because she was where she wanted to be.

> There are times when I wonder if I will be here in the morning and sometime I probably won't, but there is no future in worrying about it. I probably shouldn't be at this altitude, but what we have up here, what we enjoy [is here], and so we loath to give that up.

She further explained that she was aware of the implications of living in Montana City.

> I am aware [of the risks and concerns] because the doctors keep telling me that I probably shouldn't be at this altitude, but obviously I'm still here so that must tell you something about my attitude. It would probably be more convenient closer to the hospital and yet I don't really want to live having to be close to the hospital when friends and activities are all up here. It's more fun to be up here and have to deal with whatever happens because I shouldn't be here.

The husband of the above participant was also involved in the research project and stated,

> Well, there were a lot of concerns when this [diagnosis of pulmonary hypertension] first happened. The doctors in Denver were very concerned about us coming back here without what they considered any back up. All the patients they have treated have been with twenty minutes of the hospital and a backup. See, with primary pulmonary hypertension, the literature has showed that within 20 minutes of the prostacyclin infusion being stopped, there are severe, rebound reactions, including death in some cases. The infusion must be continuous, and if something happens, say the pump is dropped and it pulls on the catheter, or if she falls and it somehow stops, or even if the catheter gets clogged, but if the infusion is stopped for any reason, you must start another IV ... We are aware of what the doctors think and we know what it might mean to live here because of the altitude or problems with the catheter.

He further explained and defined informed risk in the following statement:

> The altitude here is a problem and the doctors really think we should move. This altitude is not good for [my wife] and the pulmonary hypertension can be worse because of it, but we know that and like I said, maybe one day we will have to move to Lackwood or whatever, but right now this where we want to be.

Another participant who also suffered from a major disease process stated,

> As far as being this far away, we have talked about it, my surgeon and I talked about it. I mean jeepers, if it is time to go in [to the hospital], it is time to go in. And if it is too late, it is too late. I don't have a concern about that at all, at all.

She further explained by stating,

> I would never move just for medical care, just simply because I love it here. I mean how can you not go out here [outside her home] and think, 'oh cool.' It is a heart song and it is a peace of heart for me to be here and that is a lot of help. It really is. I can go out there and look at the mountains and get something out of that and that makes the difference.

Another participant stated, "those of us who have been here for years, we just try to take care of ourselves without having to get any medical attention. Sometimes that is ok. We realize the risk we are taking."

Community support. Another new theme that emerged was community support. Each of the individuals made statements that the community pulls together when someone needs help. The hardy individual described previously who cared for her husband stated,

> There is a lot of people here I could have called. That is one thing about Montana City. If you ever need help, even if you are a stranger to them, you get help. That is one thing about up here. It is a great community.

Another participant shared her perception of support.

> The people in the community are great. Every time I am having a bad day all we have to do is make a phone call or stand out on the street and they are here, taking care of my boys and my business. It is incredible. It really is. They had a benefit auction for us one time when I was in the hospital. And those times too, the boys get spoiled rotten by the whole community.

Inadequate insurance. All participants had insurance. Five stated that insurance was a concern for them. Four commented it was expensive, had high deductibles, or was inadequate. One participant stated,

> Yes, we have health insurance. It is very expensive and we pay it all ourselves. That has been a real burden. And a lot of people up here do

not have health insurance, at all. I don't know if any business has health insurance and benefits, or even provides part of it. So that is a very difficult thing here. When you don't make a lot of money and the health insurance keeps going up all the time. A major part of our income goes to health insurance. That is a real burden.

Another long time resident of the community stated she had health insurance, "but it doesn't leave me much to live on. I live on about $250 a month after that."

Two retired participants brought medical insurance with them from their jobs. One stated, "we are different than a lot of people here in the community in that we brought our insurance here with us. A lot of people here do not have insurance, or do not have adequate insurance."

All participants stated their health insurance coverage did not affect how they accessed care. When I asked a long-time member of the community if her health insurance affected how she sought care, she stated,

No, I don't think so. I know it does for a lot of people here, if they don't have health insurance which a lot of them don't, I think it affects them as a choice of going to the doctor, or the hospital, or not seeking care.

Participants estimated that half to three-quarters of the members of the Montana City community did not have insurance.

DISCUSSION

The themes that emerged provided valuable information for comparison to previously identified concepts in the rural nursing literature. The primary characteristics of self-reliance included "self-reliance as learned, decisional choice, and independence" (Chafey et al., 1998, p. 162). Self-reliance as learned was demonstrated by several participants and was clearly more evident in those who had lived in the community for a long period of time. The individuals who had more recently moved into the community considered themselves self-reliant, stating that they try to take care of things themselves first. They also acknowledged that those who had grown up in the community or had lived there a long time did more for themselves than they did.

Self-reliance as a decisional choice was not as clear in the data from the Montana City participants. Participants inferred they made many choices on a daily basis, but never indicated that was of great importance to them. They all mentioned a sense of security provided by knowing a retired doctor lived in the community who was willing to provide information as they engaged in the decision-making process.

Hardiness is another theme that emerged. As previously discussed, the data from Montana City participants showed evidence of adaptability, positive attitude, and endurance, characteristics of hardiness (Wirtz et al., 1998). All participants expressed in some manner that one must "adjust to what life [has] offered" (Wirtz et al., p. 160). Two long-time residents demonstrated learned experience, an additional characteristic of hardiness, by making statements such as "the way it had always been" or "that's all we have ever known." Overall, the Montana City residents demonstrated hardiness congruent with hardiness previously described in the rural nursing literature.

Four of the themes I identified were new themes or variations of existing themes. Conscientious consumer was a theme that I identified in the Montana City data and appeared to apply in some manner to concepts previously discussed in the nursing literature. Distance played a role in where the Montana City participants accessed care for a particular injury or illness. Mileage, time, and perception are attributes of distance (Henson, Sadler, & Walton, 1998). Mileage and time are congruent with the attributes of conscientious consumer as the participants weighed these two factors when determining where to seek care for a particular health problem. For the Montana City participants, weather was a key factor that the conscientious consumer had to consider in their decision-making process.

The theme of conscientious consumer also paralleled health resources concepts (Ballantyne, 1998). Ballantyne stated, "if the client is motivated to seek health care beyond the immediate boundaries of the community, factors such as transportation, distance, inclement weather, and finances become important issues" (p. 182).

Informed risk was a new theme or perhaps a variation of an existing theme. Informed risk was not specifically found in the nursing literature. Informed risk means that individuals are aware of the risks or consequences of their decisions, but desire for quality of life outweighs the risks presented. The participants acknowledged that there may be some risks in living where they did, but they also were weighing their options when making these decisions.

Community support has been discussed in the nursing literature in a variety of ways. The concept of community support may be related to previously presented concepts (e.g., informed networks [Grossman & McNerney, 1998] and familiarity [McNeely & Shreffler, 1998]). Community support was clearly demonstrated by "rallying," "benefit auctions," "helping take care of my business and my kids."

Inadequate insurance had an impact on a number of participants. Inadequate insurance was not a concept in itself, but I identified it as a potential modifying factor for health care utilization in the community.

Although I did not identify a concept that paralleled inadequate insurance in the nursing literature, it is an issue related to resource accessibility and health care access that warrants further investigation.

IMPLICATIONS FOR NURSING PRACTICE

Informed risk affects the way health care practitioners relate to their clients. It is important that the practitioner confirm that it is truly informed risk and that individuals are able to make informed decisions. For example, it was important for the individual with pulmonary hypertension to understand the risk of being further than 20 minutes away from an appropriate medical facility and the risk she was taking with the prostacylcin infusion. It was also important for her to understand physiologically the impact altitude may have on the progression of her disease. Once practitioners are clear that their client is truly informed, then it is important to respect their decisions. Furthermore, once the decision has been made by the individual to remain in a particular environment or situation, the practitioner should work with the individual to make available the appropriate information, skills, and resources. Even if practitioners disagree with those choices, the individual's choice should be respected.

Health care practitioners should be aware of modifying factors such as time and distance that affect access to care and the health care decision-making process of conscientious consumers. The participant who was 8 months pregnant at the time of the interview provides an example.

> When they [practitioners in general] tell you "well leave your house when your contractions are five minutes part," well that could make for a child born in Gateway. They [rural doctors in Littlewood] do realize that even if you are racing it is a good two hour drive and at night you cannot go that fast.

In this example, inaccurate perceptions on the part of providers caring for pregnant clients may result in babies being born in the back seat of an automobile in the middle of nowhere. Therefore it is imperative for providers to understand conscientious consumers when making decisions relative to health care. Discussing what-if scenarios with rural clients, particularly in relation to distance, time, and weather, will help them be the best and wisest conscientious consumers.

Self-reliance and hardiness both have an impact on when, why, and how rural individuals will seek care. As with informed risk, health care providers should work with individuals in an attempt to provide the necessary information, skills, and available resources while allowing persons to be self-reliant.

Understanding the presence or lack of community support for clients in rural communities gives the practitioner insight into the availability of resources. For example, individuals who have been hospitalized and want to return home rather than stay on a transitional care unit may be able to do so with strong community support.

Inadequate insurance affected participants' use of health care. High deductible, out-of-pocket expenses, distance, and availability of services also influenced health care decision-making for these isolated rural residents. The combination of these issues warrants thorough investigation to fully understand health care access.

As indicated by Long and Weinert (1998), "continued research can provide a more solid base for the nursing theory that is required to guide practice and the delivery of health care to rural populations" (p. 16). Thus, previously identified concepts as well as newly emerging concepts or themes warrant further investigation to help health care practitioners provide the highest quality care to rural individuals.

REFERENCES

Ballantyne, J. (1998). Health resources and the rural client. In H. J. Lee (Ed.), *Conceptual basis for rural nursing* (pp. 178–188). New York: Springer Publishing.

Chafey, K., Sullivan, T., & Shannon, A. (1998). Self-reliance: Characterization of their own autonomy by elderly rural women. In H. J. Lee (Ed.), *Conceptual basis for rural nursing* (pp. 156–177). New York: Springer Publishing.

Fahlberg, L. (1983). *Nine months of winter.* Cooke City, MT: Pilot Peak.

Glidden, R. (1982). *Exploring the Yellowstone high country: History of the Cooke City area.* (2nd ed). Cooke City, MT: Ralph Glidden.

Grossman, L. L., & McNerney, S. (1998). Informal networks. In H. J. Lee (Ed.), *Conceptual basis for rural nursing* (pp. 200–208). New York: Springer Publishing.

Henson, D., Sadler, T., & Walton, S. (1998). Distance. In H. J. Lee (Ed.), *Conceptual basis for rural nursing* (pp. 51–60). New York: Springer Publishing.

Koehler, V. (1998). The substantive theory of protecting independence. In H. J. Lee (Ed.), *Conceptual basis for rural nursing* (pp. 236–256). New York: Springer Publishing.

Long, K. A., & Weinert, C. (1998). Rural nursing: Developing the theory base. In H. J. Lee (Ed.), *Conceptual basis for rural nursing* (pp. 3–18). New York: Springer Publishing.

McNeely, A. G., & Shreffler, M. J. (1998). Familiarity. In H. J. Lee (Ed.), *Conceptual basis for rural nursing* (pp. 89–101). New York: Springer Publishing.

National Geographic Road Atlas. (2000). Canada: MapQuest.com, Inc.

Rossman, G. B., & Rallis, S. F. (1998). *Learning in the field: An introduction to qualitative research.* Thousand Oaks, CA: Sage.

Wirtz, E. F., Lee, H. J., & Running, A. (1998). The lived experience of hardiness in rural men and women. In H. J. Lee (Ed.), *Conceptual basis for rural nursing* (pp. 257–274). New York: Springer Publishing.

CHAPTER SIX

Health Perceptions, Needs, and Behaviors of Remote Rural Women of Childbearing and Childrearing Age

Ronda L. Bales

Montana is a rural state characterized by vast open spaces, a sparse population, and large geographical distances between cities and towns. An estimated 70% of the state's population live in towns with fewer than 15,000 inhabitants, and 80% of Montana communities have a population of fewer than 3,000 people. Nearly 12.3% of Montanans lack access to primary care (Montana Office of Rural Health, 1999). In 2002, the Health Resources and Services Administration (HRSA) designated 35 of Montana's 56 counties as Health Professional Shortage Areas (HPSA, HRSA, 2002).

Rural health research findings suggest that health perceptions of rural individuals may also be unique as compared with perceptions of urban persons. Aspects common to rural dwellers included their definition of health as the ability to work, reliance on self and informal systems, and decreased willingness to use health care services provided by outsiders (Weinert & Long, 1990). The unique characteristics of rural dwellers may affect how and when they seek health care. Internal factors, such as self-reliance and reliance on informal support systems of family, friends, and neighbors, may lead to a delay in seeking formal health care services (Long, 1993). These factors, as well as external factors including distance and lack of adequate health care resources, may put the rural individual at increased risk for illness, disability, and premature death (Long; Veitch, 1995).

Few researchers have explored the impact of rurality on the health of midlife women or those of childbearing and childrearing age (Hemard, Monroe, Atkinson, & Blalock, 1998). Women of childbearing and childrearing age, regardless of geographic location, have common health care needs. Early detection and treatment of diseases common in women, such as breast and cervical cancer, can reduce death and disability associated with these diseases. However, access to care has been a factor that influences whether or not women participate in the screening processes for breast and cervical cancer (Wilcox & Mosher, 1993; Nuovo, Melnikow, & Howell, 2001). Although the gap is narrowing, rural women continue to have more children than their urban counterparts as well as experience their first pregnancy at an earlier age (Bescher-Donnelly & Smith, 1981). Therefore, in addition to screening for cervical and breast cancer and general health maintenance, women in this stage of life have needs for adequate birth control, family planning, prenatal care, and childbirth education.

Women of childbearing and childrearing age may experience stress as a result of multiple demands placed on them by family relationships and home and work responsibilities (Kenney, 2000; Bigbee, 1984). The number of women working outside the home has steadily risen and rural women account for a significant portion of this growth (Walters & McKenry, 1985). Rural women have less educational opportunities and less occupational choices and therefore often work at low-wage jobs (Bescher-Donnelly & Smith, 1981). Rural women working outside the home also have fewer provisions for quality child care (Bigbee, 1984). These factors, added to the primary responsibilities for home and family management intensify the multiplicity of roles experienced by rural women. Research has indicated that stress and illness may be closely related and multiple stressors can compromise the immune system therefore putting the individual at increased risk for acute and chronic illnesses (Kenney, 2000).

Women oversee their own health care as well as the health care of their family members. Rural women often act as health officers or gatekeepers of health care for the entire family (Bushy, 1993a; Hemard et al., 1998; Tevis, 1994; Ross, 1982). Therefore, the manner in which women conceptualize health is integral to the health and health practices of the family. However, women's perceptions of health have rarely been solicited (Bushy, 1993b, 1994a; Ross, 1982).

Long (1993) has emphasized the importance of providing care consistent with the way rural individuals conceptualize health. Little has been written about the health perspectives of women of childbearing and childrearing age in remote rural areas. My purpose in this study described in this chapter was to explore the health perceptions, needs, and behaviors of remote rural women of childbearing and childrearing age living in Montana for greater than 5 years. *Remote rural* was defined as

> ... a community with a population of 2,500 or less located 40 miles or further from a city with a population of 50,000 or greater. Remote rural communities do not have a hospital or medical assistance facility. A practicing physician does not reside in a remote rural community (Koehler, 1998, pp. 238–239).

METHODS

I used grounded theory approach for this study (Byrne, 2001; Chenitz & Swanson, 1986; Strauss & Corbin, 1990). Following approval by the Montana State University-Bozeman Institutional Review Board and informed consent, I conducted semistructured interviews with women of childbearing and childrearing age living in remote rural areas in Montana. I knew the initial participants personally and identified other participants through personal contacts. I obtained subsequent participants by using the snowball technique.

Sample

The convenience sample consisted of 11 women 28–49 years, who had lived in remote rural communities in Montana for greater than 5 years (age range: $M = 37.7$ years; education completed range: 12–18 years, $M = 14.7$ years). An attempt was made to vary the sample as much as possible by contacting potential participants who comprised the full age range for this study, 18 to 49 years, as well as by contacting potential participants from different geographical locations within the state.

The communities in which the participants lived had a population of 850 or less. The women had lived in their respective communities 5-40 years with an average length of time in the rural community of 17.9 years.

The sample was more educated than the general population of Montanans. Six of the 11 women (54%) held a bachelor's degree and one has a master's degree, whereas an estimated 11.7% of the general Montana population have baccalaureate degrees (U.S. Bureau of the Census, 2000).

All participants were married and had children. Two women worked full time outside the home, five worked part-time, and four women were not employed outside the home. All but one woman had children living at home at the time of the study. For the women with children at home, the number of children in the household ranged from one to five. The age of the children who lived at home ranged from 2 months to 17 years ($M = 7.7$ years).

Nine of the women had insurance and two did not have any insurance. The participants stated cost as the major factor for lack of insurance. For the nine women with health insurance, seven were part of a family involved in farming, ranching, or small business and all seven women reported that their insurance had a high deductible and premium.

Distance to emergency medical care ranged from 10-114 miles ($M = 44.8$ miles) with travel time ranging from 12 minutes to 2.5 hr, one way. The participants cited the hospital or medical assistance facility located in the nearest large town with this available service and ambulance service to the nearest town as their source of emergency care. In addition, the participants identified local individuals with medical training as a source of assistance in an emergency situation. Rural road conditions, weather conditions, geography, and road construction were some of the variables influencing travel time to emergency care.

Data Collection and Analysis

I conducted four in-person and seven telephone interviews. The questions were open-ended and intended to elicit information regarding the women's health perceptions, needs, and behaviors and how their perceptions and conceptualizations of health affected their health behaviors. I audiotape recorded interviews and later transcribed them. I analyzed the qualitative data for common themes using the methodological technique of grounded theory known as constant comparison (Strauss & Corbin, 1990).

EMERGENT THEMES

Seven themes emerged from the data: (a) distance as a way of life, (b) distance as a disadvantage in an emergency, (c) episodic evaluation, (d) children first, (e)prevention for life, (f)access within reason, and (g)holistic health.

Distance as a Way of Life

The participants identified that distance, although an inconvenience at times, was not a disadvantage. They accepted as part of everyday life that they lived some distance from health care as well as from a variety of other general services. At times it was noted to be inconvenient, but "just the way it is." The women reported "enjoying the lifestyle" that a rural environment provided and the small inconvenience that distance presented in some circumstances was worth the experience of living in a rural setting.

The women reported that distance did not deter them from seeking health care or cause a delay in seeking health care. One participant made the following comments about distance to health care:

> If we are sick, if one of the kids is sick, we are going to go to the doctor if we need to. You just get use to living out here so it doesn't make a difference. I mean you think 30 miles, you know you are going to drive there if you are sick and need the health care services or whatever. Just like you do to go out to pizza, you drive to health care.
>
> The distance, it doesn't seem very long [70 miles]. Usually we pick up grandma who is halfway and we always have something else to do, besides go to the doctor, like get groceries or something, so it doesn't seem bad.

The women did not find distance to be a significant concern in regard to their past pregnancies and impending deliveries. Although they took some precautions and thought about what the distance might mean, none of the women had specific concerns about their delivery in light of the distance that needed to be traveled to get to the hospital.

> I guess growing up 30 miles from town you know what that is like. So living 60 miles from town now, you don't think about it. It is just the way it is. You know that you have miles to travel and you can get there in around an hour and that is just the way it is. You can't worry about it. My husband wasn't concerned about having to deliver the baby if we didn't make it in time. Our big joke was that he was going to bring the calf pullers in. That is just a typical rancher. We deal with animals all the time. Calving and foaling and little animals and birthing and the whole reproductive situation. I guess it is just a natural thing. It is not something that you dwell on. You think about it, what if something happens, but like I said, you just deal with it if something happens.

When considering distance during pregnancy, factors that could cause a delay in their travel, such as weather and road construction, were recalled. "It was in the back of our mind, what if a storm comes or whatever. You think about it a little bit, but you know also realizing that comes with this lifestyle."

Another issue the women consistently identified in regard to planning for their labor and delivery was the importance of their health care providers being "in tune" to the fact that they lived some distance from the hospital and that their provider helped them plan ahead for their delivery.

The women reported that their doctor gave them advice, such as "come in when things start" or "head to town, don't just wait." The women seemed more comfortable with the distance because of their relationship with their health care providers and the fact that their providers appreciated their situation.

Two women had experienced breast cancer in recent years. Although both women had access to health care providers and a hospital within 15 miles, they were forced to travel longer distances to a larger medical center to receive care for their diagnosis. Both women traveled a distance of 60–80 miles, one way, 5 days a week for 6 weeks for radiation treatment. One of the women had to travel for chemotherapy as well. Their perspective on traveling for health care for treatment of a disease was somewhat different from the rest of the sample who only traveled for routine health care, and on a much less frequent basis. For the two women with breast cancer, traveling the longer distance was seen as even more of an inconvenience and somewhat of a disadvantage when considering access to health care. Both women discussed that although the daily travel was an inconvenience, the support of friends and neighbors in the community was an advantage that balanced out the situation for them.

> One problem is that we are kind of far away from certain medical facilities that we might need, but in my case at least making the 80 mile trip for radiation did work out really well because I had the advantage of friends and neighbors who were really helpful. I think that is one advantage of the rural situation. The more specialized things you need to go farther away for. They can handle most things locally, but if you have cancer or heart problems or something that requires more specialized care, then you have to go farther away. You are at a disadvantage in some ways because you are farther from care, but you have got good friends and neighbors to help you out too. I think that is the advantage that maybe people in a larger area wouldn't have.

Although distance was occasionally viewed as an inconvenience, all of the women were accustomed to traveling some distance for general services, routine health care services, and for the delivery of their children. If health care was needed, it was obtained. Distance to health care services did not result in a delay in seeking care, if the care was deemed necessary.

Distance as a Disadvantage in an Emergency

All the women verbalized that distance was a distinct disadvantage in the case of an emergency. They were aware that distance presented the risk of serious consequences to their health and the health of their family, or even death, in an emergency situation. In an emergency they noted, "It would take you awhile to get somewhere," and "It takes time for them to get to you." One woman stated, "You know the distance is there if something really happens." One woman recounted her concern and thought processes during an acute illness experienced by one of her children:

> We were working in the yard and I took my eyes off my son for 2 seconds. The next thing I knew he was throwing up. We took him inside and changed his clothes, but he couldn't stop throwing up and then he was finally throwing up bile and he had a horrible color, pasty white. All the color was out of his lips. I wasn't sure what he had gotten into. We called Ask A Nurse because now he has fallen asleep and we can't really keep him awake between throwing up. They told me to give it 4 hours for whatever it is to work out of his system. His breathing was rapid and shallow and he was unable to stay awake. I was taking his pulse the whole time, for 4 hours that is what I did. Then four hours went by and he woke and said, thirsty, and he was crying. But that was a long 4 hours and then I thought to myself, if he is not okay in 4 hours and they told me to bring him in, and it takes an hour and half to get there, should I leave in 2 hours to be part of that four. I really remember not liking the distance at that moment.

The issue of distance and travel time and how they would handle an emergency was considered by the women.

> With us, we live 30 miles out so it would take at least 20 minutes. I am sure they go fast and stuff, but you still can't go that fast. I would never sit with my kid in an emergency and wait for an ambulance. That is at least 45 minutes. It would be an hour by the time they came, put somebody on the stretcher, put them in the ambulance and got back to town. I couldn't sit there and calmly wait. I would get in the car and just tell them I would meet them. I think I would get them that much closer and sooner to getting help. I would call the ambulance and then I would take off.

The women had also identified individuals in their local communities with medical training who could assist should an emergency arise. They felt these people may be of great assistance in an emergency situation, especially while waiting for an ambulance to arrive.

Although they consistently identified distance as a disadvantage in emergent situations, they were well aware of the risks involved and accepted this as the one disadvantage to rural life.

> I learned early in life that things are going to happen. You are going to have accidents. You just have to deal with it when it happens, whatever the severity of it. If you have an accident, you know you are going to

have to wait for the ambulance. If you have to pack somebody up in the pickup and bring them to town, you do it. When you grow up with that and make the decision to live out here, you just take those things into consideration and that is just the way it is.

It is something you live with when you are this far out. You just know that there is always that chance that something real major, a bad emergency, could happen and your chances are a lot slimmer than if you are living right in Billings, Montana.

Episodic Evaluation

A third theme to emerge was episodic evaluation. The women used their past experience and best judgment to consider each injury or illness episode and made a decision about how to manage it. Episodic evaluation was something they did for themselves as well as their children.

For each illness episode, symptoms present, length of the illness, severity of the symptoms, and the progression or resolution of symptoms were considered. The impact of the illness on daily life, and whether or not the illness affected their ability to go to work or their children's ability to go to school, were factors that influenced their decision about whether or not to seek formal health care. All the woman began with informal care or self-care behaviors, such as home remedies and over the counter medicines, and illnesses were allowed to "run their course" unless the symptoms progressed, continued for a long period of time, or significantly affected the individual's daily activities.

> If someone gets where they are absolutely miserable for a few days and I can see they are not going to shake whatever they have, then we will go. If it is something that is affecting their everyday life or if they are missing school, then I will go see a doctor.
>
> You just kind of see how they are doing. If after a couple of days they don't get better, you take them in. You think, we are this far out, what if it gets worse. You would rather have it taken care of than have it get worse and then that is more of an emergent state. Then you think, gosh, we are 30 miles out or whatever. Then 30 miles makes a huge difference.

Most women elicited advice from their mother, sister, friend, or neighbor during some illness episodes. The women inquired about how others had handled similar situations as well as discussed what types of treatments had helped resolve a similar illness. "I talk to my mom. I trust her judgment." "I ask around, see what others have tried." Others sought advice from their health care provider over the telephone.

The women used the same type of episodic evaluation when considering whether an injury could be handled at home or if accessing professional health care was necessary. The type of injury, the quantity of blood involved, and the pain level were factors that influenced their decision to handle the injury on their own or see a health care provider.

> I have handled kids getting bucked off horses, cuts, and scrapes. You look at how deep it is and try to decide, do we need stitches, or is there a concussion or what. I guess you just assess the situation and it just depends on how bad it is.

If they had initially decided to handle an injury at home, the mothers reevaluated the injury as time went on. They sought formal health care if bleeding continued, if the pain became more severe, if the injury did not seem to be healing, or if infection seemed to be present. The women indicated they did not delay seeking care for themselves or their children if the care was deemed necessary.

Children First

The women consistently indicated that they sought health care sooner for their children than they did for themselves. They used the episodic evaluation process with their children just as they did for themselves, but reported that they took their children to a formal health care provider more readily. The woman indicated that the reason for taking their child to the doctor sooner than they would go themselves was because it was difficult to judge how someone else was feeling and how the illness was affecting them. This was especially true for younger children and infants who could not verbalize how they were feeling. As children got older, mothers were more inclined to "let things run their course" and evaluate whether to take them in based on what the child was telling them.

> I definitely take the kids in sooner. I guess because I don't want it to go on too long with them. I don't want them to get really sick. You know how you feel yourself, but you don't really know how your child feels. You only know what they tell you and what you observe. I don't like to let it get out of hand.

The women also indicated that they were the one in the family who determined whether a child was ill and if they needed to see a formal health care provider. Mothers were also consistently responsible for taking their children to the doctor. "Mom takes them to the doctor and mom sits in the waiting room." "You deal with it because you are the mom, you are the woman, and you take care of everything. They are your children." This was because that the mothers spent more time at home with the children than their spouses. "I am more tuned into it because I am with them more during the day. My husband might say, her nose is running or whatever, but I am usually a step ahead of him because I am around more."

Women stated that gauging someone else's illness or pain, particularly when the other person is a very small child, is difficult to do. Although they handled many illnesses at home without the help of a formal health care provider, they were quick to seek care if they were unsure about how their child felt or uncertain of the severity of the illness or injury.

Prevention for Life

The women indicated that routine health care and illness prevention strategies were important activities in life. They reported that it was important to detect illness or disease early so that they could be treated properly and have a better chance at a long healthy life. Ten women participated in yearly health screening activities citing prevention as the main reason for choosing to participate in health maintenance activities. Prevention for life was important for "catching things early" and "staying healthy." The women who had experienced breast cancer realized the importance of health maintenance and yearly exams and credited these activities for saving their lives.

The women verbalized they were more aware of the importance of health maintenance activities after becoming mothers because their children relied on them to be healthy and to be there to take care of them. They educated themselves on health issues through a variety of sources and actively sought out information, especially on issues of specific importance in their life. The mothers were primarily responsible for providing health education for their children. Prevention for life was a strategy practiced by the women to keep themselves and their family as healthy as possible.

Access Within Reason

All the women felt that health care was accessible within reason for the area in which they lived. Most were unable to identify any type of health care service that they wished they had available to them in their local community that was not currently available. Even when considering the disadvantage of distance in an emergency, one participant stated, "We have access. We just have to get there. It just takes time. That is the way it is out here."

Access also was seen as having the ability to obtain advice from someone over the phone, the ability to have questions answered, "flexible hours," and "getting hold of someone if I need to." One woman who did not have health insurance defined access to care as "money and insurance." However, cost was an issue for all women. Seven women who had health insurance reported high premiums and high deductibles and had to pay out-of-pocket for routine health care and office visits. Most stated that their insurance was for "major medical." However, high deductibles did not result in a delay in seeking care for these women. They obtained health care if they believed it to be necessary.

> Having to pay out-of-pocket doesn't keep us from going to the doctor. I want to keep everybody healthy and we will pay for it one way or another, so you might as well go in and get it taken care of early. It doesn't have an affect on whether I go or not just because I know I have to pay for it.

Holistic Health

Health was defined holistically. Good health included (a) a lack of major health problems, (b) minimal or no use of routine medications, (c)being mentally and physically active, and (d) having the ability to perform necessary tasks without limitations or undue stress. Good health also included being (a) physically fit, (b) eating well, and (c) having an overall sense of well-being. Poor health affected day-to-day activities, but most of the women, unless they were experiencing an acute illness episode, did not feel their health had a negative affect on their daily life.

IMPLICATIONS FOR NURSING
PRACTICE AND RESEARCH

I identified several implications for nursing practice First, although distance was perceived as a "way of rural life," health care providers should remain cognizant of the distance and time traveled for routine health care and plan follow-up care accordingly. In addition, nurses and other health care providers should educate expectant mothers on the appropriate precautions to take when traveling to a community where they will deliver their babies.

Second, concerns were raised about the time it took to access care in an emergency. This is an issue that nurses should explore with rural dwellers. The availability of emergency resources (persons, services) in their local communities should be discussed. Education regarding planning for and handling various emergencies can be addressed during routine health care visits.

Third, the women were clearly interested in maintaining their health and participating in screening activities to identify illness early in the course of a disease process. Therefore, when seen in the office, the women should be counseled regarding age-appropriate screening activities. Written information regarding preventive health and health maintenance activities for their children also should be offered at each encounter. Other strategies of delivering health education include local seminars on women's and children's health issues and providing addresses for Internet-based health information.

I also identified several implications for nursing research. Distance continues to be an interesting concept in the rural literature. Much controversy remains as to the impact of distance on health care utilization and whether individuals who live at increasing distances from health care engage in more self-care behaviors and delay seeking formal health care. Further research is warranted in regard to this concept; comparison between rural women and their urban counterparts may provide important information about similarities and differences in self-care behaviors and utilization of formal health care.

Other areas to explore include the experience of illness and the affect of stress on the lives of childbearing and childrearing remote rural women. The women in this study who suffered from breast cancer and traveled for treatment viewed distance as slightly more inconvenient than the women who traveled less frequently for routine health care. They also verbalized significant community support that counterbalanced the inconvenience of daily travel of 60 miles or more, one way. Furthermore, the women were not specifically questioned regarding their stress level. The health perceptions of women of childbearing and childrearing age who have suffered from a life-threatening illness or have experienced stress have rarely been solicited and may add valuable data to the rural health literature.

Finally, research is needed that addresses the health perceptions, needs, and behaviors of rural childbearing and childrearing women who live in different geographical areas and at varying distances from health care services. Also, the health needs of women early in their childbearing years may differ from those who are raising older children. Therefore, more research is needed to further understand the health perceptions, needs, and behaviors of women in this stage of life.

REFERENCES

Bescher-Donnelly, L., & Smith, L. W. (1981). The changing roles and status of rural women. In R. T. Coward & W. Smith, Jr., *The family in rural society* (pp. 167–186). Boulder, CO: Westview Press.

Bigbee, J. L. (1984). The changing role of rural women: Nursing and health implications. *Health Care for Women International, 5,* 307–322.

Bushy, A. (1993a). Defining rural before tackling access issues. *The American Nurse, 25* (8), 20.

Bushy, A. (1993b). Rural women: Lifestyle and health status. *Rural Nursing, 28* (1), 187–197.

Bushy, A. (1994a). Women in rural environments: Considerations for holistic nurses. *Holistic Nursing Practice, 8* (4), 67–73.

Byrne, M. (2001). Grounded theory as a qualitative research methodology. *Association of Operating Room Nurses, 73* (6), 1155. Retrieved October 22, 2001, from Expanded Academic ASAP@http://www.galegroup.com

Chenitz, W. C., & Swanson, J. M. (1986). *From practice to grounded theory: Qualitative research in nursing.* Menlo Park, CA: Addison-Wesley.

Health Resources and Services Administration. (2002). *Health Professionals Shortage Areas (HRSAs).* Retrieved April 10, 2002, from http://belize.hrsa. gov/newhpsa/newhpsa.cfm#

Hemard, J. B., Monroe, P. A., Atkinson, E. S., & Blalock, L. B. (1998). Rural women's satisfaction and stress as family health care gatekeepers. *Women and Health, 28,* 55–73.

Kenney, J. W. (2000). Women's 'inner balance': A comparison of stressors, personality traits and health problems by age groups. *Journal of Advanced Nursing, 31,* 639–650.

Koehler, V. (1998). The substantive theory of protecting independence. In H. J. Lee (Ed.), *Conceptual basis for rural nursing* (pp. 236–256). New York: Springer Publishing.

Long, K. A. (1993). The concept of health: Rural perspectives. *Nursing Clinics of North America, 28* (1), 123–131.

Montana Office of Rural Health. (1999). *Montana statistics.* Retrieved October 21, 2001, from http://healthinfo.montana.edu/ruralhealth/default.html

Nuovo, J., Melnikow, J., & Howell, L. P. (2001). New tests for cervical cancer screening. *American Family Physician, 64,* 780–786.

Ross, H. M. (1982). *Women and wellness: Defining, attaining, and maintaining health in eastern Canada.* Unpublished doctoral dissertation, University of Washington, Seattle.

Strauss, A., & Corbin, J. (1990). *Basics of qualitative research: Grounded theory procedures and techniques.* Newbury Park, CA: Sage.

Tevis, C. (1994). Partners for health and safety. *Successful Farming, 92* (8), 1–2, 57–58. Retrieved October 22, 2001, from Expanded Academic ASAP@http:// www.galegroup.com

U. S. Bureau of the Census. (2000). *Census 2000 data for the state of Montana.* Retrieved October 21, 2001, from http://www.census.gov/census2000/states/ mt.html

Veitch, P. C. (1995). Anticipated response to three common injuries by rural and remote area residents. *Social Science and Medicine, 41,* 739–745.

Walters, C. M., & McKenry, P. C. (1985). Predictors of life satisfaction among rural and urban employed mothers: A research note. *Journal of Marriage and Family, 47,* 1067–1071.

Weinert, C., & Long, K. A. (1990). Rural families and health care: Refining the knowledge base. *Marriage and Family Review, 15,* 57–75.

Wilcox, L. S., & Mosher, W. D. (1993). Factors associated with obtaining health screening among women of reproductive age. *Public Health Reports, 108,* 1–10, 76–86. Retrieved October 21, 2001, from Expanded Academic ASAP@http://www.galegroup.com

CHAPTER SEVEN

Rural and Remote Women Developing Resilience to Manage Vulnerability

Beverly D. Leipert

> If there is two-tiered medicine [health care] in Canada, it's not rich and poor, it's urban versus rural.
>
> —Health Canada, 2003

Canada is the second largest country in the world, yet 21%–30% of its population resides in rural and remote areas (Health Canada, 2003). In this vast country, health status declines as one moves farther from urban centers. Rural people have shorter life expectancies, higher death rates, higher infant mortality rates, lower incomes, higher unemployment, fewer years of education, and higher rates of smoking, alcohol consumption, and obesity than do the national average, and they often experience higher rates of crime (Health Canada, 2003; Northern Secretariat of the BC Centre of Excellence for Women's Health, 2000).

Although women's health research in Canada is increasing, research that explores the health needs and strengths of women in geographically isolated settings is limited. Much of the women's health research that exists is biomedical in nature, focuses on reproductive issues, and emphasizes quantitative methods. It does not acknowledge sufficiently the importance of health promotion and illness prevention perspectives and issues for women in rural and remote regions (Leipert, 2002; Leipert & Reutter, 1998; Sutherns, McPhedran, & Haworth-Brockman, 2004). As a result, understanding of the health of rural and remote women is limited.

Research that explores the health of women in rural and remote settings must consider the social determinants of health and their interactions (Health Canada, 1996; Northern Secretariate, 2000). Determinants of health include a variety of factors, such as physical, social, and economic environments, health services, health behaviors and skills, culture, and gender. Research that considers interactions of the health determinants helps to provide accurate and comprehensive understanding of the health of women in isolated settings. Such understanding assists health care practitioners and policy makers to be effective in advancing women's health in rural and remote settings.

PURPOSE

My purpose in this qualitative study described in this chapter was to examine how women perceive and maintain their health within geographical, social, economic, and other contexts within northern British Columbia (BC), Canada. My aims in the study were to describe women's perceptions and experiences regarding their health problems in the north and ways that women addressed these problems to maintain their health.

METHODS

In this study, I used a feminist grounded theory method as a guide. Feminist inquiry considers not only women's individual voices and experiences, but also larger sociopolitical, economic, and cultural structures that influence women's lives (MacDonald, 2001). Grounded theory is especially useful in a field of inquiry in which little is known (Stern, 1980), and where complex and hidden processes, such as those related to health, need to be identified and described in rich and dense ways (MacDonald; Morse, 2001). Feminist grounded theory seeks to generate a theory that explains how a central problem for women is resolved or processed (Keddy, Sims, & Stern, 1996). Because this was one of the first studies to examine problems related to northern women's health and northern women's process of addressing health problems, feminist grounded theory was an appropriate research method.

Setting

I conducted the study in two health regions in northern BC. Northern BC includes both urban and rural settings. Northern rural settings are characterized as rural, rural remote, and rural isolated. *Rural communities* have a population of less than 1,000 people with less than 400 people per square kilometer (Statistics Canada, 1993). *Rural remote communities* are 80–400 km or 1–4 hours transport in good weather from a major regional hospital (Canadian Association of Emergency Physicians, Rural committee, 1997). *Rural isolated communities* are more than 400 kilometers or 4 hours transport in good weather from a major regional hospital (Rennie, Baird-Crooks, Remus, & Engel, 2000). Northern BC includes only one urban center, Prince George, with a population of 70,000. In the north, both urban and rural settings are considered remote and isolated because of their distant location from health care and other resources. This is true for Prince George, which has limited health care specialists and equipment and is located several 100 kilometers from resources in southern BC. Northern urban and rural settings were both represented in this study.

Sample

Recruitment strategies included appearing for radio and television interviews about the research, publishing recruitment information in community newspapers, and posting study information in stores, auction markets, other public places, and on Aboriginal reserves. I constructed the sample by using theoretical sampling (Glaser, 1978). The study sample consisted of 25 women who had lived in northern settings for a minimum of 2 years. The women were aged 21–86 years (the majority within 41–60 years), had less than Grade 9 to university education, and had incomes of less than $10,000 ($n = 2$) to over $60,000 ($n = 5$). The women reported Aboriginal, Metis, South Asian, British, Swiss, or Canadian cultural backgrounds. The majority of the women were married or living common law, employed full-time or part-time, and in good health. Two-thirds ($n = 17$) of the study participants resided in rural and remote settings (farms, ranches) as well as in villages of less than 100 residents and in small towns, whereas the remaining one-third ($n = 8$) of the participants resided in Prince George. Each woman provided written consent to participate in the study and selected a pseudonym to protect her identity. I obtained ethical approval for the study from the University of Alberta Health Research Ethics Board and University of Northern British Columbia Ethics Review Board.

Data Collection

I collected data primarily through semistructured interviews using open-ended questions. Additional data included observational information that I collected during travels to interviews on farms and ranches and in northern communities and from written documents, such as maps, tourist guides, community histories, newspapers, and northern poetry. This information enriched my understanding of northern history, culture, and social and physical environments.

I interviewed each participant three times. The first interviews occurred in the women's communities and were 1.5–2 hours in length. Because of weather, distance, and time constraints, I conducted three-quarters of the second interviews and all third interviews by telephone. These interviews were .5–1 hour long. I tape recorded first and second interviews and then transcribed the tapes and imported them into the NVIVO (1999) computer program for analysis. I also incorporated as data notes taken during third interviews and memos containing reflections subsequent to interviews.

Data Analysis

I conducted analysis concurrently with data collection and used the constant comparative method of grounded theory (Glaser, 1978, 1992). With the assistance of the NVIVO (1999) computer program, I reviewed interview transcripts line by line and coded them for categories. Participants clarified, elaborated upon, and verified emerging categories, subcategories, and relationships in second and third interviews. I conducted a fourth interview with three participants for verification of the final theory. Analysis and data collection ceased when no new information or insight was forthcoming about the categories and their relationships, and when the theory seemed to be elaborate in complexity and clear in its articulation of the central problem and the process used to address it (Glaser, 1978).

Limitations

Limitations of the study include the exclusion of non-English speaking women; limited representation of various groups of women, such as very remote women, lesbian women, and women who live in extreme poverty; and by recruitment from two rather than all four northern health regions in BC. Nevertheless, data analysis revealed a theory rich in complexity and grounded description of northern women's health problems and processes.

FINDINGS

The intent of grounded theory is to generate a theory that explains a process of how individuals respond to a main concern or problem (Glaser, 1978). The main problem for the women in this study was vulnerability to health risks. The health risks that the women were vulnerable to were physical health and safety risks, psychosocial health risks, and risks of inadequate health care. Women responded to these health risks by developing a process of resilience which included strategies of becoming hardy, making the best of the north, and supplementing the north (see Figure 7.1).

Becoming hardy for northern women involved taking a positive attitude, following spiritual beliefs, developing fortitude, and establishing self-reliance. Women made the best of the north by participating in northern activities, making decisions about health care services, seeking education and information, seeking and receiving social support, and working on financial and work issues. Supplementing the north involved being political and leaving the north, temporarily or permanently. As a result of developing resilience, women experienced consequences of thriving, surviving, and declining in behavioral, cognitive, and emotional domains. The degree to which women thrived, survived, or declined was dependent upon their abilities to develop and use strategies of resilience. Women's locations within the northern context, the degree of vulnerability they experienced, and the personal resources they had available affected the degree to which women could develop and use resilience in response to vulnerability. Personal factors were relevant in that women who were healthy, young, educated, financially secure, experienced in isolated settings, and who desired to be in the north experienced less vulnerability and were better able to be resilient.

The Northern Context

Aspects of the north emerged as significant contextual variables. The historical location of the north included a history of resource-based exploitation, impoverishment of indigenous populations, and lack of control of northern destiny by northerners (Coates & Morrison, 1992). The physical environment, which included challenging terrain, long distances, and lengthy cold winters with little sunlight, contributed to physical and mental health issues. For example, Leah noted that "Winter is so depressing here.... Half the town has seasonal affective disorder." Because communities may be several 100 kilometres apart, women have limited ability to access social support and health resources that could help them.

Because of distance, sparse populations, and diverse cultures, the sociocultural environment included elements of isolation, lack of resources,

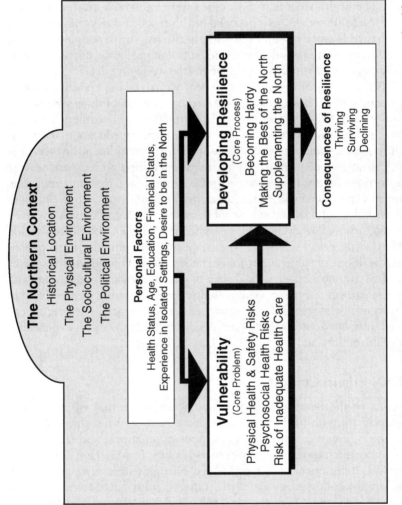

Figure 7.1. Developing resilience to manage vulnerability: Northern Canadian women's health.

overfamiliarity, and inequity. For example, goods such as diverse clothing and fresh food, if they exist in northern communities, were "either low quality stuff or you're paying top dollar" (Linda). Cultural, educational, and employment options for women were very limited and often existed only in larger communities. Overfamiliarity discouraged women from accessing health resources because, as Marie noted, "I'd have to go out of town to keep my anonymity." Throughout small communities in the north, activities were focused on male interests, such as rodeos, hockey, hunting, and ranching. To access woman-friendly activities, such as women's clothing stores and women's organizations, northern women often needed to travel to distant locations. Travel, especially in winter, could be dangerous and was always time consuming and costly. Thus, inequitable access to local resources meant that women needed to forgo access altogether. Forgoing access limited women's opportunities and compromised women's access to health and quality of life resources.

Politically, the north is undervalued and given little real political power and support outside the north. Signe, an elderly woman who lived a long time in the north, perhaps expressed it best when she stated:

> ... people [in the south] think that Prince George [the largest city in northern BC] [is] a little one horse town where the horse died. They put the cancer clinic in Kelowna [a city in the south]. Well HELLO! Who is that good for? Prince George would have made a whole lot more sense. But we go with this political attitude that everything's down there.

The political environment, when combined with the northern physical and sociocultural environments, created problems for people within the north. Participants experienced isolation from women, from men, and from the community. The few women's centers that existed in the north were often stigmatized and underresourced, thus discouraging women from contacting them for help. Women's isolation from men occurred because, "There's this macho male camaraderie and it excludes women" (Marie) and "There's this idea that men and women are on different sides ... there isn't easy mixing between the sexes here" (Eileen). Women new to a community could be isolated because they were considered outsiders, and as such, their access to employment and social resources could be limited. Leah explained, "People know that they didn't grow up here ... you have to be friends with someone to 'get in'."

The northern context often caused women to occupy a less powerful role. Rosie commented, "I hate to say it in this day and age but women don't feel that they have lot of power in a lot of rural [northern] communities." Gender segregation, dogmatic religious beliefs, and the marginalized status of the north were perceived by participants as contributing factors to northern women's limited power. Limiting women's power limited their ability to control their lives and to maintain and promote their health. Participation in research was valued by several participants as important for northern women in gaining power, control, and voice, as Signe stated:

> I think what you're doing is really valuable. This [research] needs to be done because men have been in control for so long and women have just had to go along with it. They've had no say. They've had no say at all.

Vulnerability to Health Risks

The core problem that emerged in this study was vulnerability to three health risks: (a) physical health and safety risks, (b) psychosocial health risks, and (c) risks of inadequate health care. Women's locations within the northern context and personal factors (health status, age, and financial status) affected women's experiences of these risks.

Physical health and safety risks. Vulnerability to physical health and safety risks resulted from climate, geography, wildlife, employment in the physical environment, and pollution from resource-based industries. Climate and geography made travel hazardous, especially in winter, and the decreased number of daylight hours (less than 6 hours in winter) increased challenges of driving. Climate and geography risks caused some women to postpone access to health care, as Christine advised, "Put it [travel to distant health care] off until spring when traveling's easier." Delaying or cancelling care compromised women's ability to maintain their health, and was especially problematic for older women, women with acute conditions, and women who had waited a long time for health care appointments. In addition, climate and geography risks hindered health promotion efforts, as women would forgo attendance at education, health screening, and other events if the weather or roads were impaired.

Wildlife posed risks to northern women's health in urban as well as rural and remote locations. Several women remarked that they needed to be aware of bears and moose in their environments, especially in spring and fall. In addition, outdoor employment exposed women to occupational hazards that were not as prevalent or that did not exist in warmer, southern, urban environments. As Christine explained, "I've been stepped on ... bit ... squashed ... thrown off horses into fences, over fences, off of tractors (laughter), off the hay wagon ... I've broken my baby fingers three times." Because northern communities were often located near employment in resource-based industries such as pulp mills, women remarked that respiratory problems increased when they moved north. As a consequence of vulnerabilities to these physical risks, northern women were at risk of injury, illness, and even death.

Psychosocial health risks. Vulnerability to psychosocial health risks included threats of abuse and social and mental health issues. Isolation, the long cold winters, expectations of women, and limited sociocultural and educational options combined to create unhealthy psychosocial situations for northern women. Christine noted that "old school and settler" attitudes that "women are for birthing children, working on the farm, and that she's yours, you own her" are still "very much alive." Alice commented, "Isolation brings more abuse—a woman is kind of trapped," and Elizabeth noted that she was limited in her ability to deal with a threatening incident in a small, isolated community because, "How do you get away from these people ... where are you going to go?"

Social and mental health issues, such as boredom, loneliness, and depression, were common. Women are often in the north as a result of their husband's employment and thus did not have the support of family and friends. Limited social and cultural opportunities compounded this problem. Leah observed, "In Victoria [a city in the south], anything you want to join, you can join. Here I don't see a lot of choices for women." The couples and children-oriented nature of northern communities especially affected the mental health of single women and women without children. Elizabeth noted that, "As a single person, you don't quite fit in," and Casey felt more included in community events because she and her husband adopted a child. As a result, single women and women with interests other than children often left the north, and women who stayed were vulnerable to environments that put their psychosocial health at risk.

Risks of inadequate health care. Diagnostic, treatment, and health promotion and prevention services either did not exist or were limited in northern settings. The northern physical environment combined with women's personal situations, such as their health needs and financial status, created additional difficulties accessing appropriate and timely health care. Resources that did exist were often inadequate and inappropriate. Few women physicians practiced in the north, and recent health care reform had compromised public health nursing practice (Leipert, 1999). Anonymous confidential care, which is difficult to access in small communities, was particularly problematic for stigmatized mental health services. Inappropriate attitudes on the part of physicians, especially lack of respect for women's experiences and desires, were evident in this study. For example, Christine remarked:

> I've had doctors tell me that my problems are all in my head, when they've only just met me and know nothing about me. That's probably true in southern latitudes, as well, but you have more choices for doctors there.

Elizabeth, a young unmarried woman, detailed her experience of a physician's attitude that resulted in inadequate care:

> That man was brutal, rough, but he was the only gynecologist ... and he says to me, "If you're going to have kids, you better have them now." And I said, "Well, I'm not into being a single parent." [He says] "Well, what's the matter? Good looking girl like you, you should be able to find a man." I would have asked to go somewhere else but there was nowhere else to go ...

Outcomes of these risks included women's avoiding care, experiencing inability to obtain care in a timely and appropriate manner, living with disease and illness longer, experiencing increased complications of treatment, and experiencing compromised recovery.

Developing Resilience

In response to vulnerability to health risks, women in the study engaged in a core process of developing resilience. This process involved strategies of becoming hardy, making the best of the north, and supplementing the north.

Becoming hardy. Becoming hardy for northern women involved taking a positive attitude, following spiritual beliefs, developing fortitude, and establishing self-reliance. Taking a positive attitude helped women put northern challenges into perspective and deal with them, thereby enhancing their commitment to northern life. Spiritual beliefs provided personal comfort, meaning and balance, opportunities for cultural and social connections, and a sense of peace, control, care, and belonging. Spirituality included religious and cultural beliefs, as well as friendships, personal reflection, and communing with nature. Establishing self-reliance increased women's confidence, courage, and skills to tackle new and difficult challenges. Examples of self-reliant strategies included learning to drive, using various strategies to defend oneself against wildlife and threatening humans in isolated settings, and learning to suture wounds if women lived in remote locations.

Women were better able to develop hardiness if they were healthy and motivated to be in the north, could address isolation and other northern context issues, were able to learn about and purchase resources, and had a social support network. Women who were ill, in low income or remote situations, worked outdoors, or traveled on isolated or winter roads were especially challenged in becoming hardy. Adequate personal and social resources were essential in becoming hardy. Carmen noted, "You have to have an upbeat attitude. What makes you hardy is the fact that you don't dwell on the fact that you're living where it's cold and remote," Lilac recommended "having things to amuse you at home in winter," and Gert valued "the company of women."

Making the best of the North. Making the best of the north meant that women used and developed available resources and opportunities. These included participating in northern activities, making decisions about health care services, seeking education and information, seeking and providing social support, and working on financial and work issues.

Women participated in northern activities by (a) enjoying the ready access to outdoor activities, such as camping and hiking; (b) developing indoor interests, such as quilting, painting, and computer use; and (c) volunteering for community groups. Sometimes making the best of the north through participation required a conscious effort. Carrmen explained, "When you live in more remote areas, you have to make yourself be positive. It's not something that just happens." For example, Carmen planned trips to Prince George for entertainment and "to do something different."

Study participants made a variety of decisions about health care. They tried to circumvent inadequate care by seeking a second opinion from another physician or by changing their physician. These circumventions were not always possible because of a scarcity of physicians and physician refusals in small communities to provide advice to patients of colleagues. Women also sought the more accessible and sometimes more appropriate services of public health nurses. Public health nurses were valued because they were "approachable" and took a "holistic approach to health" (Rosie), and because they accorded time, education, and respect to women. Other times, women sought health care in another northern community or outside the north. However, women with low incomes and women who were elderly, ill, or disabled often had to put up with care provided locally. To supplement the limited health care in the north, and because alternative therapies were believed to be legitimate in their own right, women also made decisions to use alternative health care such as massage and naturopathic options. Health needs, age, cultural and educational backgrounds, economic circumstances, available time, and their knowledge about care accessibility and quality influenced women's decisions about health care

Women also developed resilience by seeking education and information from nurses, physicians, universities, community colleges, and distance education programs. Education and information helped to change attitudes, enhanced job and career opportunities, increased knowledge and abilities regarding health and health care, and enriched quality of life. Factors that affected women's ability to access educational resources included women's geographic location; their access to finances for tuition and travel; time for study and travel; and access to technology, such as electricity, telephones, computers, roads, and automobiles.

Social support provided women with instrumental (practical), emotional, affirmational, and informational resources (House & Kahn, 1985). Marie explained, "When people in the north go out of town shopping, they always ask their friends, 'Is there anything you want me to pick up for you?'" Signe noted that it was important "to find somebody to talk to, to ease the loneliness of the long dreary winters." Frequently, northern residents had left extended family to seek employment in the north. Thus, friends often took the place of family. In addition, social support, especially by women, helped women who were new to a community become an insider and thus better able to secure friends, information, support, employment, and other resources.

Financial and work issues included limited employment options for women, lack of child care, male attitudes about what women can and should do, inadequate remuneration, lack of respect, sexual harassment at work, and reluctance of communities to employ women who were new to the community. The boom and bust nature of northern resource-based economies compromised job prospects for men, with resultant financial implications for their female partners. Study participants addressed these limitations by engaging in diverse full-time and part-time employment in both the public and private sector. Part-time work decreased risks by decreasing travel in dangerous climates and terrains and helped women maintain control and make the most of their talents, interests, and opportunities. However, part-time employment also decreased women's incomes.

Nevertheless, women in the study illustrated that through resourcefulness, assertiveness, and effective decision making, part-time and full-time work sometimes improved their financial and employment situations. For example, Casey capitalized on her computer and ranching resources and developed part-time employment "helping a friend do a seed catalogue, babysitting, baking, I [have] eggs and we have hay…" Ruhi developed assertiveness skills to deal with harassment at her restaurant job, and other women made decisions to work part-time, change jobs, or do volunteer work to address employment situations. With adequate incomes, women were better able to access health resources both near and far.

Supplementing the north. Supplementing the north involved being political (personally and for the community) and leaving the north, temporarily or permanently. Supplementing the north included adding to, as well as changing, what presently existed in the north, thereby enriching northern resources and minimizing vulnerability.

The main mode of political action used was that of advocacy, speaking out for themselves and others. Leah advised, "It's important to learn to advocate for yourself with your doctor," and Casey believed that "being your own advocate will take you far." Women engaged in community advocacy to increase awareness about and access to resources. Community advocacy activities included participating in Take Back the Night walks, subscribing to and writing for a regional publication that focused on northern women's interests, and serving as a member of a community committee that met with the Premier of the province about local health matters. Participation in this research was also seen as a political act. Eileen explained, "Women up here feel disempowered, under, and invisible … this research will help women become more visible to themselves and that's part of becoming more empowered." Women needed time and finances, as well as commitment, courage, assertiveness, and tact to be successful as political activists in and for northern communities.

Leaving the north temporarily was a strategy that every participant used to decrease exposure to vulnerabilities and to supplement resources. Obtaining health care in southern locations increased the quality, timeliness, and appropriateness of care, and for women who required special or more diverse care, their ability to obtain any care at all. Goods and services obtained from southern locations increased women's quality of life by increasing choices and decreasing costs of living in the north. Women who were able to travel to vacations and events outside the north brought back expertise and experiences that enriched their lives and the lives of other northerners. Women who were poor, ill, or very geographically isolated often had greater need to leave the north; however, their ability to leave was also compromised by their needs and circumstances.

Leaving the north permanently was a resilient strategy because it required courage and self-assertion to leave friends and family and an established life in the north. Leaving permanently was a strategy that was considered especially salient for single women and for women who wanted enriched education, employment, and sociocultural options. Eileen, a single mother, was considering leaving because she felt that people in her community "look at single moms as having made mistakes, not quite fitting in, as being peripheral." Marie, a single retired woman, was looking forward to leaving the "redneck rough crude" north to lead "the quality of life I want to lead." Leah, a young single woman, was moving south where "all my friends are" and where she could access desired education. Although leaving permanently may increase women's resources and quality of life, their leaving would mean that the north would lose vital resources—women with an informed vision of how northern women's health could and should be advanced.

Women's location within the northern context, the degree of vulnerability they experienced, and personal factors (age, health and financial status, and cultural background) affected the degree to which women could develop and use resilient strategies. Although elderly women and women who were isolated, ill, or poor experienced greater vulnerability to health risks and a greater need for resilience, their ability to be resilient was compromised by their situations. Thus, those with the greatest needs were often the least able to address their needs.

CONSEQUENCES OF RESILIENCE
FOR NORTHERN WOMEN

Women's strategies for developing resilience resulted in three main consequences for northern women's health and quality of life: (a) thriving, (b) surviving, and (c) declining (See Table 7.1). *Thriving* represents growth and includes the development of physical, intellectual, and psychological abilities that enhance health. *Surviving* implies stability and the ability to sustain physical, intellectual, and psychological health. *Declining* is the deterioration of physical or emotional health or cognitive abilities and interests. Thriving, surviving, and declining were manifested in three domains: (a) behavioral, (b)cognitive, and (c) emotional. Study participants experienced these consequences according to their degree of vulnerability, their ability to use strategies of resilience, and their personal needs and resources.

Northern women experienced thriving, surviving, and declining in various configurations. For example, a woman may have thrived behaviorally, survived cognitively, and declined emotionally. In addition, the three domains were interrelated. For example, cognitive thriving may have enhanced thriving in behavioral and emotional domains. Moreover, the consequences of resilience may have varied over time and in response to different situations. For example, a woman who was thriving during the warm summer months may have declined when winter arrived.

The data show that the more resilient a northern woman was, the less vulnerable she was to health risks, and the better able she was to survive and thrive. However, the study revealed a new finding in that, counterintuitively, resilience could also lead to declining. For example, although resilience could result in short-term thriving or surviving, resilience could also result in long-term declining because thriving or surviving in one domain could have led to declining in another. One participant's situation illustrated this finding. Signe, an elderly woman who was waiting for surgery in the south, enjoyed significant social support that helped her develop resilience, thrive emotionally, and survive cognitively. However,

Table 7.1: Consequences of Resilience

	THRIVING (Growth)	SURVIVING (Stability)	DECLINING (Deterioration)
BEHAVIORAL	The development of enhanced physical abilities and behaviors that help women participate in activities and "fit in" with community.	The ability to achieve physical stability and endure, especially during adversity when physical health is compromised.	Physical and behavioral deterioration.
COGNITIVE	The ability to develop intellectual interests and abilities using local and distant resources.	The ability to sustain intellectual abilities and interests with local resources.	Deterioration of intellectual abilities and interests due to limited resources or limited access to resources.
EMOTIONAL	Enhanced psychological coping so that greater self-confidence, independence, positive self-esteem, and happiness result.	The ability to psychologically cope with day-to-day stresses, to "get by."	Deterioration of the ability to fulfill expectations and achieve a happy life.

Signe's resilience also led her to become more accepting of the delay for surgery and thus to decline behaviorally (physically). These findings about the negative consequence of declining were mentioned only minimally in the literature (Fraser, Richman, & Galinsky, 1999; Wright, 1998). Thus, the findings of this study extend researchers' understanding of how resilience can result in both positive and negative health outcomes for women in rural and remote settings.

IMPLICATIONS AND RECOMMENDATIONS FOR NURSING

Implications of the research for health care practice and health-related policy indicate that services must be expanded in northern communities to include more diverse and enriched health care providers and services that address health promotion and illness prevention as well as diagnostic and treatment needs. Although findings revealed that northern women were indeed resilient, their resilience does not absolve society of responsibilities to strengthen system deficiencies and enrich health care resources. Increased efforts must be made to recruit and retain health care professionals who can provide respectful and appropriate care in northern settings.

Northern health care professionals must be comfortable living and working in small northern communities that are underresourced and culturally diverse, where lack of anonymity prevails, where isolation and distance are facts of life, and where newcomers are regarded as outsiders (Leipert, 1999; Rennie, Baird-Crooks, Remus, & Engel, 2000). In addition, health care practitioners must include empowerment, advocacy, community development, and coalition-building approaches in their practices. These approaches are particularly important to help make the most of resources in sparsely populated communities and to increase support and power for northern women.

Implications for women's health research indicate that more feminist qualitative research is needed in isolated settings, particularly regarding the health issues and resilience of women who were not well represented in this study, such as women in very remote settings and elderly and disabled women. Additional qualitative and quantitative research could expand and test components of the theory revealed in this study in other rural and remote settings. Research that explores aspects of resilience, such as the negative consequence of declining and resilience at the community level would provide important information for health care practice and policy.

This study revealed important new knowledge about the northern context, northern women's vulnerability to health risks, and northern women's resilience. The theory revealed in this study will be useful in informing health care practice and policy in rural and remote settings, and in stimulating further research and theory elaboration and testing relevant to rural and northern women's health.

REFERENCES

Canadian Association of Emergency Physicians, Rural Committee. (1997). *Recommendations for the management of rural, remote, and isolated emergency health care facilities in Canada.* Ottawa, Ontario: Author.

Coates, K., & Morrison, W. (1992). *The forgotten north: A history of Canada's provincial norths.* Toronto, Ontario: James Lorimer.

Fraser, M., Richman, J., & Galinsky, M. (1999). Risk, protection, and resilience: Toward a conceptual framework for social work practice. *Social Work Research, 23*(3), 131–143.

Glaser, B. (1978). *Theoretical sensitivity.* Mill Valley, CA: Sociology Press.

Glaser, B. (1992). *Basics of grounded theory analysis: Emergence vs. forcing.* Mill Valley, CA: Sociology Press.

Health Canada. (1996). *Towards a common understanding: Clarifying the core concepts of population health.* Ottawa, Ontario: Author.

Health Canada. (2003). *Rural health in rural hands.* Retrieved July 23, 2003, from http://www.hc.sc.gc.ca/english/ruralhealth/rural_hands.html

House, J., & Kahn, R. (1985). Measure and concepts of social support. In S. Cohen & S. Syme (Eds.), *Social support and health* (pp. 83–108). Orlando, FL: Academic Press.

Keddy, B., Sims, S., & Stern, P. (1996). Grounded theory as feminist research methodology. *Journal of Advanced Nursing, 23,* 448–453.

Leipert, B. (1999). Women's health and the practice of public health nurses in northern British Columbia. *Public Health Nursing, 16,* 280–289.

Leipert, B. (2002). *Developing resilience: How women maintain their health in northern geographically isolated settings.* Unpublished doctoral dissertation, University of Alberta, Edmonton.

Leipert, B., & Reutter, L. (1998). Women's health and community health nursing practice in geographically isolated settings: A Canadian perspective. *Health Care for Women International, 19,* 575–588.

MacDonald, M. (2001). Finding a critical perspective in grounded theory. In R. Schreiber & P. Stern (Eds.), *Using grounded theory in nursing* (pp. 113–157). New York: Springer Publishing.

Morse, J. (2001). Situating grounded theory within qualitative inquiry. In R. Schreiber & P. Stern (Eds.), *Using grounded theory in nursing* (pp. 159–175). New York: Springer Publishing.

Northern Secretariate of the BC Centre of Excellence for Women's Health. (2000). *The determinants of women's health in northern rural and remote regions.* Prince George, BC: University of Northern British Columbia.

NVIVO. (1999). QRS NUD*IST VIVO. Melbourne, Australia: Qualitative Solutions and Research Pty. Ltd.

Rennie, D., Baird-Crooks, K., Remus, G., & Engel, J. (2000). Rural nursing in Canada. In A. Bushy (Ed.), *Orientation to nursing in the rural community* (pp. 217–231). London: Sage.

Statistics Canada. (1993). *Census of agriculture: Selected data for Saskatchewan rural municipalities.* Ottawa, Ontario: Government of Canada.

Stern, P. (1980). Grounded theory methodology: Its uses and processes. *Image: Journal of Nursing Scholarship, 12,* 20–30.

Sutherns, R., McPhedran, M., & Haworth-Brockman, M. (2004). *Rural, remote, and northern women's health: Policy and research directions.* Winnipeg, Manitoba: Centres of Excellence for Women's Health.

Wright, M. (1998). Resilience. In E. Blechman & K. Brownell (Eds.), *Behavioral medicine and women: A comprehensive handbook* (pp. 156–161). London: The Guilford Press.

CHAPTER EIGHT

Strategizing Safety: Perinatal Experiences of Rural Women

Katharine S. West

The health of mothers and infants is of critical importance to a community. Health statistics related to maternal and infant morbidity and mortality reflect the current health status of women and serves as a predictor of health of the next generation (Centers for Disease Control [CDC], 2000). Maternal-child statistics are also considered to closely mirror the general health of the community and its prevailing socioeconomic conditions. To support maternal-child health and thereby the health of the community, health care programs must respond not only to the biological needs of and risks to mothers, but also to their beliefs and customs and to the social fabric of their lives (Hoffmaster, 1986).

Maternity care must not only be available, but also accessible and acceptable to clients (Bushy, 1994). Availability refers to the existence of a particular service, including the necessary personnel to provide that service. *Accessibility* refers to whether a person has logistical access to services, including the resources to pay for them. *Acceptability* refers to whether the service offered is a good fit with the values and beliefs of the client (Bushy). Women living in rural areas have limited access to receiving available prenatal services that are acceptable to them (Conrad, Hollenbach,

The author acknowledges the assistance of Barbara Artinian, PhD, Professor of Nursing, Azusa Pacific University for her assistance with this study.

Fullerton, & Feigelson, 1998; Gertler, Rahman, Feifer, & Ashley, 1993; McManus & Newacheck, 1989). A lack of appropriate care can contribute to poor perinatal outcomes (Hoffmaster, 1986). Thus, it is likely that the experiences of rural women differ from urban or suburban women.

The nursing community may benefit from a better understanding of what it is like for mothers to have a baby when living in a rural area, identifying what internal and external factors influence their experiences, and what strategies the mothers use to optimize birth outcomes. At a time when disparities in service delivery between metro and nonmetro areas are increasing, both federal and state governments acknowledge the importance of providing standardized services (California Department of Health Services, 2000a, b, & c; CDC, 2000). One way to accomplish this is to provide client-specific information to the local public health nursing service. Assessing what mothers know, and specifically what rural mothers know, is important to improve acceptability of health care services. Incorporating women's knowledge and values into community plans to meet state and federal health goals is critical for developing successful plans, and ultimately, improving birth outcomes. Mothers may have different definitions and concerns than the government has regarding birth services, and it would be prudent to investigate this. It is also desirable to tap into the creative solutions that mothers may have developed for themselves and further develop these ideas for the rural community.

The study described in this chapter contributes information related to access, support systems, perceptions, and expectations. Furthermore, the results of this study promote public health nursing through the increased knowledge and assessment of the community of rural pregnant women. Kuehnert (1991) stated that nursing interventions enable and empower communities to change public policy affecting accessibility, availability, and affordability of health services, and other social conditions underlying many health problems. The public health nurse who provides maternal–child health care addresses the particular needs of mothers and children, may improve patient outcomes by influencing policy development, and may provide policy advocacy in partnership with the community, thus improving pregnancy outcomes for rural women.

Purpose

I designed this qualitative descriptive study to discover how pregnant women living in a rural area seek and experience perinatal health care. My second purpose was to give a voice to rural women and their ways of knowing and functioning during the perinatal period.

In this study I focused specifically on experiences of women having babies while living in Mariposa County, California, to understand and identify internal and external factors that influenced their experiences and pregnancy outcomes. The findings show how mothers viewed their interactions with the health care team and their experience of having a baby in a rural area, behaviors and emotions that typified a mother's response to managing her pregnancy, and factors that influenced these interactions and experiences.

METHODS

Symbolic interactionism is a conceptual framework that provides a way to focus on human behavior, how people define the events in their lives (their beliefs), and how they act in relation to their beliefs (Chenitz & Swanson, 1986). Humans ascribe definitions and meaning to events in their lives through an understanding of self and through shared social interaction. Interaction with the health care system is only one factor describing the rural client's engagement with the health care system. When there are many factors present, the symbolic interactionist approach allows the researcher to conceptualize behavior in complex situations in a new and different way. Through this approach I gained insight and clarification for what is important to the women in this study and what strategies they employed during pregnancy while living in a rural area. I used the discovery mode of grounded theory (Chenitz & Swanson) with this study to focus on women's concerns, as no known prior descriptive research had been done on this specific topic. Research findings from this study provide a description of the core variables or the basic social process underlying the experience of the subjects. Grounded theory is especially suited to studying rural women and their pregnancies because there are few theories to explain or predict the behaviors of this special population.

Setting

Mariposa County is a mountainous county located in the western Sierra Nevada range near the center of the state of California. In 2001, the county encompassed an area of 1,455 square miles with an estimated population of 15,950. There were no incorporated cities. Half of the county was classified as nonmetro-rural and the other half as nonmetro-frontier.

The setting for the study was the area south of the Merced River. The western portions of this region encompassed rolling foothills dotted with oaks and pines and ranch land with some of the richest grazing areas in the state. The majority of county health care services were located in the county seat, Mariposa, the largest town with an estimated population of 1,900. Transportation had been a point of concern relating to health care services in all of Mariposa County, as there had been limited public transportation through the years. Because of the large geographic area and the minimum driving distance of 40 miles to the next major metropolitan area, it has been a significant challenge to deliver comprehensive perinatal health care to the residents of the county (Mariposa County Health Department [MCHD], 1999).

With a steady birth rate of approximately 130 babies per year, the majority of Mariposa mothers delivered in one of three neighboring counties because no physician provided delivery services within Mariposa County. Regular local obstetrical services were discontinued in 1982 when the town's general practitioner retired. A local clinic provided childbirth classes and offered prenatal care every other week by a visiting family practice physician from the next county. High-risk obstetrical care was only available by traveling to one of four neighboring counties. Most women drove a minimum of 1–2 hours one-way for prenatal appointments and to reach the hospital of delivery (MCHD, 1999).

Data Collection

The inclusion criteria for the study were women who (a) had current residence in Mariposa County, (b) were currently pregnant at the time of the interview or delivered within the county since 1982, and (c) provided written consent to participate in the research study. I obtained a convenience sample from referrals by family ministries at churches in the county. I obtained demographic data at the time of consent. I interviewed study participants until no new information was forthcoming (data saturation).

Collectively, at the time of the interviews, the 9 interviewees had been pregnant 32 times, with 22 pregnancies completed and one in progress. Eighteen of the pregnancies qualified for inclusion in this study because they occurred in Mariposa County after in-county deliveries had ceased. Prenatal care was started at an average of 8 weeks gestation with a range of 4–16 weeks. Four women's babies were delivered by an obstetrician-gynecologist (OB-GYN), one by a perinatologist, two by a midwife in a hospital setting, and one by a midwife at home. Five women delivered babies in Fresno County, two in Merced County, and one at home in Mariposa County. The newborns weighed an average of 2,679 (range: 816–4,196 grams). There was one preterm infant less than 27 weeks gestation who received care in a regional neonatal intensive car unit. The women each had between one and eight living children aged 8 months to 32 years, including one set of twins, and one term infant who died in the post-neonatal period from complications as a result of a congenital birth defect.

Using an interview guide allowed me to explore the women's experiences to better understand what it is like to be pregnant in a rural county.

I used carefully worded questions to encourage the women to share their experiences and to identify what factors influenced their pregnancies. Because attitudes are difficult to measure, overt questions about attitudes were not asked. Rather, attitudes were allowed to emerge from answers regarding social interactions. In a similar manner, concerns were not directly addressed but allowed to emerge from the data.

Data Analysis

I audiotaped the interviews and then transcribed them. I analyzed the transcriptions by using QSR N-Vivo™ (2000), which facilitated the recognition and understanding of information presented in the interviews. The constant comparative method required that I code interviews initially to reflect the substance of what was said and then compare them with subsequent interviews for similarities and differences. I then compared, clustered, and labeled the codes until a category for those codes emerged (Chenitz & Swanson, 1986). Analysis ultimately revealed a basic social process of strategizing safety.

FINDINGS

Pregnant women in Mariposa County were confronted with the same decisions as pregnant women everywhere: They had to (a) select a caregiver, (b) choose behaviors that support a healthy pregnancy, (c) prepare for labor, and (d) experience a successful delivery. But women in Mariposa County had one significant difference: They must also come to terms with at least 1 hr of travel during active labor when they and their health care provider must meet for the birth. The women all voiced concerns about an unattended precipitous delivery.

One category that emerged from the study data revealed the basic social process of strategizing safety. The women strategized safety to manage their specific worry about delivering en route to a distant caregiver. Delivering on the highway with its potential complications and problems was the mothers' primary concern, and strategizing safety was the core variable that continually worked to resolve that concern. Strategizing safety best explained the large amount of variations apparent in the data. In one way or another, every person volunteered concern about the distance and the plans she made to cope with this concern. One mother explained, "It's just the travel distance and having to make alternate plans that most people wouldn't have to make. We had kind of a mock OB [obstetrical] kit in the car just in case."

The Basic Social Process: Strategizing Safety

The basic social process of strategizing safety has four phases (Figure 8.1): (a) seeking information, (b) choosing, (c) following through, and (d) fine-tuning. For the Mariposa women in this study, strategizing safety in pregnancy commenced upon confirmation of the pregnancy and concluded with the birth. The first phase, *seeking information,* involved fact-finding about the various types of obstetrical care that were available, locally or at a distance. Interpretation of the facts was filtered through personal beliefs and previous experience. The second phase, *choosing,* included deciding on a caregiver for the pregnancy—either a physician or a midwife or combination of the two. In making her choice for caregiver, a woman committed herself to a location for delivery. The third phase, *following through,* began with the initiation and continuation of prenatal care. As pregnancy progressed, changes in circumstances or development of complications sometimes required an alteration in decisions. Coping with the pregnancy was managed with the help of the woman's social support network and her own inherent abilities. The fourth phase, *fine-tuning,* included preparation for labor and the experience of delivery. The labor experience included getting to the right place for delivery at the right time and was the

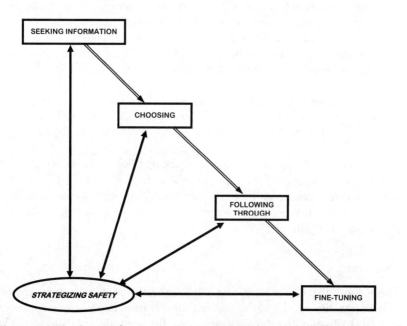

Figure 8.1. Basic social process: Strategizing safety and the four phases of seeking information, choosing, following through, and fine-tuning.

core of the basic social process. Stressors and circumstances unique to the peripartum dictated changes in plans at this phase. Medical interventions were sometimes guided by the need to resolve what one mother termed "the one hour of worry" because of the distance involved.

Seeking Information

> [My last baby] was kind of a surprise. My first thought was, "Oh dear. Moved up to this place where I don't know anybody. There are no OB-GYNs listed in the phone book. How am I going to find a doctor?"

The first phase of strategizing safety is seeking information. Initially a woman had "... a suspicion about being pregnant. And then I went looking for a doctor to confirm it." Sometimes they found the physician or midwife through friends or relatives or current health care providers: "I got my referral through my sister and her midwife." "And then I just went with that group because everybody, you know, [the midwife] just delivered all the babies, so I just went with them."

A woman pregnant for the first time sought additional information about types of health care providers and possible delivery options. Being a primipara and the newcomer in town, she did not have a relationship with an obstetrical caregiver and required information before she could make her choices.

Personal history influenced to some degree the kind of information that participants wanted to obtain. For example, one participant gathered information about home delivery because she was born at home.

> My grandma had [her] children here, most of them at home.... I think I liked the idea [of a home delivery] because, well, my mom had ... her children at home, and I thought if she can do it, surely I could do it.

In this first phase, the women were seeking information based on what they knew from people they knew, or where they believed they might find obstetrical services. From the very beginning, they were already considering the 1 hour of worry. This became more evident in the next phase as they made their choice.

Choosing

The second phase of strategizing safety is choosing. Choosing is accomplished as a direct result of the information obtained in phase one. Elements and facts surrounding the circumstance influence individual choices. The meaning and importance of the decision to the person making the choice also influence choice.

In the case of the experience in Mariposa County, women chose between a physician and a midwife, and both types of providers were available to attend hospital deliveries in neighboring counties. However, few
midwives were available to attend home births in Mariposa County.

> My sister-in-law had a baby at home … . I asked her if her midwife
> would come over here, but she doesn't travel that far. But then I asked
> for a referral. That's how I found out about the midwife here. The
> reason I wanted to do that, I was a little, I mean part of you is a little
> nervous because you don't know if something could go wrong. I did
> have a doctor for back up if there were problems.

Other women made their choices by first deciding on the location for
delivery and then finding a caregiver on staff at that location. This was
sometimes influenced by the report from other women:

> I called around. I asked people for names and I called around and asked
> the offices questions. I had made the decision that I didn't want to go to [a
> particular town]. I didn't want to deliver [there].… because I heard a lot of
> bad stories, that they didn't like it. They didn't like the doctors there. They
> didn't feel comfortable in the hospital. They didn't like the nurses. They
> didn't like either one of the hospitals [there]. I don't think I've ever heard a
> success story … . So, I knew that I wanted to deliver in [another] area.

In addition, prenatal visits were available at the midwifery clinic in a
nearby town where "At least that's a compromise. You still have to travel
in labor, but you can have your visits closer." Finally, there were visits
offered at physicians' offices outside of Mariposa County: "And that's
exactly what we do when we came down for my prenatal visits. We'd
usually plan them for early in the morning, get that done first, and then
we'd go shopping and go eat lunch, you know."

Ultimately, choosing hinged on several factors, but time and distance
were always the major influences of the final decision. Mariposa women
weighed all these options in their minds, balancing the pros and cons of
travel considerations for prenatal care with considerations for delivery.
Travel concern was the constant factor, with the main point being to
resolve fear and worries. The 1 hour of worry was the compelling factor
that guided their choosing.

Following Through

Following through, the third phase of strategizing safety, occurs after
information has been obtained and a choice has been made. Following
through is evidenced by the woman's behaviors as related to the specific

circumstance for which safety must be strategized. Coping and adaptation behaviors that enable one to follow through during this phase are derived from a combination of personal experience, self-care, and social support from friends and family.

During the perinatal experience of the Mariposa women, following through was contingent on the distance the women must travel to reach their caregiver or the distance the caregiver must travel to reach the patient. For instance, the resolve to keep her appointments was reflected by the mother who admitted,

> I had to go. What choice did I have really? Some days I was just plain tired. But I think that was the hardest part, and being so far away. The one time that I was spotting, I was thinking, "What am I going to do"? I could have gone to [a nearby hospital] but I don't know any of those doctors, and I want my own doctor.

The health care provider sometimes shared the travel burden with the mother. "Actually [for] my exams, the doctor would come up to a clinic up here. But [for my other pregnancies], I'd just go to her office in town."

Women frequently combined their prenatal visits with other activities. "I would usually go after ... work in the morning, and then I would go in the afternoon to the midwife. So it worked out okay that way." Sometimes, alternative plans were developed in conjunction with the women's support networks and health care provides. One woman was offered an option when "... people from church came up and told me that they work in [town], and that they'd be more than happy to take me in."

Fine-Tuning

Fine-tuning begins with final preparation for the event that indicated a need for safety in the first place. Fine-tuning may come about from actions of the person who is strategizing safety or may result from the actions of others. Fine-tuning may also be imposed on the situation by the environment. Stressors may develop leading to further fine-tuning. Similar coping skills that were useful in the following-through phase may become significant in this phase as well. Social support from family and friends continue to help the person achieve a conclusion to the event.

For pregnant women in Mariposa County, fine-tuning was the phase that was synonymous with labor and delivery. It was the onset of labor when the 1 hour of worry was most acutely experienced and fine-tuning was implemented.

> Our plan was that if I had a long labor, we were going to get a hotel room down the street from the hospital and labor in a hotel. They had

suites just down the road from the hospital. And so the plan was to labor at the hotel, and then when [contractions] got closer, to go to the hospital.

Distance and travel needs were foremost in their thoughts. Mariposa's families constantly weighed the odds during the phase of fine-tuning: "The only hard thing is the emergency. [Emergency services are] not really worth much at all.... it's kind of just a helipad and a band-aid dispenser." The experience of labor proved whether their particular strategy for safety was adequate. Labor in the right place attended by the right people and a successful birth was the outcome for which the woman sought information many months previously. The variables concerning the details of her labor guided her choice of caregiver and influenced the steps she followed throughout her pregnancy.

Once labor began for the rural woman, getting there was the observable critical behavior during the 1 hour of worry. Getting there sometimes involved more than just transportation; sometimes getting there required fine-tuning by coming up with an alternative route:

> We were a little concerned with the road conditions and you have to go up this one grade called Briceberg. We were a little concerned what the weather was going to be like. Sometimes they just close the roads and they won't let you go through.

Because some of the roads could be covered with snow, the winter season demanded a different sort of fine-tuning. One family who lived between Mariposa and Yosemite had to plan for a winter due date. The mother reflected that had the road to town been snowed over, "We could go up to Yosemite, although they don't really have those kind of services, they do have a clinic there. They have a hospital, and probably the doctor could have helped us there."

The original plan sometimes included an alternative labor support person in the event that the woman could not contact her preferred labor support.

> We had my mom who lives next door, so if I was here, and [my husband] wasn't here, then my mom was to drive. If [my husband] were here, then of course he would drive me. And we had back-up plans with neighbors.

However, if the woman found herself in early labor, and already at or near to the planned location of delivery, the 1 hour of worry sometimes resulted in fine-tuning the labor plan. One woman was in early labor at the hospital when she fine-tuned her plans:

[We all] talked about that openly. [My doctor], the nurses, myself and my husband said, "If you had someplace to go here, I would just send you home. But since you live so far away," and he just had to think about us going to a hotel. He just didn't agree with that. That was an issue. So ... had we been up here, I think that it would have been a different ending.

The birth itself sometimes demanded immediate fine-tuning as described by the mother who delivered along the highway on the way to the hospital.

Well, you've got your gurney, which is not wide. Actually, I just got on all fours and really, that's not a bad way to have a baby. Because there was nothing to hold on to or anything. Actually, I ... just kind of squatted down and held on because there was nothing. There was no way to really get comfortable.... And I was pretty upset to think [an emergency medical technician was going to do the delivery] because I wasn't sure what his skills were. So they didn't have to do anything really. Just catch the baby, but they did fine.

Fine-tuning concluded with the birth of the infant. With the arrival of the newborn, strategizing safety was completed with all the corresponding fears of an unattended delivery; the 1 hour of worry had ended.

Summary

The identified social process in this study, strategizing safety under the circumstance of rural perinatal care, was completed with the infant's birth. For Mariposa women, the safe arrival of the newborn was the result of 9 months of their strategizing to optimize the situation surrounding the 1 hour of worry. Although the same is certainly true that urban women seek safe delivery for their infants, urban women's concern for safety during travel in labor does not usually manifest, if it manifests at all, until the final weeks of pregnancy. On the other hand, women in Mariposa County strategized safety from the beginning of pregnancy, throughout pregnancy, occasionally during that significant hour of travel, and sometimes even after arriving at the planned location for delivery. One mother summed up the situation:

I would love to have my babies where I wouldn't have to travel fifty-five or sixty miles. Maybe because I have healthy pregnancies and deliveries, I don't have that worry so much, but I just think a clinic or someplace to go to have my babies. I don't like traveling in labor.... Like I said, I do have healthy pregnancies, but I think it would be wonderful to have a place up here to have my babies.

CONCLUSIONS

Research about the inner world of the pregnant woman has been published in the nursing and psychological literature since the middle of the 20th century. Much of the field of maternal–child nursing is based on the work of Rubin (1961, 1967a, 1967b, 1975). According to Rubin's long-accepted seminal research (1975), there is a sequence to the psychological tasks of pregnancy and a different focus during each phase. According to Rubin, the mother's focus is inwardly aligned and the fetus is interpreted as being a part of her physical self. Nesting behaviors and thoughts of delivery help her prepare for birth, including solving logistical issues such as transportation at the time of labor. Only in the final weeks of a full-term pregnancy does she begin to prepare for the trip to the hospital with thoughts toward alternative plans or contingencies. Rubin (1975) called this set of behaviors *safe passage.*

More recently, Patterson, Freesen, and Goldberg (1990) conducted research to explore how women utilized health care during pregnancy. The major concern of women was identified as seeking safe passage throughout pregnancy and childbirth by means of several processes that were described as largely psychological, or internal, in nature. Patterson et al. also stated that seeking safe passage might consist of a single approach with the ultimate outcome being the enrollment in prenatal care.

Some similar processes were also identified in this study of rural women with one notable difference. Women in Mariposa County were specifically concerned with the external environment and the attendant implications for safe passage throughout pregnancy and ending with delivery. Mothers in Mariposa began to prepare for the trip to the hospital, at least mentally, immediately upon confirmation of pregnancy. These thoughts pervaded their entire pregnancy. Specifically, it was the 1 hour of worry—the concern with delivering en route to the hospital—that influenced all of their decisions and choices. Seeking safe passage was found to be far more than an internal exercise at the beginning of pregnancy. Strategizing safety was the process by which the women attempted to bring control to their external environment throughout their pregnancy in anticipation of the birth.

DISCUSSION AND IMPLICATIONS

One approach for improving rural access to obstetrical services might be to implement a public health nursing care pathway for maternity support services managed through the rural health department. "First Steps" was a legislated program first established in Washington that implemented such a maternal health care pathway (Olds, 1997). The results were well received by both health care team and family members when the maternity care path brought prenatal care services directly into the community.

Another way to increase the accessibility of the health care team might be to increase the utilization of the advanced practice nurse in the rural area. In California, rural communities have considered using certified nurse midwives to meet their maternity care needs (Nesbitt, Connell, Hart, & Rosenblatt, 1990). In addition, expanding the staff of local county health departments could supplement rural health care teams by including Maternal-Child Clinical Nurse Specialists to work in partnership with preexisting perinatal programs. Legislation was passed in California in 1996 that allowed the certified clinical nurse specialist to directly bill MediCal for prenatal care (Minarik, 1997).

Commentary

Ultimately it is the family's choice to live in the rural area with its advantages and disadvantages. Because of this choice, women know they are responsible to strategize their own safety and that of their babies. Even though their 1 hour of worry influences their decisions for 9 months, the women in this study believed the trade-off was worth it. "It's like having your own path to heaven" to live in a rural area according to one mother. Another described the reasons she chose to have her children in a rural area when she said:

> It's just a joy to see a child go outside and entertain himself all day long with the grass, the rocks, the trees, and the animals rather than something artificial, and not to have to be entertained by something artificial all the time. Although we own all of those things. I mean we have the Nintendo's and the Game Boys and whatever else, but just the opportunity to experience God-given entertainment. It's worth it to me. It doesn't mean it's wrong or right for anybody else, but to me that makes it all worth it.

Finally, to sum it up, another mother affirmed:

> But I think I just love being up here so much better then, looking back, it's still worth it. The drive is still worth it. I wouldn't move down there just to get closer to medical care because I think all the benefits are worth it. But it would be nice if we had ... it would be wonderful if we had someplace close to go for prenatal and postpartum care here at our hospital.

REFERENCES

Bushy, A. (1994). When your client lives in a rural area, Part I: Rural health care delivery issues. *Issues in Mental Health Nursing, 15,* 253–266.

California Department of Health Services. (2000a). *Comprehensive perinatal services program (CPSP)*. Retrieved December 24, 2000, from http://www. dhs.ca.gov/prp/mchb/Comprehensive_Perinatal.htm

California Department of Health Services. (2000b). *Federal performance measures*. Retrieved December 24, 2000, from http://www.dhs.ca.gov/prp/mchb/Federal_Performance_Measures.htm

California Department of Health Services. (2000c). *Outcomes measures*. Retrieved December 24, 2000, from http://www.dhs.ca.gov/prp/mchb/Outcomes_Measures.htm

Centers for Disease Control (CDC). (2000). 16–Maternal, infant, and child health. *Healthy People 2010*. Retrieved September 7, 2004, from http://health.gov/ healthypeople/document/pdf/Volume2/16MICH.pdf

Chenitz, W. C., & Swanson, J. M. (1986). *From practice to grounded theory: Qualitative research in nursing*. Menlo Park, CA: Addison Wesley.

Conrad, J., Hollenbach, K.A., Fullerton, J.T., & Feigelson, H.S. (1998). Use of perinatal services by Hispanic women in San Diego County: A comparison of urban and rural settings. *Journal of Nurse Midwifery, 43*, 90–96.

Gertler, P., Rahman, O., Feifer, C., & Ashley, D. (1993). Determinants of pregnancy outcomes and targeting of maternal health services in Jamaica. *Social Science Medicine, 37*, 199–211.

Hoffmaster, J. E. (1986). Rural maternity services: Community health nurse providers. *Journal of Community Health Nursing, 3*, 25–33.

Kuehnert, P. L. (1991). The public health policy advocate: Fostering the health of communities. *Clinical Nurse Specialist, 5*(1), 5–10.

Mariposa County Health Department. (1999). *Family Health Outcomes Project (FHOP) report*. Mariposa, CA: Author.

McManus, M. A., & Newacheck, P. W. (1989). Rural maternal, child, and adolescent health. *Health Services Research, 23*, 807–848.

Minarik, P. (1997). Medicare reimbursement for nurse practitioners and clinical nurse specialists passes; States' Legislative and Regulatory Forum II. *Clinical Nurse Specialist, 11*, 274–275.

Nesbitt, T. S., Connell, F. A., Hart, L. G., & Rosenblatt, R. A. (1990). Access to obstetric care in rural areas: Effect on birth outcomes. *American Journal of Public Health, 80*, 814–818.

Olds, S. (1997). Designing a care pathway for a maternity support service program in a rural health department. *Public Health Nursing, 14*, 332–328.

Patterson, E. T., Freese, M. P., & Goldenberg, R. L. (1990). Seeking safe passage: Utilizing health care during pregnancy. *Image—the Journal of Nursing Scholarship, 22*, 27–31.

QSR N-Vivo™. (2000). Qualitative data analysis software program (Version 1.2) [Computer software]. Melbourne, Australia: QSR International Pty Ltd.

Rubin, R. (1961). Basic maternal behavior. *Nursing Outlook, 9*, 683–686.

Rubin, R. (1967a). Attainment of the maternal role: Part I. Processes. *Nursing Research, 16*, 237–245.

Rubin, R. (1967b). Attainment of the maternal role: Part II. Models and referrants. *Nursing Research, 16*, 342–346.

Rubin, R. (1975). Maternal tasks of pregnancy. *Maternal-Child Nursing Journal, 4*, 143–153.

CHAPTER NINE

Rural Family Health: Enduring Acts of Balancing

Sonja J. Meiers, Sandra K. Eggenberger, Norma K. Krumwiede, Mary M. Bliesmer, and Patricia A. Earle

Rural families are unique in how they respond to the expectations of the modern health care system, which requires families to be actively involved in the care of their family member. The rural family, as a unique inter-related system, has health beliefs and utilizes health care in ways that are distinctly different from urban dwellers (Bushy, 2000). Our focus in the study described in this chapter was to understand the health experience of families in a rural mid-western setting. Our specific aims were to (a) define rural family health and (b) describe the process that families in a particular rural setting employ in creating health.

BACKGROUND AND SIGNIFICANCE

Professional nurses have historically acknowledged the relationship of family to health (Hanson, 2001; Nightingale, 1858; Whall, 1986; Whall & Fawcett, 1991). However, nursing science with a focus on caring for the family-as-a-whole has received little attention until the last decade (Hanson & Boyd, 1996; Meister, Bell, & Gilliss, 1993; Wright & Leahey, 1994). Family-focused research in psychology, psychiatry, counseling, medicine, family science, and nursing has predominantly resulted in overview texts and periodicals regarding the family system, the family life cycle, family interaction, and family coping (Duvall, 1979; Hill, 1949, 1958; Olson, Russell & Sprenkle, 1989; Rosenblatt, 1994; Walsh, 1993; Wright & Leahey). Nurse researchers have suggested that nursing care emphasis should be placed on providing instruction, support, and relief to family members and neighbors who are often the primary care providers for sick and disabled people (Lee, 1998). Therefore, knowledge development in the emerging field of family nursing, with a focus on caring for and with the entire family, is in its infancy. A key emphasis in this knowledge development process must be to identify the foundational concept of family health.

Clarity regarding what is meant by family health for nursing is necessary as it is of central concern to the development of theory and practice, a worthy focus since the need for family care is increasing in all settings. Individuals in rural areas define health, access health care, and engage in treatment for illness in unique ways (Lee, 1998). Rural families tend to define health as being able to do work, and as a result, symptoms that do not decrease the ability to be active and work may be ignored until absolutely necessary. Rural individuals and families tend to be more self-reliant than their metropolitan counterparts and not as easily accepting of others, especially those with positions of power and status, such as health care providers (Bigbee, 1991).

Research regarding how the rural family unit manages its health is minimal and an investigation using a theoretical framework created deliberately for use in a rural nursing context is extremely rare (Cody, 2000; Denham, 1999; Winstead-Fry, 1992). In a study of rural Appalachian families, health was identified by Denham as a "dynamic and complex construct consisting of multiple member interactions within and across the boundaries of households nested within social contexts" (p. 133). To enhance the understanding of rural family health, the research question focus for this study was "How do rural families create family health?"

METHODS

We used a qualitative design with grounded theory methodology to guide the study. This research explored the family social process of creating health and described the dimensions of this interactive process, thereby contributing to theory development (Glaser & Strauss, 1967).

Setting and Participants

In this study, we used the definition of rural from the Office of Management and Budget (2005). Families who lived in an economically and socially integrated area of less than a 50,000 person population in south central Minnesota were eligible for the study. We recruited families who were not dealing with an active health problem to establish a baseline understanding of the nature of family health. We used this study as preparation for future studies with families dealing with acute or chronic illness. Family membership for this study was self-defined.

We obtained approval for the study from the Institutional Review Board of Minnesota State University, Mankato, prior to recruitment of participants. Prior to interviews, adult participants signed consent forms, and children, 9 years and older, signed assent forms. We assured all participants confidentiality and anonymity.

Theoretical Sampling

We used a theoretical sampling technique simultaneously with the process of data collection. We identified the initial family as an eligible family from the professional network of one of the researchers (N. Krumviede). This family had been articulate regarding health issues in community conversations where the researcher was involved. We identified additional families through a snowball sampling technique. As the analysis proceeded, we enrolled families who could further illuminate the family process of creating health. For instance, as the category of transitions evolved, we made a strategic decision to enroll a family that could be assumed to be experiencing transitions. This sampling technique resulted in data being obtained from 12 families identified as A–M over a 24–month period of sampling and analysis (see Table 9.1). The sample included 39 individuals ranging in age from 1–78 years with a median family income between $50,000 and $59,999.

Data Collection

We invited all family members to participate. All research members conducted interviews at one time or another. Two members of the research team conducted each interview with the family as a family group in the family home. In all instances, they interviewed minor children in the presence of their parents; all members were present at the interview with the exception of one family in which the research members interviewed the college-aged son separately because of scheduling conflicts.

Each of the two researchers present interacted with the family to enhance comfort and conversational style. We used a semistructured format with audiotaped interviews lasting 1–2 hours. We used the following probes to enhance interaction: (a) Describe your family for us, (b) What is your definition of family health? and (c) Describe good times and bad times for your family.

Prior to transcription, we completed preparation of data, including subject identification, and instructions to the transcriptionist regarding how to notate pauses or laughter. The interviewers recorded facial expressions

Table 9.1. Family Descriptions

Family	Age of female adult	Occupation of female adult	Age of male adult	Occupation of second adult	Ages and gender of children
A	39	RN	40	County worker	19m, 18m, 15m, 9m
B	44	Bookkeeper	45	Mechanic	18m
C	37	Cosmetologist			9f, 12m
D	44	Medical secretary	45	Farmer	21f, 18m, 15f, 11m
E	68	RN	70	Skilled laborer	34m, 33m, 16m
F	41	Education Paraprofessional	42	Agribusiness	13m, 15f
H	30	RN	32	Sales	1m, 3f
I	37	Homemaker	38	Health Care Administrator	9f, 7f, 5f
J	66	Retired Sales	78	Retired Mechanic	
K	45	RN	46	Business Consultant	24f, 2f
L	46	Farmer	47	Farmer	19f, 18f, 15f, 11m, 10f, 8m
M	53	Counselor			
	42	Professor	—	—	21m

Note. RN = registered nurse; f = female, m = male.

and body movement as audio field notes. The transcriptionist transcribed these notes and included them as an addendum with each interview to provide the interview context for analysis (Sandelowski, 1995). The interviewers verified the accuracy of the interview transcription by listening to the original audiotapes while simultaneously reading the transcripts.

DATA ANALYSIS

We analyzed interview data following the process described by Strauss and Corbin (1990). Each of us open coded the verbatim transcripts to determine phenomena that comprised the family health experience as a social process. We worked in pairs to review the conceptual labels and validate interpretations. We then reviewed these interpretations as a team and began to assemble the labels into categories of processes. We identified properties and dimensions of the category. We subsequently reviewed all transcripts according to this process until we analyzed 375 pages of data text.

We then subjected the data to the process of axial coding, a set of procedures whereby data are put back together in new ways to make connections between categories (Strauss & Corbin, 1990). As the analysis proceeded, we identified similarities and differences of categories. Finally, we identified a core category, the central phenomena around which all other categories were integrated.

Trustworthiness. We directed our attention toward establishing rigor in this qualitative study through the measures of transferability, credibility, dependability, and confirmability as detailed by Lincoln and Guba (1985). Our use of exemplars in reporting findings enhances the possibility that other researchers can judge the appropriateness of transferring the study findings to another setting. We achieved credibility by reviewing data text in dyads followed by team analysis to clarify and confirm categories. In addition, conducting family interviews in the naturalistic setting of the home enhanced the credibility of the data. We achieved dependability by the use of audiotape recorded, transcribed verbatim interviews. We all discussed the core category and reached consensus on a hypothesis statement regarding relationships between categories. Empirical grounding of the study is evident in the findings as the categories and labels are directly linked to the data. Such empirical grounding is necessary so that the discipline of nursing can determine usability of the resultant theory (Strauss & Corbin, 1990). We established confirmability by recording the decision-making process in determining codes, categories, and themes. In addition, we used ongoing critique of the decision-making process and consultation with an expert grounded theory researcher (Lincoln & Guba, 1985).

FINDINGS

Rural Families Creating Health

These rural families created health in an ongoing process of enduring acts of balancing in response to the inevitable transitions that occurred in family life (see Figure 9.1). The core category, enduring acts of balancing, is demonstrated as adjustment to times of transition. Balancing was needed between (a) work and family, (b) inside and outside commitments, (c) individual and family needs, (d) resources and lack of resources, and (e) time and lack of time. Family health was integrated into the enduring acts of balancing in this rural sample. Family health was strengthened by the family's commitment to work through challenges and differences to form a safe, comfortable, caring environment of unity and uniqueness. The family was considered healthy as long as no one was taking medication. Families, with their unique and ongoing identity and relationships managed times of transition to maintain their sense of unity and integrity. Families engaged in the process of enduring acts of balancing to manage the challenge posed by specific transitions. Examples of specific balancing acts included (a) partnering and sharing essential work roles to manage the family farm, (b) being present for each other during good and bad times, (c) prioritizing family time and work time, (d) creating space for the other family member in the busy day, (e) making family decisions about economic priorities, and (f) modifying family rituals during times of transition. The outcomes of these acts of balancing were continued family work and family caring. In the following section, selected exemplars from family interviews demonstrate aspects of the core category and its related concepts.

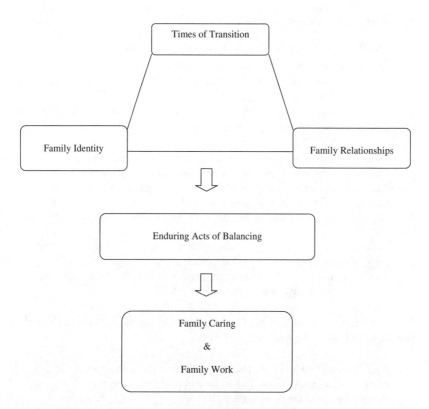

Figure 9.1. Enduring acts of balancing: Rural family health.

Source: Family Nursing Research Team, Minnesota State University, Mankato.

Enduring Acts of Balancing

The process of partnering and sharing essential work roles to manage the family farm (a uniquely rural situation) demonstrated a commitment to family of origin:

> Father: "... we [referring to brother] had a partnership and ... I was doing all the work with the hogs and he was there for his share of the check ... And I thought 'Well this is not working', so I don't know if that fueled some resentment. I says [sic] that's it, you commit one way or the other and I had the backing of my oldest brother. He said, years later, 'Yeah it wouldn't have worked'. And I still feel that there are some of the brothers and sisters who still think they are entitled to something because their roots are here too [the family farm].... And if we had been naive enough to go along with what they [the siblings] were going to decide, I don't think we would be here because we were to the point I had talked to a realtor about moving to Iowa ... It wasn't worth it, it was not worth it. It really has an impact on you. Not only your economics, but your family."

> Mother: "It took awhile for some [referring to extended family members] to really be able to even talk among themselves and there was bitterness.... I think it has gotten better over the years."

Actively prioritizing family time over work time demonstrated commitment to family needs while recognizing individual needs:

> Mother: "I just work part-time as a teacher's aide and I don't make great money, but the hours are good. I have the summer off and then I can make my family a priority. I would like to have a career, but I don't think that I would like to be stretched that way ... So, we kind of made that decision that we are fine to live without the two full time incomes."

> Father: "... that is one of the reasons that I [changed jobs]. I [changed jobs] when she [daughter] started kindergarten ... I just realized that it was not going to work ... [with my previous job's] time requirements. It just did not fit into what I wanted for my family life."

A teenage son described the benefit of creating space for the other family member in the busy day:

> Son: "I mean you will never be able to do that [have the perfect family] because life always throws you a curve ball and you know you have got to take the good times with the bad times ..."

> Mother: "If you can do that."

Son: "If you can work through it and see another person's point of view and what they are trying to bring to the family conversation..... "

Times of Transition

Conditions that prompt the use of enduring acts of balancing in rural families included planned and unplanned transitions associated with family life. These transitions centered on additions and subtractions of persons and things within rural family life as well as situations affecting family security. Additions included births, growing independence of adolescents, and gaining of new family members through marriage. Subtractions included deaths and losses. Family members lost jobs, functional ability, relationships through separation and divorce, and financial security through events such as crop-related disasters. Families reported facing different challenges throughout the developmental, economic, and social spectrum of their lives together. Family life followed a trajectory from formation to reformation through losses, additions, and changes in levels of dependence and interdependence.

Transitions were sometimes related to rights of passage with growth. For instance, parents of a teenager about to receive her driver's license detailed feelings about their daughter's growing independence.

Mother: "So, yes and no. I don't want the responsibility of having to be there [to drive their teenage daughter], but on the other hand it makes me nervous to think that she can do it [drive] on her own."

Father: "And I predict that we will have several differences of opinions when, where and how."

Mother: "But, she already understands, I think, her expectations are not going to be met, which then she will need to take into consideration."

Transitions were also influenced by the environment surrounding families. For instance, one father described the threat to financial security that bad weather causes and its influence on the emotional climate of the family.

Oh, I think I get all stressed out [when the weather is bad and the markets react in a way that is related to family income] and am not going to show it and the ones closest are the ones who are going to feel it. They are going to hear it, it all relates back to income and providing.

Family Identity

At time of transitions, families are challenged to adjust their family identity within the context of their evolving world. Family identity is created through a dynamic process of internal and external feedback. Internal feedback is derived from each family's experiences of life and their perceptions. Family perception is the filter through which the family views its identity. External feedback is derived from the family's experiences of connection to the greater community. Family values, structural and qualitative family definitions, family relationships to the community, and the ability of families to seek information were all examples of identity challenge during times of transition. Children in the sample shared their impressions quite freely in response to the statement, "Describe your family for me."

A father described a situation surrounding a life-altering accident in the family's past that illuminated a conflict between family values and legal rights that challenged family identity.

> ...we didn't even go after the insurance company. We could have. I mean later when he was 21 ... But, I didn't really feel right taking it when the Lord gave him his life ... maybe we shouldn't...

A mother and daughter shared their thoughts about how family identity adjustment was somewhat based upon relationships within the community.

> Mother: "When I think of family, I think of these four and my parents ... and sometimes it extends to people at work.... "

> Daughter: "Like older people ... we have a lot of people that we have known over the year that we could go to ... I don't argue with them ... I help them around the house ... helping them.... "

One son described his family in comparison with other families:

> I've heard some of my friends and the way their families are and I consider my family probably the best out of half the families I know. They gave me everything I needed and probably more, but we've had problems at times, too.

Other children described their families as:

> "We are like three people renting a house together [intergenerational family]." "Big, weird, argumentative, talkative, A little larger than the typical family of the Midwest. Driving to town, never home, letting the house be a mess—everyone is always coming and going. Helping with church things and community things—there's a lot ... going on."
>
> "I guess we're all kind of flamboyant, outgoing, the family as a whole is family oriented and we like to do things together."

Family Relationships

The process of negotiating relationships within the family to adjust their sense of family identity was multifaceted. Families negotiated forming and reforming of relationships through communication. Connections and coalitions were realigned within the family communication process. For instance, power and control issues were negotiated and boundaries and roles were clarified. The family often came to a common view of a crisis event while working together to understand its impact. Such processes of negotiation may not have been intentional but evolved as a reflection of historic family patterns. A father described the unique family process of negotiation through communicating during a time of growing adolescent independence.

> We had a great conversation about two years ago, didn't we [name]? For probably an hour screaming at each other and I mean ... we were just kind of taking shots at each other and there is nothing wrong with that because I was fueling the fire constantly. I just wanted to see how far I could get him to go and he was testing his old man to the max.... No violence or none of that, it was just a good scream session.

Another significant time of transition requiring active negotiation of relationships was the time of family formation. A mother described the process she went through to achieve comfort with different levels of family connections:

> I've learned a lot from marrying [name] because they are very family oriented and very close ... and my family loves each other but we never spent this much time together ... there is always someone to turn to ... someone always around ... It was hard at first because I am very independent and I felt like if it was mine then I would do it ... I would feel bad if someone came in and helped me, because it was mine and I was supposed to do it.

Finally, a family member described the process of negotiating care responsibilities with her sister. She and her sister were sharing the work of caring for their elderly mother. This process illustrated the constant formation and reformation of family that is influenced by family values.

> My sister and I were taking turns keeping her [mother] and keeping her out of the nursing home as long as we possibly could ... she has gone down hill and is in a nursing home now.

Family Caring

Through the process of enduring acts of balancing, families continue the work of caring for their family member in newly negotiated ways. Families reported that the work of caring involved discipline, support of each other, listening, ensuring safety, planning for the future, and monitoring member actions. Members maintained contact with each other through the work of caring by enacting coalitions, worrying about each other, and ensuring access to each other. The work of caring was also supported by extended family and employers. A family described their attention to safety issues as a way of caring.

> ... before we went to the county fair, my husband [name] talked to her about not talking to strangers ... and then I think she did not want to go.

> Father: I discussed it on the way home one night, and I felt bad because then she [daughter] said that she did not want to go to the fair anymore ... I just wanted to have it in the back of her mind about not talking to strangers ... We are more worried [than our parents] because there is more of an alarm because they are our kids....

A father told the story of learning the importance of holding back and working to support his son during a frightening experience. He also detailed the incorporation of the event into the foundation of family discipline.

> He says I rolled the pick-up in the ditch. At that point I wanted to go right through the phone and grab him and start choking him for doing that. But, it's clicking that fast I am going "wait a minute he is stand-ing there talking to me telling me he just rolled this thing in the ditch," maybe I better just mellow out here, dad, and we will go take and look and see ... there are those scary things with kids and yet you want to react intact because, dang it, why did you do that and yet thank God, for once the brain kicked in before all the excitement did ... But some of those were the bad times that actually probably turn out to be good because he didn't actually get hurt and yet you're thankful that somebody ... learned a pretty valuable lesson.

Families anticipated the inevitable letting go while acknowledging the good feelings of family times and the differences in family members. They incorporated knowledge of the influences of events in their family history on family growth. A father described a history of family counseling that has aided family growth as he states, "We take everyone's feelings into consideration ... about five years ago we had some family counseling on some issues and I think that has helped us a lot..."

A wife described how she and her husband seek connections in everyday experiences and are influenced by their families of origin in their choice of activities, "... we like to watch birds, go for walks, go for hikes ... since we come from such large families, we enjoy being together with our families and our friends."

Family Work

Essential family work is accomplished through shared decision making and shared roles within the demands of rural life to facilitate getting the work of family done. Decision making about health, priorities, and activities was accomplished by seeking information and focusing on the future. A 13-year-old boy described getting the inevitable work of cleaning done, "[Bad times are] ... when we have to clean ... every time something's happening ... It's sometimes not even that dirty."

A father described the pull of family work and the daily grind of home maintenance integrated with childrearing tasks.

> When I'm at work, I think about what all needs to be done at home, like mowing the lawn ... it take about 8 hours and I would like to be inside helping her with the dishes or washing clothes or picking up the tens of thousands of toys that are laying around...

These families created health in an active process of experiencing and interacting with each other and the environment. The social process of enduring acts of balancing is an active process of creating health in the environment, evolving and changing through interactions. Enduring acts of balancing is the ongoing process of creating family health. Consequences of the process of enduring acts of balancing are the continued work of caring, getting the daily work of family done, and facilitating growth and development of individual family members.

DISCUSSION

Rural Families Creating Health

Our purpose in this study was to advance researchers understanding of the process rural families use to create health. Rural family health is created in an ongoing process of enduring acts of balancing in response to the inevitable transitions of family life in the context of family identity and family relationships. Outcomes of this process are continued family work and family caring. Creating family health involves actively managing everyday life experiences by working together and attending to the evolving family identity.

Times of Transition

Family life theorists have done much work regarding family transitions (Bengtson & Allen, 1993). Generally, transitions in the life course of families are used as key markers of social change in family life. Transitions are viewed as normal or abnormal and are measured by the successful accomplishment of developmental tasks (Carter & McGoldrick, 1989; Duvall, 1957), with abnormally timed transitions viewed as problematic for families. Denham (1999), for example, referred to transitional time surrounding death as a central dimension of the family's experience while caring for their dying member. Other authors have indicated that serious acute or chronic illnesses present significant transitions that challenge coping and developmental processes (Wright & Leahey, 1994). Families in this study indicated that transitions occur almost constantly and are related to factors beyond those traditionally identified by family life course theory: (a) exit from school, (b) entry into the labor force, (c) departure from family of origin, (d) marriage, and (e) establishment of a separate household (Modell, Furstenberg, & Hershberg, 1976). An important aspect of transition for these families included multiple examples of moving between independence and dependence within the family. Possibly their movement is significant because, according to rural nursing theory (Long & Weinert, 1998), rural families are self-reliant and more independent as groups than urban dwellers. This may lead to a family that is more interconnected, lending to a more difficult experience during evident transitions toward independence even if it does not mean separation.

Family Relationships and Family Identity

Communication theorists state that family relationships, rules, and roles are worked out through interaction over time and result in the family's unique identity and creation of health (Fitzpatrick & Ritchie, 1993). In addition, through the course of family development, fundamental and enduring assumptions about the world result from significant interactions within the family and between the family and the environment. Rural families hold an identity within the greater rural community. This identification is often linked to the components of old-timer–newcomer in relationship to the length of time the family or extended family has lived and been a part of the rural community (Long & Weinert, 1998). Findings in this study suggest that the daily processes families use to create family health may be related to ongoing formation of the family paradigm being formed within the rural community context (Reiss, 1981).

Study findings support the premise that family health is inextricably intertwined with the pattern of family relations so that family health itself is part of the vital fabric of family life (Pratt, 1976). Certainly the family is more than a context for health occurrences. The family is a living, processing, adjusting, coping, and stabilizing entity. The family health experience is an active process of living in the environment, evolving and changing through interactions. These families detailed a process whereby they are conscious of their past but are constantly moving toward the future, supporting the notion that the family health experience is necessarily created through highly interactive processes considering family members and the environment, a concept similar to Newman's (1994) expanding consciousness. The participants emphasized that interactions between family members and between the family and the environment, (e.g., specifically weather, extended family and community) influence expanding consciousness.

Family Work and Family Caring

The families in the current study were able to identify a set of beliefs about the importance of getting the work of family done. Work was essential to the family and best experienced when doing the work together. The self-reliance of the rural family was often linked to a sense of pride in work accomplished to care for their own. Families identified being healthy until one of its family members required taking a medication. In addition, family caring beliefs were identified.

Family caring included insuring that family members were safe and received adequately provision. The ability of each member to serve and fulfill a role within the family allows the family to grow and develop while doing the work of family. The tight bonds and intimacy of the family often challenges the individual's need for privacy while maintaining the connected caring for family members as individuals and family as a whole.

Implications and Recommendations for Nursing

The empirically grounded framework that emerged from the data analysis in this study can serve as a framework for a future, larger study. Future research is needed to consider the conceptual relationships within the framework and to test components of the framework. For instance, Is the family's sense of the ability to get family work done related to the degree of threat to family identity? or How does the closely interconnected rural family manage inevitable transitions toward independence or increased dependence in a rural community in one geographical region as compared with another?

Nurses engaged in rural nursing practice can learn a great deal from listening to the family's discussion of their daily experiences regarding how they create health. Asking the family to respond to the following question may be helpful in initiating family-level care: What kinds of things does your family normally do when you sense a challenge in your family life? Nurses who are aware that their interactions with families in the rural setting are critical to evolving family identity, can enhance the family's ability to create health. Nursing practice that recognizes the significance of transitions in the life of a rural family will guide families to prepare and manage their life of transitions. Nursing practice in the rural setting that acknowledges and supports the acts of balancing in a family will also foster family health. Praising the work of family, along with the individual family member's work, supports the family as a whole in the rural environment.

Pedagogy necessary to stimulate this level of practice would necessarily focus on techniques to enhance interaction between nurses and families. Nurse educators who live and serve in rural settings can influence the quality of care provided to rural families through the use of frameworks and pedagogues focused specifically on rural practice. Nursing students need continued practice with healthy families in the rural setting to continue developing an understanding of family life and processes in this setting.

REFERENCES

Bengtson, V. L., & Allen, K. R. (1993). The life course perspective applied to families over time. In P. Boss, W. J. Doherty, R. LaRossa, W. R. Shumm, & S. Steinmetz (Eds.), *Sourcebook of family theories and methods: A contextual approach* (pp. 469–504). New York: Plenum.

Bigbee, J. L. (1991). The concept of hardiness as applied to rural nursing. In A. Bushy, (Eds.), *Rural nursing* (Vol. 1, pp. 39–58). Newbury Park, CA: Sage

Bushy, A. (2000). *Orientation to nursing in the rural community.* Thousand Oaks, CA: Sage.

Carter, B., & McGoldrick, M. (1989). *The changing family life cycle.* Boston: Allyn & Bacon.

Cody, W. (2000). Nursing frameworks to guide practice and research with families: Introductory remarks. *Nursing Science Quarterly, 13,* 277.

Denham, S. (1999). Family health in an economically disadvantaged population. *Journal of Family Nursing, 5,* 184–213.

Duvall, E. (1957). *Family development.* New York: Lippincott.

Duvall, E. (1979). *Marriage and family development* (5th ed.). Philadelphia: Lippincott.

Fitzpatrick, M. A., & Ritchie, L. D. (1993). Communication theory and the family. In P. Boss, W. J. Doherty, R. LaRossa, Shumm, W. R., & S. Steinmetz (Eds.),

Sourcebook of family theories and methods: A contextual approach. (pp. 565–589). New York: Plenum.

Glaser, B., & Strauss, A. (1967). *The discovery of grounded theory.* Chicago: Aldine.

Hanson, S. M. H. (2001). *Family health care nursing: Theory, practice, and research.* Philadelphia: Davis.

Hanson, S. M. H., & Boyd, S. T. (1996). *Family health care nursing: Theory, practice, and research.* Philadelphia: Davis.

Hill, R. (1949). *Families under stress: Adjustment to crisis separation and reunion.* New York: Harper & Row.

Hill, R. (1958). Social stresses on the family: Genesis features of families under stress. *Social Casework, 39,* 139–158.

Lee, H. (1998). *Conceptual basis for rural nursing.* New York: Springer Publishing.

Lincoln, Y., & Guba, E. G. (1985). Establishing trustworthiness. *Naturalistic Inquiry* (pp. 289–331). Beverly Hills, CA: Sage.

Long, K. A., & Weinert, C. (1998). Rural nursing: Developing the theory base. In H. J. Lee (Ed.), *Conceptual basis for rural nursing* (pp. 3–18). New York: Springer Publishing.

Meister, S. B., Bell, J. M., & Gilliss, C. L. (Eds.) (1993). *The nursing of families: Theory, research, education, practice.* Newbury Park, CA: Sage.

Modell, J., Furstenberg, F., & Hershberg, T. (1976). Social change and transition to adulthood in historical perspective. *Journal of Family History, 1,* 7–32.

Newman, M. A. (1994). Paradigms of health. In M. A. Newman (Ed.), *Health as expanding consciousness* (2nd ed., pp. 1–14). New York: National League for Nursing Press.

Nightingale, F. (1858). *Notes on matters affecting the health, efficiency, and hospital administration of the British army.* London: Harrison & Sons.

Office of Management Bulletin No. 05-02. Update of statistical area definitions and guidance on use of statistical area definitions. Washington, DC: Government Printing Office.

Olson, D., Russell, C., & Sprenkle, D. (1989). *Circumplex model: Systemic assessment and treatment of families.* New York: The Hawthorne Press.

Pratt, L. (1976). *Family-structure and effective behavior: The energized family.* Boston: Houghton Mifflin.

Reiss, D. (1981). *The family's construction of reality.* Cambridge, MA: Harvard University Press.

Rosenblatt, P. C. (1994). *Metaphors of family systems theory: Toward new construction.* New York: Guilford.

Sandelowski, M. (1995). Rigor or rigor mortis: The problem of rigor in qualitative research revisited. *Advances in Nursing Science, 16*(2), 1–8.

Strauss, A. L., & Corbin, J. (1990). *Basics of qualitative research.* Newbury Park, CA: Sage.

Walsh, F. (1993). *Normal family processes.* New York: Guilford.

Whall, A. L. (1986). The family as the unit of care in nursing: A historical review. *Public Health Nursing, 3,* 240–249.

Whall, A. L., & Fawcett, J. (1991). *Family theory development in nursing: State of the science and art*. Philadelphia: Davis.

Winstead-Fry, P. (1992). Family theory for rural research and practice. In P. Winstead-Fry, J. C. Tiffany, & R. V. Shippee-Rice (Eds.), *Rural health nursing* (pp. 127–147). New York: National League for Nursing Press.

Wright, L. M., & Leahey, M. (1994). *Nurses and families: A guide to family assessment and intervention* (2nd ed.). Philadelphia: Davis.

PART III

The Rural Dweller and Response to Illness

The first chapter in this part is Buehler, Malone, and Majerus-Wegerhoff's chapter from the first edition of *Conceptual Basis for Rural Nursing*. The authors describe patterns of responses to symptoms by rural persons; the title is "The Symptom-Action-Time-Line (SATL) Process." Next, O'Lynn updates the SATL process through an extensive literature review and recommends a revision of the process.

The experience of chronically ill rural women and the use of an online support group intervention is the focus of Winters and Sullivan in the part's third chapter. Last, Shreffler-Grant provides insight on the acceptability of health care providers in rural locales having critical access hospitals.

Patterns of Responses to Symptoms in Rural Residents: The Symptom-Action-Time-Line Process

Janice A. Buehler, Maureen Malone, and Janis M. Majerus-Wegerhoff

INTRODUCTION

How people identify, evaluate, and respond to symptoms is an important determinant of their health and illness behavior (Lenz, 1984). An increasing amount of literature addresses health behaviors of rural people (Lee, 1991; Long, 1993; Long & Weinert, 1989; Moon & Graybird, 1982; Weinert & Long, 1990). However, little information is available on the patterns of responses of rural people to symptom occurrence signifying actual or potential health problems. In addition, there is a paucity of information on health behaviors of certain rural groups, specifically, women and Plains Indians.

Although actual processes of health-seeking behavior are not delineated in most research of rural health behaviors, some patterns are evident. A survey of health risk prevalence in rural Montana (Moon & Graybird, 1982) revealed that participants believed in self-responsibility for health. Lee (1991) noted that the quality of hardiness may be responsible for some rural dwellers' delay in seeking assistance from the professional health care system when symptoms of illness appear. Rural people were viewed as delaying health care until they were very ill, thus often needing hospitalization at the point care was sought (Long, 1993; Long & Weinert, 1989; Rosenblatt & Moscovice, 1982; Weinert & Long, 1990).

Studies on responses to symptom occurrence, not specific to rural people, have been conducted by behavioral and social scientists. Mechanic (1960) stated that possible responses to illness include discretionary inaction, the use of medicines, seeking professional care, and using a lay network. Suchman (1966) described individual responses to symptom occurrence as proceeding in this sequential pattern: (1) the Symptom Experience Stage, (2) Assumption of Sick Role Stage, (3) Medical Care Contact Stage, and (4) Dependent Patient Role Stage.

Segall and Goldstein (1989) noted that lay persons clearly do routinely self-evaluate and self-treat many of their health problems as a part of daily living and that the nature and extent of these self-care practices are not well understood. They concluded it is not clear whether self-care behavior is equally prevalent among different social groups, whether self-care is used for both health maintenance and the treatment of illness, and whether self-care is used only in response to selected symptomatic conditions.

METHODS

The qualitative method of grounded theory was used in this study (Glaser & Strauss, 1967). Grounded theory provides a means of understanding behavioral patterns from the perspective of the participants. It enables learning about their world and the interacting influences of personal, social, and cultural characteristics without imposing the cultural biases of the interviewer (Chenitz & Swanson, 1986). Grounded theory allows for the direct examination of the world of rural residents in a naturalistic way (Schatzman & Strauss, 1973).

The convenience sample was composed of 16 rural or frontier Montana women, 8 of whom were Native American women living on a federal reservation and 8 of whom were Caucasian farm or ranch women. Elison (1986) defines rural as a population density of more than 6 but less than 100 per square mile and a driving distance to a hospital of at least 30 minutes. "Frontier" is defined as a population density of less than 6 per square mile and driving time to a hospital of either 60 minutes or severe geographic and/or seasonal climatic conditions.

The eight Caucasian farm or ranch women were married and had at least two children. Six of them were self-employed, actively farming and ranching with their husbands. Two were employed in a small city 60 miles from their homes. Four of these women lived in rural locations and four in frontier locations. Their nearest neighbors lived one-fourth mile to 8 miles away. One informant's nearest neighbor was 5 miles away but did not have a phone. For emergencies, this informant would travel 12 miles to the nearest neighbor with a telephone. The primary means of paying for health services for these women was through private pay and individual health insurance.

Of the eight Native American women, seven were classified as rural and one as frontier. Five of the informants lived on small ranches and three lived in one of two towns each with populations of less than 200 (U.S. Bureau of Census, 1987). Seven of the informants have lived on the reservation all of their lives. Three of the women were unemployed and on Aid to Families with Dependent Children, two considered themselves full-time homemakers, and the remaining three were employed in local towns. Five of the Native American women were married, two were single, and one was divorced. All informants had children, with an average number of 2.3 children per household and a range of 1–6 children per household. Five informants lived with extended family members, and three lived with only their children and husbands. All eight women used the Indian Health Service which provided free health care as entitled by treaty.

Face-to-face focused interviews were conducted in the homes of the participants. Open-ended interview questions and probes were used to stimulate free responses (Woods & Catanzaro, 1988). Topics included describing the steps used when someone in the home becomes ill, examples of when self-treatment would be used or of when someone would be consulted, signs indicating illness, examples of home remedies, length of time before seeking help, and reasons for deterrence in obtaining care from professional health resources.

The grounded theory data analysis for this study revealed a basic social process (BSP) termed the *symptom-action-time-line process* (SATL).

FINDINGS

Both Native American and Caucasian farm/ranch women used the symptom-action-time-line process to respond to symptoms of actual or potential health problems. The process consists of four stages in which symptoms are identified and actions are taken to move to a desired state of health. The stages are (a) symptom identification, (b) self-care, (c) lay resources, and (d) professional resources. Each stage has a time period (time-line) in which the participant takes actions in response to a symptom, evaluates the effectiveness of the actions in resolving the symptom, and decides whether to go on to the next stage. Time periods during stages are dependent on the intensity, duration, and amount of interference in function caused by the symptom and may be minutes, days, or years. The first stage, symptom identification, is the stimulus leading to the other stages.

Symptom Identification Stage

Symptom identification was preceded by symptom occurrence and included assessment of conditions or signs perceived as being an undesired alteration in the person's usual state of health that required actions to move the person to his or her desired state. Participants identified their desired state as being the way they were before the symptom occurred. The symptoms had three properties: physical signs and sensations, degree of interference in the ability to function, and intensity and duration. Physical signs included "fever," "vomiting," "pain," "pulling at ears," "broken bones," "hard to breathe," and "losing blood." Interference in function included "not being able to do ordinary things like housework," "I couldn't move my finger," and "unable to eat or play." Intensity and duration of symptoms were the degree and rate of change in a symptom, onset of new symptoms, and length of time they persist. Examples included "temperatures over 102 degrees for 3 days" and "a bloody nose that couldn't be stopped after 2 hours." After the symptoms were assessed, they were given meaning, and a decision was made whether to take action. This was dependent on knowledge and past experience with illness, intensity and duration of the symptoms, and degree of interference with normal functioning. A Native American woman stated, "Whenever my girl pulls at her ears and is fussy, I know from before that she probably has an ear infection and we should go in (to the clinic).... The first time (she was sick), I waited until she had a fever, and it went so high it really scared me." Participants in both groups stated they noticed most symptoms within minutes to a few hours after occurrence.

Variation noted between Caucasian and Native American women in symptom identification was due to meanings given to symptoms. For example, one of the Native American women, after getting no relief from headaches through use of medications prescribed by a physician, attributed her headaches to supernatural origins and sought care from a medicine man. Both groups of women described lower thresholds of tolerance for duration and intensity of symptoms in their children. This resulted in shorter symptom-action-time-line processes for children.

Self-Care Stage

The second stage of the SATL process was characterized by the initiation of self-care. Self-care involved those activities self-initiated and performed for self or family members in response to symptoms. Examples of self-care listed by respondents ranged from "getting extra rest," "slowing down," "waiting for more symptoms" to more complicated activities such as "soaking my foot three times a day." The time-line described by both groups of women for starting self-care after symptom identification was seconds for intense symptoms to a "couple of days" for minor symptoms.

The self-care stage was also characterized by using self-care tools, those items used by the respondent to resolve symptoms on their own. Both groups listed such items as nonprescription medications, leftover prescription medicine, teas, thermometers, heating pads, disinfectants, and reference books. The majority of the Native American women used traditional self-care tools to treat certain symptoms. These included sage, sweet-grass, and medicine bundles. One Native American woman used a first aid book for reference whereas half the Caucasian ranch women regularly referred to their "family health textbooks." One informant in this group stated, "I looked up symptoms my daughter had, and the book told me what I could do for her at home or if I needed to see a doctor." Another informant added, "Everyone in my family knows how to look up their illnesses in our health book." All of these informants live in the frontier area. Another self-care tool mentioned only by these frontier women was "animal" ointments to treat hand rashes resulting from feeding lambs.

Actions for this stage included initiating self-care; evaluating its effectiveness based on a decrease in the duration, intensity, or the amount of interference in the ability to function; and deciding to seek help if self-care was ineffective. A typical response, for both Native American and Caucasian informants, regarding the decision to seek help was, "I tried taking Tylenol but after two days I still had a fever, so I called my mother for advice."

Lay Resources Stage

In this, the third, stage, the participants involved their informal network of family, friends, and neighbors, that is, their lay resources, by describing the symptoms and obtaining assistance to alleviate symptoms. Properties of this stage included symptom validation, asking advice for self-care or self-care tools, receiving physical care, or seeking emotional support—particularly for deciding to go to a physician. Time-lines for consulting lay resources after symptom identification ranged from 1–3 days for both groups. Both groups had usually initiated a self-care activity before they consulted their lay resources.

Ranch women stated their most frequently used lay resources were their mothers, but they also consulted with neighbors. Two frontier ranch women described how they had become aware of each other having similar joint pain of the great toe. They compared their symptoms over the phone while referring to their health textbooks that guided them to diagnosing themselves as having gout. They then verified these symptoms and information with another lay resource, a neighbor who was a registered nurse. Ranch women also described an organized informal lay network of volunteer farmers and ranchers who acted as first responders to emergencies. They were called for such symptoms as "chest pain," "losing blood," and "broken bones."

Organized, volunteer networks of lay resources were not described by Native American women. The majority identified their mothers as their primary source of help. A few consulted only with their husbands, stating that they had no relatives or friends living in the area for them to contact. Participants stated they would usually consult a relative before they would consult a neighbor who was not a relative. The majority of the Native American women also consulted their lay network for advice on the use of traditional healing practices. The following described this use of a lay resource.

> My son (nine-months-old) had been fussy for two days; he was not taking his bottle and had cold sweats. Tylenol didn't seem to be helping, so my mother suggested that I take him to my aunt because he might have colic. My aunt massaged him and blew smoke in his ear. He went to sleep and was O.K. after that.

Actions for this stage included contacting a lay resource; evaluating whether there was a decrease in the symptom's intensity, duration, or interference with function; and deciding whether to take further action. Varying degrees of self-care continued throughout this stage.

Professional Resources Stage

Seeking help from professional resources occurred when there was failure to alleviate symptoms through the use of self-care or lay resources, or when symptoms intensified, or when new symptoms developed. Professional resources listed by both groups included physicians, registered nurses, dentists, and chiropractors. Both groups stated they consulted professional help when "nothing else helped," "there wasn't anything I could do," or "for emergencies." Nurses were sometimes consulted for advice about whether symptoms required immediate attention or could wait awhile longer. Nurses were frequently used as lay resources in this instance, since they were called at their homes when off duty. Physicians were usually not called at home unless the participant had been under physician care for a specific condition.

Time-lines, from the symptom identification stage to the professional resource stage in situations other than emergencies, were 4–7 days for rural women and 1–2 weeks for frontier women. Time-lines for Native American women ranged from 2–5 days in both rural and frontier areas.

Time-line variations occurred for children and in emergencies. For children, total time-line durations were much shorter, ranging from less than 1 day to 3 days. Each stage within the time-line process was shorter; lay resources were consulted sooner and often used only to help transport the child to the professional resource. Barriers to seeking professional care were minimized so that time and distance became less important for children than for adults. In emergencies, individuals tended to bypass self-care and lay resources and go directly to professionals. Barriers were minimized according to the urgency of symptom occurrence.

If symptoms were not alleviated after going to a professional resource, participants either returned to the same professional or went to a different professional. At times, symptoms were simply "tolerated." Several Native American women sought alternative care by contacting a medicine man. This occurred because they believed physicians had not helped. The medicine man was described by these participants as another type of professional. The most frequently identified barriers to professional resources were distance and transportation. Other barriers mentioned were fear of "bad news," a lack of women doctors, and the time required to see a professional, especially time spent in waiting rooms.

IMPLICATIONS

The symptom-action-time-line process clarifies response patterns rural women display when confronted with symptoms of actual or potential health problems. The process provides a framework for health care professionals that is client centered, and therefore, has powerful implications for intervention and health education; promotes culturally sensitive planning and provision of health services; and adds to the body of literature on rural use of health resources.

The SATL process provides a systematic framework for health care providers to assess patterns of response to symptoms and to develop interventions to facilitate rural residents' responses to their symptoms. For a full understanding of what actions a rural client will use to alleviate a health problem, each stage in the process must be carefully assessed on an individual basis.

CONCLUSION

Findings in this study suggest that rural residents use several indicators to identify and evaluate their symptoms. These indicators can be clarified by using the properties of the symptom identification stage as an assessment guide, which will yield information on what signs and sensations prompted symptom identification, tolerance levels for symptoms, amount of interference caused by symptoms, knowledge levels about symptoms, meanings of symptoms, and the time-line and conditions necessary for taking further actions. With these baseline data, health care providers can determine a client's capability to accurately interpret a symptom and take appropriate actions. Corresponding interventions may be aimed at increasing the client's knowledge of indicators of disease processes and the preferable time period in which to initiate an action.

Through assessment of the self-care stage of a client's symptom-action-time-line, information can be elicited regarding the client's self-care patterns. This includes the conditions under which self-care is activated and the variety of self-care tools that are available and employed by the client. Interventions can be directed at expanding a person's access to more effective self-care tools or adapting health care to the tools already available to the person. Findings in this study suggest that assessment of self-care resources leads to an evaluation of a client's lay resources, since self-care tools are often shared with a network of relatives or neighbors. Knowing whom a rural client most often relies on for symptom validation provides valuable information about functional support systems actively used by rural/frontier people. Interventions with a rural client may be more effective if key people in these networks are included.

Assessment of the professional resource stage provides information about the conditions necessary for an individual to seek professional care, appropriateness of time-lines, and barriers that prevent access to care. For example, if clients are seeking professional care for conditions that could be handled at home, interventions can be aimed at making a client's response pattern clear to both the provider and the client by using the SATL process. With this information, the client and provider can identify which response in the process is deficient and mutually determine a more appropriate response.

The multidimensionality of the SATL process increases health professionals' awareness of the dimensions and complexities involved in caring for people from diverse cultural and geographical backgrounds. A health care provider can identify cultural views of health and illness by using the SATL process. These beliefs are deeply entwined within traditional customs and culture. By gaining insight into the traditional attitudes that people have toward health and illness, health care providers can become more sensitive to the issues surrounding health care and the cultural health beliefs of the consumer, thereby providing more comprehensive health care.

Finally, the symptom-action-time-line process has important implications for research. Although research studies appear in the literature on self-care, use of lay or informal health resources, and use of formal health services, these studies tend to focus on single health resource utilization. The SATL process begins to explicate how various types of health resources are used in an integrated manner by actual rural/frontier residents. Furthermore, the preponderance of literature on consumer use of health resources focuses on urban rather than rural populations. Further research is needed to validate the use of the SATL process among rural and urban subpopulations.

REFERENCES

Chenitz, W., & Swanson, J. (1986). *From practice to grounded theory.* Menlo Park, CA: Addison-Wesley.

Elison, G. (1986). Frontier areas: Problems for delivery of health care services. *Rural Health Care, 8*(5), 1, 3.

Glaser, B., & Strauss, A. (1967). *Discovery of grounded theory.* Chicago: Aldine.

Lee, H. J. (1991). Relationship of hardiness and current life events to perceived health in rural adults. *Research in Nursing and Health, 14,* 351–359.

Lenz, E. (1984). Information seeking: A component of client decisions and health behavior. *Advances in Nursing Science, 6*(3), 59–72

Long, K.A. (1993). The concept of health: Rural perspectives. *Nursing Clinics of North America, 28*(1), 123–130.

Long, K. A., & Weinert, C. (1989). Rural nursing: Developing the theory base. *Scholarly Inquiry for Nursing Practice: An International Journal, 3*(2), 113–131.

Mechanic, D. (1960). Illness behavior and medical diagnosis. *Journal of Health Social Behavior, 1,* 86–94.

Moon, R., & Graybird, D. (1987). *High risk prevalence: A report card for Montana.* Helena, MT: Montana Department of Health and Environmental Sciences.

Rosenblatt, R., & Moscovice, I. (1982). *Rural health care.* New York: Wiley.

Segall, A., & Goldstein, J. (1989). Exploring the correlates of self-provided health care behaviour. *Social Science Medicine, 29*(2), 153–161.

Schatzman, L., & Strauss, A. (1973). *Field research.* New Jersey: Prentice-Hall.

Suchman, E. (1966). Health orientation and medical care. *American Journal of Public Health, 56*(1), 97–105.

United States Bureau of Census. (1987). *Statistical Abstract of the United States: 1988* (108th ed.). Washington, DC: U. S. Government Printing Office.

Weinert, C., & Long, K. A. (1990). Rural families and health care: Refining the knowledge base. *The Journal of Marriage and Family Review, 15*(1–2), 57–75.

Woods, N. F., & Catanzaro, M. (1988). *Nursing research: Theory and practice.* St Louis, MO: Mosby.

CHAPTER ELEVEN

Updating The Symptom-Action-Time-Line Process

Chad O'Lynn

In chapter 10, an important study was reprinted from the first edition of this book (Buehler, Malone, & Majerus, 1998). The Buehler et al. study is important because the authors proposed an initial model detailing how rural dwellers recognize health symptoms and the process rural dwellers go through in relieving those symptoms. As Buehler et al. noted, the significance of such a model is the provision of a framework from which health care providers can better assess an individual's interpretation and response to symptoms. Health care providers can work with individuals to more accurately interpret symptoms and choose responses that optimize health outcomes. In addition, the model provides health care providers a framework to better assess all resources available to individuals (such as self-care or lay resources) that might be tapped to resolve health problems and provide emotional support during illness. Buehler et al. recommended that further research be completed to validate the use of their Symptom-Action-Time-Line (SATL) process model for rural dwellers.

The study completed by Buehler et al. (1998) was small in scope and limited to a small group of rural Montana women. To appropriately transfer the model for use in other studies, further examination of the model is warranted. My purpose in this chapter is to provide part of this examination. In this chapter, I report the findings of a recent literature review designed to examine the level of support for the SATL process model. On the basis of these findings and a discussion of the model's limitations, I recommend revisions to the SATL process model. The revisions may enable the model to be used with other populations.

REVIEW OF THE SATL PROCESS

I refer the reader to chapter 10 for details on the derivation of the SATL process through grounded theory methodology. However, I present a brief review and graphic depiction of the SATL in this section.

The SATL process comprises four phases: (a) symptom identification, (b) self-care, (c) lay resources, and (d) professional resources. The process is preceded by the occurrence of a symptom, and unless that symptom is recognized by an individual (symptom identification), the process does not continue. It is important to note that Buehler et al. (1998) defined a *symptom* as a negative entity (e.g., a person identifies a symptom as an alteration in the usual state of health that requires some sort of action). This definition is crucial in prefacing the SATL process as one of resolving a problem.

Symptoms have three general components: (a) physical signs and sensations, (b) degree of interference with the person's usual or desired level of functioning, and (c) intensity and duration of the symptom (Buehler et al., 1998). These three components, in addition to an individual's prior experience and knowledge of the symptom, are used in developing meaning of the symptom for the individual. On the basis of this meaning, an individual will decide whether or not to take action. Generally, the first action taken after identifying a symptom is one of self-care.

Self-care includes activities that are initiated and performed by the individual experiencing the symptom in the hope of alleviating the symptom (Buehler et al., 1998). For individuals dependent upon others for health needs (e.g., children, dependent elders), family members would be responsible for initiating activities to address an identified symptom. Self-care activities are variable and include taking over-the-counter medications, taking home and herbal remedies, or reading reference books to learn more about the symptom and symptom resolution. Self-care activities, as well as all other actions taken in the SATL process, are evaluated by the individual in terms of efficacy, and a decision is made whether to proceed or not through the SATL process, alter actions, or cease activities.

If self-care activities do not resolve a symptom to the individual's satisfaction, or if assistance is needed, lay resources are tapped. Lay resources comprise family, friends, neighbors, or support persons and are used to provide (a) validation of symptom interpretation, (b) advice and emotional support, and (c) physical care (Buehler et al., 1998). Although not specifically defined by Buehler et al., lay resources differ from professional resources in that lay resources are not financially reimbursed for their services. If symptoms do not resolve, if symptoms intensify, or additional symptoms occur, professional resources are then sought. If professional resources do not lead to symptom resolution, individuals may seek other professional resources.

The time one takes to progress through the SATL process is variable (Buehler et al., 1998). The amount of time to act generally depends upon the intensity and duration of a symptom and how much the symptom interferes with usual functioning. When a symptom is particularly intense or greatly interferes with usual functioning, actions occur more quickly. In addition, if children are involved, or if the symptom is interpreted to constitute an emergency, actions occur relatively quickly and may bypass phases of the SATL process altogether, prompting the individual to use a professional resource immediately upon identifying a symptom. However, if one progresses through the SATL process completely, the time taken to go from symptom identification to self-care can take up to 2 days, from symptom identification to lay resources can take from 1–3 days, and from symptom identification to professional resources can take from 4–14 days. Decision points within the SATL process, and how individuals progress through the SATL process, have great implications for health care providers and researchers. A graphic depiction of the SATL process is located in Figure 11.1.

METHOD FOR LITERATURE REVIEW

Much of the literature pertaining to rural health care focuses on disparities in health for rural dwellers as compared with nonrural dwellers, description of the health of rural dwellers, barriers to accessing health care services for rural dwellers, and the experiences and demographics of health care providers in rural areas. None of these broad areas of literature address directly the SATL process of identifying symptoms and actions to resolve them, with the possible exception of access barriers. Buehler et al. (1998) discussed access barriers only secondarily, more specifically in that additional effort is made to overcome access barriers if symptoms involved children or were deemed emergent. This secondary focus is reasonable in that access barriers more than likely modulate the SATL process rather than serve as foundational antecedents in determining the components of the process itself. As such, literature examining specific barriers for rural dwellers in accessing health services was not deemed appropriate for inclusion in the literature review.

In July 2004, I conducted a search of peer-reviewed resources contained in the Cumulative Index to Nursing & Allied Health Literature (CINAHL), MedLine, and PsychInfo databases to locate research-based support for the SATL process model. Using the keyword of *rural* and its associated keywords of *rural health, rural environment,* and *rural populations,* the CINAHL database from 1982 through July 2004; the MedLine database from 1966 through July 2004; and the PsychInfo database from

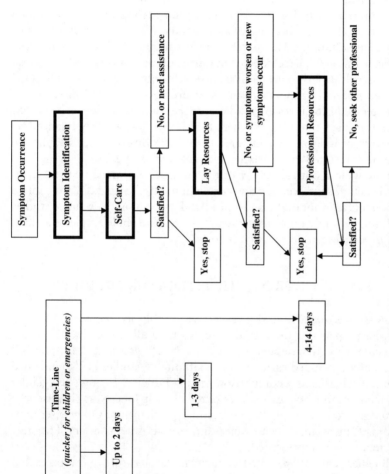

Figure 11.1. The Symptom-Action-Time-Line (SATL) Process (developed from model described in Chapter 10 by Buehler, Malone, & Majerus, 1998)

1985 through July 2004. Rural keywords were the primary sorting category to ensure that the literature would be salient to rural dwellers, although use of the SATL process may be present in nonrural populations as well. I then combined the rural keywords with other keywords suggestive of the SATL process including *self-care, decision-making, self-assessment, alternative therapies, complimentary medicine,* and *home remedies* based on available keyword search options within each database. I excluded dissertation abstracts because of the difficulty of obtaining full texts of multiple dissertations. The search yielded a total of 155 journal articles.

From this yield, I excluded review articles, case-studies, and anecdotal reports resulting in a new pool of research-only reports. In addition, I excluded all articles reporting studies occurring outside the United States. This latter exclusion is reasonable because the study by Buehler et al. (1998) occurred in the United States where health care is so heavily financed by nongovernmental sources compared with most other developed countries. These steps resulted in 60 articles available for review.

Following a critical review of the 60 articles, I made further exclusions. I excluded intervention and correlational studies that did not address components relevant to the SATL process. Furthermore, I excluded studies which focused only on health care providers. The final sample of articles for review included 36 research reports.

FINDINGS FROM THE LITERATURE REVIEW

The 36 studies included in this review were published between 1991 and 2004. Participants in these studies represented all regional areas of the continental United States except the desert Southwest and California. All of the studies included rural dwellers, although 6 studies (17%) included urban participants as a comparison group. Table 11.1 shows the gender and racial or ethnic characteristics of the participants. Notably absent in the studies were Asian or Pacific Islander participants. Otherwise, non-Hispanic Caucasian, African American, Native American, and Hispanic participants were represented.

Buehler et al. (1998) noted a paucity in the literature of resources that describe the process rural individuals undertake in managing symptoms once they have been identified. Generally, I confirmed this paucity in the present literature review. Of the 36 studies reviewed, 8 (22%) minimally supported the tendency to use self-care and lay resources before going to a health professional for nonemergent symptoms experienced by adults (Congdon & Magilvy, 2001; Davis et al., 1992; Grubbs & Frank, 2004; Horner et al., 1994; Johnson, 1994; Lee & Winters, 2004; Roberto & Reynolds, 2002; Sellers, Poduska, Propp, & White, 1999). However, none

Table 11.1. Participants' Gender and Racial/Ethnic Characteristics
(N = 36 studies)

Characteristic	n	%
Gender		
All female	10	28
Mixed	25	70
All male	1	3
Race/Ethnicity		
All non-Hispanic White	4	11
Mixed	27	75
All minority	2	6
Unknown	3	9

of these studies described or tested a comprehensive process of symptom identification and action.

The majority of the studies I reviewed confirmed the use of self-care strategies to treat symptoms (T. A. Arcury, Quandt, McDonald, & Bell, 2000; T. Arcury, Quandt, Bell, & Vitolins, 2002; Armer, 1996; Bennett & Lengacher, 1999; Boyd, Taylor, Shimp, & Semler, 2000; Burman, 2001; Canales & Geller, 2003; Congdon & Magilvy, 2001; Davis et al., 1992; Engberg, McDowell, Burgio, Watson, & Belle, 1995; Ganther, Wiederholt, & Kreling, 2001; Gaskins & Lyons, 2000; Grubbs & Frank, 2004; Horner et al., 1994; Johnson, 1994; Lee & Winters, 2004; Long & Curry, 1998; Moore & Johnson, 1993; Rabiner et al., 1997; Roberto & Reynolds, 2001, 2002; Rohrer, Kruse, Borders, & Kupersmith, 2003; Sellers et al., 1999; Stoller, Gilbert, Pyle, & Duncan, 2001; Sullivan, Weinert, & Cudney, 2003; Vallerand, Fouladbakhsh, & Templin, 2003, 2004; Vitolins et al., 2000; Wallace, Tuck, Boland, & Witucki, 2002). Many of these studies supported the self-care strategies described by Buehler et al. (1998) including taking over-the-counter medications, herbal remedies, and family remedies; referring to health information sources, such as books and television; and using physical treatments (e.g., heating pads, stretching, or yoga). However, a number of studies discussed the value of prayer and spirituality as self-care strategies (T. A. Arcury, Bernard, Jordan, & Cook, 1996; T. A. Arcury et al., 2000; Bennett & Lengacher, 1999; Congdon & Magilvy, 2001; Gaskins & Lyons, 2000; Johnson, 1999; Roberto & Reynolds, 2002; Wallace et al., 2002). These strategies were not discussed by Buehler et al. In some of the studies that compared rural and nonrural dwellers, researchers noted that rural dwellers were more likely to use self-care strategies to treat symptoms than nonrural dwellers (Boyd et al., 2000; Ganther et al., 2001; Moore & Johnson, 1993; Rabiner et al., 1997).

I also found support for the use of lay resources in managing symptoms in the studies reviewed. Primarily, researchers reported the strategies of soliciting the assistance and support of friends and family in managing symptoms and in using formal support groups (T. Arcury et al., 2002; Bennett & Lengacher, 1999; Boyd et al., 2000; Burman, 2001; Canales & Geller, 2003; Congdon & Magilvy, 2001; Gaskins & Lyons, 2000; Gross & Howard, 2001; Grubbs & Frank, 2004; Hines et al., 1999; Horner et al., 1994; Johnson, 1998; Long & Curry, 1998; Roberto & Reynolds, 2001, 2002; Stafford, Szczys, Becker, Anderson, & Bushfield, 1998; Sullivan et al., 2003; Vallerand et al., 2004; Wallace et al., 2002). However, in only a few of the studies I reviewed did researchers discuss the progression to lay resource use after self-care had failed or the use of lay resources prior to the use of professional resources (Davis et al., 1992; Horner et al.,1994; Lee & Winters, 2004; Roberto & Reynolds, 2002; Sellers et al., 1999).

Generally, the results of the studies support the finding from Buehler et al. (1998) that professional resources are utilized after self-care or lay resources are used. Some of the studies I reviewed included the use of complementary or alternative therapies to manage symptoms (T. A. Arcury et al., 1996; T. A. Arcury et al., 2000; T. Arcury et al., 2002; Bennett & Lengacher, 1999; Canales & Geller, 2003; Congdon & Magilvy, 2001; Gaskins & Lyons, 2000; Johnson, 1999; Long & Curry, 1998; Vallerand et al., 2003; Wallace et al., 2002). Complementary therapies included spiritual interventions as noted earlier, but also included the use of professional resources such as those provided by a masseuse, acupuncturist, naturopath, chiropractor, and herbalist. Other results supported the finding that professional resources are utilized if symptoms persisted (Horner et al., 1994; Roberto & Reynolds, 2002).

None of the researchers of the studies I reviewed provided specific time frames for utilizing resources as described by Buehler et al. (1998). However, research results did support basic timeline tenets within the SATL process particularly those referring to the use of professional resources: Progression to and direct utilization of professional resources was quicker if symptoms involved children (Gross & Howard, 2001; Strickland & Strickland, 1996) or were perceived as emergent or crisis in nature (Congdon & Magilvy, 2001; Lee & Winters, 2004; Long & Curry, 1998; Sullivan et al., 2003). In addition to these situations, some researchers noted that the progression to professional resource utilization was quicker if the individual perceived a need for a prescription to treat the symptom (Johnson, 1994; Lee & Winters, 2004) or if the symptom would result in the individual missing work (Lee & Winters; Sullivan et al.) Buehler et al. did not note these latter two situations.

Buehler et al. (1998) reported that if professional resources were not effective in relieving symptoms, participants continued to work with the professional, seek another professional (particularly a provider of alternative therapy), or accept the symptom's nonresolution. In the studies I reviewed researchers did not address this specific decision point in the same fashion. However, a number of researchers reported that participants used multiple strategies concurrently (T. A. Arcury et al., 1996; Bennett & Lengacher, 1999; Burman, 2001; Canales & Geller, 2003; Johnson, 1999; Roberto & Reynolds, 2001; Stafford et al., 1998; Vallerand et al., 2004). Many of these studies pertained specifically to the use of complementary or alternative therapies.

DISCUSSION

The literature reviewed supports aspects of the SATL process used by rural dwellers. Although none of the researchers contradicted the model proposed by Buehler et al. (1998), no researcher discussed or tested a comprehensive process for symptom identification and action. It should be noted, however, that the number of studies I reviewed was small. Most of the studies were cross-sectional and descriptive in design, limiting the ability to confirm the SATL process model within individuals over time. Moreover, most of the studies I reviewed had small sample sizes, focused on elderly populations, and did not include participants residing outside the United States.

With the exception of the Asian or Pacific Islander communities, the literature I reviewed represented racial or ethnic diversity. In addition, the literature represented geographic diversity. I recommend that studies examining rural Alaskan, Hawaiian, and Southwest communities be conducted to provide additional information about the SATL process.

In terms of gender, women were well represented in the sample of studies I reviewed, including 10 studies in which women were studied exclusively. In only one study (Sellers et al., 1999) researchers examined men or men's health exclusively. This limitation is significant because Sellers et al. noted that although both men and women may rely on self-care and lay resources before utilizing professional resources, men may interpret symptoms very differently and delay use of professional resources as long as possible (Levant & Habben, 2003; Sabo & Gordon, 1995; Sellers et al., 1999). Consequently, men may incorporate very different time frames for actions. I recommend that additional men's studies in rural communities be conducted to validate the SATL process.

Despite the general support in the literature for the SATL process as described by Buehler et al. (1998), the SATL process model has some limitations. Foremost is its difficulty in describing actions taken for multiple symptoms, particularly those associated with chronic illness. The model, with its emphasis on sequential progression through the SATL phases, is best-suited for single problems or injuries, such as a fever, flu, or fractured bone. Such problems are readily identified, given meaning, and subjected to treatment. Chronic conditions, such as diabetes or congestive heart failure, are characterized by recurring and multiple symptoms with varying degrees of intensity and duration. Initial presentation of symptoms may indeed lead an individual through the customary SATL process. However, as individuals become more familiar and educated regarding how to interpret symptoms when they recur, previous experience may influence whether or not they bypass self-care and lay resources completely and proceed directly to utilizing professional resources.

Although not stated by Buehler et al. (1998), one may infer from the model that when one progresses linearly through the SATL process, previous strategies may be abandoned because of unsatisfactory outcomes. The literature I reviewed did not support this inference. On the contrary, researchers described the concurrent use of multiple modes of symptom treatment. This concurrent use of strategies suggests a more circular model. With a more circular model, one can more readily explain how an individual might use prayer, hot packs, support from friends, prescription drugs, and physical therapy concurrently to manage an illness or injury, with varying use of these strategies over time as symptoms wax and wane.

Another limitation of the SATL process model is Buehler et al.'s (1998) failure to discuss symptoms that are recognized as problematic but ignored. For example, one may recognize a self-limiting symptom such as a strained muscle, but choose no action to relieve the strain. One could consider the act of ignoring a recognized symptom as a type of self-care action. The act of ignoring symptoms may be characteristic of rural men (Levant & Habben, 2003; Sellers et al., 1999). Also, Buehler et al. described a symptom as a physical sign or sensation. This definition excludes psychological symptoms, such as those typically seen in depressive and anxiety disorders, that may be readily recognized by the individuals experiencing them. Inclusion of these symptoms is key because mental health services are often unavailable or poorly implemented in rural communities (DeLeon, Wakefield, & Hagglund, 2003; Dobalian, Tsao, & Radcliff, 2003; Haard & Anderson, 2004; Kane & Ennis, 1996; National Institute of Nursing Research, 1995).

The emphasis on the time-line aspect of the SATL process model is problematic, in that it suggests a rather linear progression through phases of symptom identification and resultant actions. Buehler et al.(1998) noted that time frames for action were influenced by whether or not the symptoms were associated with children or with emergent conditions. As noted previously, others have suggested that time frames for action are also influenced by whether or not symptoms required a prescription or caused one to miss work (Johnson, 1997; Lee & Winters, 2004; Sullivan et al. 2003). In addition, it is reasonable to assume that barriers in accessing health resources for rural dwellers as described widely in the literature will influence how quickly or slowly one may adopt actions to address symptoms. As such, time frames are descriptive outcomes resulting from contextual variables. In one of the studies I reviewed (Strickland & Strickland, 1996), the researchers wondered whether or not self-care and lay resources were used based on preference and efficacy or whether access barriers slowed or prevented the utilization of professional resources. Consequently, time frames should be discussed in terms of how contextual variables for rural dwellers influence actions responsive to symptoms, rather than presented as a fundamental component of an action process itself.

Still another limitation of the SATL model is that it focuses on problem-solving and does not account for activities to prevent problem occurrence. In other words, the model does not explain actions taken to prevent illness and promote health. These actions constitute a growing proportion of health activities and expenditures and form the foundation for a variety of health initiatives. In addition, rural people find these activities important and engage in them (Davis et al., 1992; Meadows, Thurston, & Berenson, 2001; Pullen, Walker, & Fiandt, 2001; Vitolins et al., 2000).

RECOMMENDATIONS FOR REVISION OF THE SATL PROCESS MODEL

To address the limitations of the existing SATL process model and better reflect the literature reviewed, I make the following recommendations for revision:

1. Expand the definition of symptom to include psychological symptoms.
2. Expand the definition of symptom to be more reflective of a *health need* so that measures one takes to prevent illness or promote health are included.
3. Recognize that intentional disregard of a symptom is a type of self-care action.
4. Embed the model within an environmental context external to the decision tree to account for variables such as gender, culture, race or ethnicity, socioeconomic status, family or social role, residential location, barriers in accessing resources, etc.

5. Reassign the time-line aspect of the process to a descriptive outcome, rather than a component of the action process itself.
6. Design the model to be more circular in nature.
7. Rename the model, The Symptom-Action Process (SAP).

Figure 11.2 shows a graphic depiction of the revised model.

In the revised model, the action process is embedded in an external context. After symptoms are identified, individuals may incorporate various types of actions: (a) self-care, (b) lay resources, or (c) professional resources in a sequential or concurrent fashion. The context will influence which action, or combination of actions, is taken. The sloping nature of the action types reflects the propensity to progress from self-care to lay resource use to professional resource use. The double arrows between action types account for fluid movement among aspects of the model and concurrent use of types of actions. New to this model are the arrows leading from the action types back to the symptom occurrence aspect of the model. These arrows close the circle of the process and account for symptoms that might recur, new symptoms that develop, or new information requiring new action resulting from previous actions taken by an individual.

Both the SATL process model and the revised SAP model describe a process in which an individual identifies a problem or need and takes

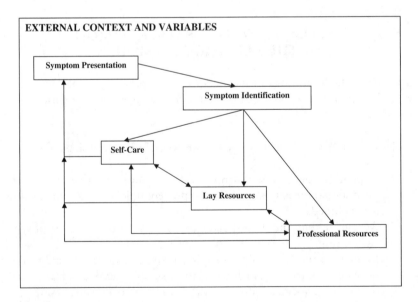

Figure 11.2 Symptom-Action Process: A revision of the Symptom-Action-Time-Line Process.

action(s) to address it. As such, these models may describe the behaviors of all individuals, including nonrural dwellers, although how actions are taken may differ across populations. I recommend that research be conducted to evaluate how well the revised model is empirically supported. If the revised model is well supported, then it may serve as an ideal framework for comparison studies examining health behaviors across participant demographic variables.

CONCLUSION

Buehler et al. (1998) derived the SATL process model from a grounded theory study in which they described the process a group of rural Montana women used to respond to health symptoms. I conducted a current literature review to determine the level of support for this model. I reviewed 36 research studies located in the CINAHL, MedLine, and PsychInfo databases that focused on the process rural dwellers use to respond to health symptoms. Those studies provide general support for aspects of the SATL process model, although in only 8 studies researchers described a sequential process of how rural dwellers respond to health symptoms.

Despite the general support for the SATL process model, I noted several limitations of the model. To address these limitations and maintain support from the reviewed literature, I proposed a revised model titled SAP. The revised model may provide a better framework in examining the health behaviors of various subgroups of rural dwellers, as well as assist in comparing the behaviors between rural and nonrural dwellers. Examination of how and why these health behaviors are manifested may enhance the understanding among health professionals and policy makers. The SAP model will aid professionals in assessing the health needs of rural dwellers and in planning how to best meet those needs with policies and services. I recommend further research with rural men and rural Asian or Pacific Islander participants to determine the support for the revised model. In addition, examination of studies completed outside the continental United States should occur to determine whether or not the revised model has broader relevance to rural dwellers across the globe.

REFERENCES

Arcury, T., Quandt, S. A., Bell, R. A., & Vitolins, M. Z. (2002). Complementary and alternative medicine among rural older adults. *Complementary Health Practice Review, 7,* 167–186.

Arcury, T. A., Bernard, S. L., Jordan, J. M., & Cook, H. L. (1996). Gender and ethnic differences in alternative and conventional arthritis remedy use among community-dwelling rural adults with arthritis. *Arthritis Care Research, 9,* 384–390.

Arcury, T. A., Quandt, S. A., McDonald, J., & Bell, R. A. (2000). Faith and health self-management of rural older adults. *Journal of Cross Cultural Gerontology, 15*(1), 55–74.

Armer, J. M. (1996). An exploration of factors influencing adjustment among relocating rural elders. *Image: Journal of Nursing Scholarship, 28,* 35–39.

Bennett, M., & Lengacher, C. (1999). Use of complementary therapies in a rural cancer population. *Oncology Nursing Forum, 26,* 1287–1294.

Boyd, E. L., Taylor, S. D., Shimp, L. A., & Semler, C. R. (2000). An assessment of home remedy use by African Americans. *Journal of the National Medical Association, 92*(7), 341–353.

Buehler, J., Malone, M., & Majerus, J. (1998). Patterns of responses to symptoms in rural residents: The Symptom-Action-Time-Line process. In H. Lee (Ed.), *Conceptual basis for rural nursing* (pp. 318–328). New York: Springer Publishing.

Burman, M. E. (2001). Family caregiver expectations and management of the stroke trajectory. *Rehabilitation Nursing, 26,* 94–99.

Canales, M. K., & Geller, B. M. (2003). Surviving breast cancer: The role of complementary therapies. *Family & Community Health, 26,* 11–24.

Congdon, J. G., & Magilvy, J. K. (2001). Themes of rural health and aging from a program of research. *Geriatric Nursing, 22,* 234–238.

Davis, D. C., Henderson, M. C., Boothe, A., Douglass, M., Faria, S., Kennedy, D., et al. (1992). Health beliefs and practices of rural elders. *Caring, 11*(2), 22–28.

DeLeon, P., Wakefield, M., & Hagglund, K. (2003). The behavioral health care needs of rural communities in the 21st century. In B. Stamm (Ed.), *Rural behavioral health care: An interdisciplinary guide* (pp. 23–32). Washington, DC: American Psychological Association.

Dobalian, A., Tsao, J. C., & Radcliff, T. A. (2003). Diagnosed mental and physical health conditions in the United States nursing home population: Differences between urban and rural facilities. *Journal of Rural Health, 19,* 477–483.

Engberg, S. J., McDowell, B. J., Burgio, K. L., Watson, J. E., & Belle, S. (1995). Self-care behaviors of older women with urinary incontinence. *Journal of Gerontological Nursing, 21*(8), 7–14.

Ganther, J. M., Wiederholt, J. B., & Kreling, D. H. (2001). Measuring patients' medical care preferences: Care seeking versus self-treating. *Medical Decision Making, 21*(2), 133–140.

Gaskins, S., & Lyons, M. A. (2000). Self-care practices of rural people with HIV disease. *Online Journal of Rural Nursing and Health Care, 1*(1).

Gross, G. J., & Howard, M. (2001). Mothers' decision-making processes regarding health care for their children. *Public Health Nursing, 18,* 157–168.

Grubbs, L., & Frank, D. (2004). Self-care practices related to symptom responses in African-American and Hispanic adults. *Self-Care, Dependent-Care, and Nursing, 12*(1), 4–9.

Haard, L., & Anderson, E. (2004). Factors related to depression in rural and urban noncustodial, low-income fathers. *Journal of Community Psychology, 32*(1), 103–119.

Hines, S. C., Glover, J. J., Holley, J. L., Babrow, A. S., Badzek, L. A., & Moss, A. H. (1999). Dialysis patients' preferences for family-based advance care planning. *Annals of Internal Medicine, 130,* 825–828.

Horner, S. D., Ambrogne, J., Coleman, M. A., Hanson, C., Hodnicki, D., Lopez, S. A., et al. (1994). Traveling for care: Factors influencing health care access for rural dwellers. *Public Health Nursing, 11,* 145–149.

Johnson, J. E. (1994). Sleep and alcohol use in rural old-old women. *Journal of Community Health Nursing, 11,* 211–218.

Johnson, J. E. (1998). Older rural adults and the decision to stop driving: The influence of family and friends. *Journal of Community Health Nursing, 15,* 205–216.

Johnson, J. E. (1999). Older rural women and the use of complementary therapies. *Journal of Community Health Nursing, 16,* 223–232.

Kane, C. F., & Ennis, J. M. (1996). Health care reform and rural mental health: Severe mental illness. *Community Mental Health Journal, 32,* 445–462.

Lee, H. J., & Winters, C. A. (2004). Testing rural nursing theory: Perceptions and needs of service providers. *Online Journal of Rural Nursing and Health Care, 4*(1). Retrieved June 1, 2004, from http://www.rno.org/journal/issues/Vol.4/issues/Lee_article.htm

Levant, R., & Habben, C. (2003). The new psychology of men: Application to rural men. In B. Stamm (Ed.), *Rural behavioral health care: An interdisciplinary guide* (pp. 171–180). Washington, DC: American Psychological Association.

Long, C. R., & Curry, M. A. (1998). Living in two worlds: Native American women and prenatal care. *Health Care for Women International, 19,* 205–215.

Meadows, L. M., Thurston, W. E., & Berenson, C. A. (2001). Health promotion and preventive measures: Interpreting messages at midlife. *Qualitative Health Research, 11,* 450–463.

Moore, J. F., & Johnson, J. E. (1993). Over-the-counter drug use by the rural elderly. *Geriatric Nursing, 14,* 190–191.

National Institute of Nursing Research. (1995). *Chapter 2: Rural America: Challenges and opportunities.* Retrieved April 9, 2003, from ninr.nih.gov/ninr/research/vol7/chapter2.html

Pullen, C., Walker, S. N., & Fiandt, K. (2001). Determinants of health-promoting lifestyle behaviors in rural older women. *Family & Community Health, 24,* 49–72.

Rabiner, D. J., Konrad, T. R., DeFriese, G. H., Kincade, J., Bernard, S. L., Woomert, A., et al. (1997). Metropolitan versus nonmetropolitan differences in functional status and self-care practice: Findings from a national sample of community-dwelling older adults. *Journal of Rural Health, 13,* 14–28.

Roberto, K. A., & Reynolds, S. G. (2001). The meaning of osteoporosis in the lives of rural older women. *Health Care for Women International, 22,* 599–611.

Roberto, K. A., & Reynolds, S. G. (2002). Older women's experiences with chronic pain: Daily challenges and self-care practices. *Journal of Women & Aging, 14*(3–4), 5–23.

Rohrer, J. E., Kruse, G., Borders, T., & Kupersmith, J. (2003). Realized access to physician services among the elderly in West Texas. *Journal of Rural Health, 19,* 72–78.

Sabo, D., & Gordon, D. F. (1995). Rethinking men's health and illness. In D. Sabo & D. F. Gordon (Eds.), *Men's health and illness: Gender, power, and the body* (pp. 1–22). Thousand Oaks, CA: Sage.

Sellers, S. C., Poduska, M. D., Propp, L. H., & White, S. I. (1999). The health care meanings, values, and practices of Anglo-American males in the rural midwest. *Journal of Transcultural Nursing, 10,* 320–330.

Stafford, D., Szczys, R., Becker, R., Anderson, J., & Bushfield, S. (1998). How breast cancer treatment decisions are made by women in North Dakota. *American Journal of Surgery, 176,* 515–519.

Stoller, E. P., Gilbert, G. H., Pyle, M. A., & Duncan, R. P. (2001). Coping with tooth pain: A qualitative study of lay management strategies and professional consultation. *Special Care in Dentistry, 21,* 208–215.

Strickland, J., & Strickland, D. L. (1996). Barriers to preventive health services for minority households in the rural south. *Journal of Rural Health, 12,* 206–217.

Sullivan, T., Weinert, C., & Cudney, S. (2003). Management of chronic illness: Voices of rural women. *Journal of Advanced Nursing, 44,* 566–574.

Vallerand, A. H., Fouladbakhsh, J. M., & Templin, T. (2003). The use of complementary/alternative medicine therapies for the self-treatment of pain among residents of urban, suburban, and rural communities. *American Journal of Public Health, 93*(6), 923–925.

Vallerand, A. H., Fouladbakhsh, J. M., & Templin, T. (2004). Self-treatment of pain in a rural area. *Journal of Rural Health, 20,* 166–172.

Vitolins, M. Z., Quandt, S. A., Case, L. D., Bell, R. A., Arcury, T. A., & McDonald, J. (2000). Vitamin and mineral supplement use by older rural adults. *Journal of Gerontology: Medical Sciences, 55A*(10), M613–M617.

Wallace, D. C., Tuck, I., Boland, C. S., & Witucki, J. M. (2002). Client perceptions of parish nursing. *Public Health Nursing, 19,* 128–135.

CHAPTER TWELVE

The Chronic Illness Experience of Isolated Rural Women: Use of an Online Support Group Intervention

Charlene A. Winters and Therese Sullivan

Chronic illness is a major public health problem (Marks, 2003) affecting more than 90 million Americans (Centers for Disease Control [CDC], 2003; Husaine & Moore, 1990; Jensen, 1991; Stuifbergen, 1995). Seven of every ten Americans who die each year, or more than 1.7 million people, die of a chronic disease (CDC, 2003). Effective self-management is instrumental to a person's ability to adapt successfully to their illness and maintain a quality life. Education, support from family, friends, and health care providers, and the ability to manage uncertainty are important factors in chronic illness self-management (Strauss et al., 1984).

The context within which chronic illness occurs has a significant impact on how the chronically ill arrange for services and support. Persons living in sparsely populated rural areas have few health care providers, hospitals, and other resources (Gesler, Hartwell, Ricketts, & Rosenberg, 1992; *Agency for Health Care Policy & Research,* 1996). Living in rural areas with few health care resources may complicate an individual's ability

This research was funded by the Center for Research on Chronic Health Conditions in Rural Dwellers (Grant NIH/NINR IP20 NR 07790-01). The authors acknowledge Dr. Clarann Weinert for her assistance with this study.

to manage their illness. Nearly one fourth of America's population lives in rural areas (*Agency for Health Care Policy & Research,* 1996), yet little is known about how rural persons experience chronic illness (Scott, 2000). Our purpose in the study reported in this chapter was to explore the chronic illness experience of isolated rural women living with arthritis, fibromyalgia, cancer, diabetes, and multiple sclerosis (MS).

Arthritis and other rheumatic conditions, cancer, diabetes, and MS are common among Americans, affecting nearly 75 million persons. Recent national figures indicate that arthritis and other rheumatic conditions alone affect nearly 49 million persons and continue to be the leading causes of disability in the United States. Cancer continues to be the second leading cause of death in the U.S. and more than 9.6 million people are living with a history of cancer. Diabetes mellitus (DM) affects 18 million Americans and is the leading cause of new cases of blindness, kidney failure, and lower extremity amputations. Just having DM greatly increases a person's risk for heart attack or stroke (*Chronic Disease Prevention,* 2002). In 2004, more than 400,000 persons living in the Untied States had MS and 200 new cases were diagnosed each week (*About MS,* 2004). MS is most common in the northern states and occurs mostly in women of northern European ancestry aged 20–50 years.

Disparities in health among rural dwellers are well documented. Living in sparsely populated rural areas is in itself a health risk factor because of numerous conditions that can negatively influence health (Eberhardt et. al., 2001). Rural residents tend to have more chronic illnesses, have lower rates of health insurance, and have limited access to health care services and health care providers (Meit, 2004). For example, in Montana, a person may need to travel 120 miles one-way to a health care specialist (Winters, 1999) or 320 miles round-trip to an illness-related support group, and in many areas, public transportation is inadequate or nonexistent.

Management of chronic illness requires persons to recognize and control symptoms, implement prescribed treatments, adjust to changes in the course of the disease, prevent medical crises, attempt to normalize daily life, fund medical care, and confront emotional, marital, and family problems (Benet, 1996; Hwu, 1995; Robinson, 1993; Strauss et al., 1984; Winters, 1997, 1999). An individual's adaptive behaviors, psychosocial outcomes, and ability to provide self-care are influenced by uncertainty about the meaning of symptoms and treatment outcomes (Mast, 1995; Mishel, 1993; Strauss et al., 1984; Weiner, 1975). Uncertainty occurs when people lack the information or knowledge needed to understand their illness and is influenced by resources available to assist persons in the interpretation of illness-related events. Resources include relationships individuals have with their health care providers, cognitive ability, and social support (Mast, 1995; Mishel, 1984). How rural persons experience chronic illness in the face of limited access to resources is not fully known. We designed this qualitative descriptive study to explore the illness experiences of chronically ill isolated rural women.

METHODS

We conducted a secondary analysis of existing data from one cohort of participants in the Women to Women Project (WTW). WTW is a large-scale, multiphase intervention study that provides online peer-support and health education via computer and the Internet to isolated rural women living with chronic illness. The overall goal of WTW is to evaluate the impact of participation on psychosocial health. In Phase I of WTW, a purposive sample of 120 chronically ill women from one western U.S. state were randomized into four cohorts of 30 women. Each cohort had 15 women with computers and 15 women without computers. The computer groups participated in an online support group using an asynchronous chat room and structured education sessions spanning a period of 5 months. The noncomputer groups did not participate in the computer-based activities and continued to use their usual sources of support and information. All participants received a three-ring binder containing a description of the study and articles on a variety of health issues pertinent to women with chronic illness. Each participant completed written questionnaires to measure psychosocial outcomes over a 10-month period (Sullivan, Weinert, & Cudney, 2003; Weinert, 2000). Although WTW addressed psychosocial health, the study we describe in this chapter specifically focused on the experiences of living with chronic illness shared by the women in one computer group. The Montana State University-Bozeman Human Subjects Committee approved this study.

Sample

Eligible participants in WTW were women diagnosed with cancer, DM, rheumatoid diseases, or MS who lived at least 25 miles from an urbanized area (12,500 persons or more). All women in WTW were required to read and speak English, have sufficient dexterity to communicate using a computer keyboard, and have a telephone in their home. The women were recruited to participate via word of mouth and with the help of voluntary agencies, state agricultural extension services, schools of nursing, parish nurses, nursing students, health professionals, public and professional libraries, newspapers, and public television announcements.

Participants in the study we report in this chapter came from one computer group ($n = 15$). We close this cohort because it was the first cohort to complete WTW. We included all women in the computer group in the sample. Fourteen of the women were Caucasian and one was Native American. All the women were from rural areas and lived on farms or in small towns. Eight of the women worked full-time outside the home; two were full-time homemakers; five were unemployed. The women reported their primary health problem to be cancer ($n = 2$), MS ($n = 5$), rheumatoid arthritis or fibromyalgia ($n = 5$), and DM ($n = 3$). Mean age was 47.2 years and the average time between illness diagnosis and the beginning of the study was 5.29 years.

Data Collection

We analyzed qualitative and demographic data collected for WTW. We made no direct or indirect contact with the participants during this study. The qualitative data consisted of 453 messages posted to the online support group chat room by the women over a 22–week period. The messages were conversations held between group members on topics of their choice. They had been stored verbatim in the end-user database then downloaded by the WTW research assistant for analysis. Although all the women participated in the discussions, the number of messages posted and their lengths varied. The number of postings ranged from 4–118 ($M = 57.18$; $SD = 39.30$) and the time spent online ranged from 346–3239 minutes ($M = 1370.23$; $SD = 873.37$) indicating that women were spending time online even if they were not posting.

The quantitative data analyzed for the study consisted of demographic information. The data were collected as part of the screening interview to determine eligibility for participation in WTW. Electronic and printed copies of the data were provided to us by the WTW project manager under the direction of the principal investigator for WTW.

Data Analysis

We checked a printed copy of each chat room conversation for accuracy with the electronic data then analyzed the conversations for common themes using methods described by Miles and Huberman (1994). We analyzed chat room conversations specifically by (a) reading each conversation completely to get a sense of the whole, (b) dividing conversations into units denoted by a change in subject matter or activities described, and (c) labeling individual units from each conversation using a word or words that represented the unit topic (descriptive codes) and writing them in the margins of each printed copy. We also wrote theoretic memos (thoughts about the connections between the codes) in the margins. We continued coding until we classified all of the data. After coding by hand on the hard copy, we entered the electronic file of each conversation into QSR NUD-IST (Version 4), a software program designed to manage qualitative data. We then entered the codes for each conversation and with other coded conversations to identify common themes among them. To confirm and validate findings, we linked all initial codes, theoretic memos, and the emerging themes to primary data sources. We discussed emerging themes until we achieved consensus.

We analyzed quantitative data to provide a description of the participants and to provide context for the qualitative findings. We displayed all data using Statistical Package for the Social Sciences (Version 11.5) and analyzed the data using descriptive statistics to determine item frequencies and measures of central tendency.

FINDINGS

It was clear from the qualitative data that the women in the computer group felt positively about the intervention. They were pleased to have access to information about their illness and to other women facing similar challenges. Many expressed feeling a "connection" with group members. Some women referred to the group as their "cyber friends," exchanged phone numbers, and made plans to meet offline. In addition to talking about their illnesses, the women shared stories about their families, exchanged recipes, described vacations, and told jokes. They offered words of support, prayer, and hope for "better times" for their online peers and their family members. As the computer intervention was nearing conclusion, the women expressed sadness about loosing the connection with their newly made friends. They spoke of "going through withdrawal" and having a "hard time" giving up the program. One participant wrote:

> I will miss visiting with you all. There have been times when I felt too crummy to type anything, but I could always read. My last exacerbation would have been ten times worse if I had not been able to hear your words of wisdom, jokes, and suggestions for better health.

Common Themes

We identified six common themes from analyzing the online support-group conversations.

1. Uncertainty/Searching for answers
2. Physical and emotional isolation
3. Maintaining balance

4. Others first
5. Vigilance: Financial, physical, emotional
6. Ways of coping

Uncertainty/searching for answers. The women experienced uncertainty throughout their illness experience. Before diagnosis, uncertainty was related to not knowing what was happening to them and the inability of their health care providers to provide an immediate explanation of their symptoms. A long diagnostic process was common requiring trips to more than one doctor before the correct diagnosis was made. One woman wrote, "I can't even count how many things I went to the doctor for over the years that I am now told are symptoms of this hateful illness." The average time from onset of symptoms to diagnosis was 9.7 years (range = < 1–32 years). Frustration and an erosion of trust in their physician's judgment accompanied uncertainty while women who were quickly diagnosed thought of their health care provider as "good."

Diagnosis did not put an end to the uncertainty. New or changing symptoms were common as were new treatments with unfamiliar outcomes and side effects. Uncertainty prompted a search for information, explanations, and answers. The women read about their illnesses and asked questions of their health care providers. During the intervention, the women asked others in the group if they had similar experiences to their own and were relieved to hear that they did. One woman expressed surprise and relief at the similarities of the experiences described by the women. She had felt alone and doubted her "stability" thinking that she must have been "making things up in her head" because "doctors couldn't seem to find a reason" for her symptoms.

Physical and emotional isolation. The women lived in rural communities or on farms, in areas of few health care resources and had little contact with other chronically ill women. The women felt emotionally isolated, afraid to talk about their illness with persons who were not ill for fear of alienating them and straining their relationship. They wrote of not being able to tell nonill persons how they really felt for fear they would tire of hearing from them and "walk away." Although they had the support of family and friends, not being able to share feelings about their illness with others who were not ill potentially decreased the support they received and promoted their sense of emotional isolation. As one woman wrote, "This disease accomplishes one thing. It isolates."

Maintaining balance. This theme referred to the women's roles, responsibilities, and their need to balance activities and energies to maintain each role. Eight of the 15 women worked full-time outside the home. One commented, "I need to say NO to more things and not get so upset over things that haven't gotten done. I know this but I need to remember it." Limited or no access to health care providers, pharmacies, and other health care services sometimes strained the women's ability to maintain balance. The need to travel to distant cities for specialized health care sometimes required an overnight stay and the driving assistance of a family member or friend. Time away from home and work affected the delicate balance the women were trying to achieve.

Others first. The women in this study put the needs of their community, employer, and family before their own. They found time to provide community service and participate in civic activities, spend time with friends, and assist neighbors in need. The women worked long hours at home, and for employers, while still finding time to see to the needs of their spouses and children, whether the children were living at home or not. The women wrote about accompanying family members and friends to various activities that often involved long hours in the car. Putting *others first* affected their ability to maintain balance in their lives by draining their energy and exacerbating their symptoms. Although sometimes uncertain about how their activities would affect them, over time the women learned that they would "pay the price" if they did too much. However, knowing this did not guarantee that they would pull back. Often times they would continue their activities and suffer the consequences.

> I need to share with you ... maybe it is like true confessions ... how I didn't accept responsibility for my recent exacerbation. My employer needed ... my church needed ... my students needed ... and all the time I was getting more tired and nauseated but I kept on going until I was really sick.

Vigilance. We used this theme to describe the alert watchfulness the women displayed toward their physical, emotional, and financial health. Prior to diagnosis, the women actively sought meaning for their symptoms. After diagnosis, the women were alert for any changes that might indicate improvement or deterioration in their condition, the onset of new problems, or treatment side effects. During the intervention, the women discussed at length their symptoms, queried others to see if they were experiencing similar problems, and shared strategies used to manage them. The most common physical symptoms discussed were pain, sleeplessness, and fatigue. The most common emotions expressed were frustration, depression, and stress.

The cost of care was a frequent topic of discussion among the women. Many shared that they were stressed by the financial burden of health care and uncertain about how they would pay for their care. The women spent a considerable amount of their time dealing with this issue. Online, the women shared strategies to cut costs, finance care, and navigate the bureaucratic red tape of the programs that assist persons with chronic illness. Some expressed their appreciation for health insurance and concern for those who did not have coverage. They welcomed assistance from husbands who would "handle all that."

Ways of coping. We used this theme to describe several methods used by the women to cope with their illness. Common methods included information gathering and self-care. The women took an active role caring for themselves by learning about their illnesses through reading, attending informational sessions presented by experts in the field, and asking questions of their health care provider. As one woman wrote, taking an active role in her health care and not waiting for the doctors to "tell her what to think and do" provided a sense of "control over her illness." The women participated in their prescribed treatments but also tried new things, such as herbs and special diets, with the hope of improving their well-being. They frequently shared self-care strategies with their online peers. Good communication and a positive relationship with their health care provider were viewed as essential to their ability to cope with their illness. Women who felt that they were "heard" by their health care provider evaluated them as "good" and "caring." A good relationship with their health care provider was important enough to prompt some women to change doctors.

Faith and humor were frequently used as coping mechanisms. The women's conversations frequently included references to scripture, prayer, and faith. Funny stories, anecdotes, and jokes were also common and well received. The women commented on several occasions how good it was for them to laugh and asked their peers to "Keep the jokes coming."

Keeping busy, even though activity could exacerbate their symptoms, was a common strategy used by the women. Participants attempted to maintain normalcy in their lives by maintaining their usual routines and activities. The women tried to balance their activities with rest periods but often did more than they should have done. Maintaining normalcy also involved not talking about their illness with persons who were not ill.

The support network of family and friends was an important coping mechanism. Although persons without illness may not fully understand what the women were going through, their help was needed and appreciated. Contact with other chronically ill persons was seen as especially helpful. The women expressed a great deal of appreciation for their online peers. One woman wrote, "I have gotten so used to talking to all of you! It's different than talking to anyone else, because we can 'let it all hang out' and everyone understands. Thanks for listening to me and encouraging me." Reaching out and providing support to others was also important. The women shared information, gave advice, and demonstrated concern and compassion for members of the online group and their families.

DISCUSSION AND IMPLICATIONS

The findings from the qualitative data support what is already known about chronic illness and add knowledge specific to living with chronic illness in a rural setting. The data confirmed that chronically ill persons strive to understand their illness, recognize and control symptoms, implement prescribed treatments, adjust to changes in the course of the disease, deal with uncertainty, attempt to normalize daily life, find ways to fund medical care, and confront emotional and physical problems (Strauss et al., 1984). The findings also corroborate that difficulty in achieving a diagnosis can lead to uncertainty and an erosion of faith in the physician (Mishel, 1988, 1993; Mishel & Braden, 1988). The findings support the emotional isolation commonly felt by persons with chronic illness (Davies & Sque, 2002) and the importance of support, understanding, and a sense of collaboration between patient and health care provider (FitzGerald, Pearson, & McCutcheon, 2001).

The findings specific to managing chronic illness in a rural setting were experiences related to physical isolation and limited access to others with a similar condition. The emotional isolation the women in this study experienced may have been complicated by their physical isolation. Distance, weather conditions, and geographical constraints affected the woman's access to health care providers and health care resources and potentially decreased the support available to them. For example, some of the women in this study traveled hundreds of miles to reach the closest health care specialists, not because they were the "best" but because they were the closest to them. It was also common for those who attended presentations by health experts to have to travel 3 or more hours to a distant city to attend the seminar.

Distance is an accepted part of rural living (Long & Weinert, 1989). However, traveling can be arduous for ill persons, physically and financially, and often involves careful planning. A trip to the specialist sometimes meant an overnight stay, required the driving assistance of a family member or friend, as well as additional trips for diagnostic testing and follow-up care. Effective time management and advanced planning were essential components of the women's illness management strategies. Health care specialists can help decrease the physical and financial burden of chronic illness with thoughtful scheduling, effective communication, and careful collaboration with the women's local health care provider when appropriate. In some circumstances, the use of telemedicine may be an appropriate alternative to a trip to a distant health care specialist.

The women had the support of family members; however, some lived a distance away. They were also physically isolated from other persons living with similar health problems. The women believed that persons who were not ill were less able to understand what they were going through. They also worried that "compassion fatigue" would become a problem for family and friends who were nearby. As a result, the women "put on a happy face" and "didn't let others know how they felt" and experienced emotional isolation. Health care providers can help their patients cope with their illness by encouraging what has worked; in this case, faith, humor, and keeping busy. Facilitating a phone number or e-mail exchange between interested patients or recommending one of the many professional organizations that have online support groups can be empowering (Burrows, Nettleton, Pleace, Loader, & Muncer, 2000) and should be considered. Given the positive experience of the 15 women in this study, an online chronic illness support group appears to be a viable solution to the problem of isolation. However, additional research is needed to examine the value and health benefits of virtual communities (Eysenbach, Powell, Englesakis, Rizo, & Stern, 2004).

The women were frustrated by delayed or difficult diagnosis, professionals who "didn't listen," and the high cost of care. The women desired to be understood, to understand what was happening to them, and to be able to implement appropriate self-care strategies. Clear, open, and frequent communication with clients may help to decrease frustration and uncertainty while providing the basis for a positive relationship. Health care providers can help their patients to implement self-care strategies by providing both verbal and written information and recommending reputable online information resources. Providing "virtual office hours" where rural patients can contact their health care provider via e-mail might also be helpful. Although information can decrease uncertainty (Mishel, 1993), health care providers should remind their patients that uncertainty is part of chronic illness.

Although the findings add to our understanding of the chronic illness experiences of rural women, questions remain. For example, Do isolated rural women with other diagnoses experience chronic illness differently? Do younger or older women and teens manage their illness differently than middle-aged women? Furthermore, more research is needed regarding the role nurses play in the experiences of chronically ill rural women. The women were referring to physician providers in their chat room conversations and never mentioned nurses in their postings. More research is needed to understand the role nurses play in the illness experience of rural women.

SUMMARY

Using a computer and the Internet was a manageable and accepted method of providing peer-support to a group of isolated rural women with chronic illness. With proper instruction and assistance, even the most novice computer user was able to navigate the computer and participate in online conversations with a group of their peers. The women's illness experiences support the findings of others and illustrate commonalities found among persons living in rural areas. Recognizing the common problems and uncertainties experienced by these women is an important step in planning effective care. Further exploration is needed to understand the complex and multifaceted chronic illness experiences of isolated rural women.

REFERENCES

About MS. (2004). Retrieved July 2, 2004, 2004, from http://www.nationalms-society.org/about%20ms.asp

Agency for Health Care Policy & Research. (1996). *Improving health care for rural populations. Research in Action fact sheet.* (AHCPR Publication No. 96–P040). Washington, DC: U.S. Government Printing Office.

Benet, A. (1996). A portrait of chronic illness: Inspecting the canvas, reframing the issues. *American Behavioral Scientist, 39,* 767–776.

Burrows, R., Nettleton, S., Pleace, N., Loader, B., & Muncer, S. (2000). Virtual community care? Social policy and the emergence of computer mediated social support. *Information, Communication and Society, 3* (1), 95–121.

Centers for Disease Control. (2003, October 27). *Chronic disease overview.* Retrieved July 15, 2003, from http://www.cdc.gov/nccdphp/overview.htm

Chronic disease prevention: The burden of chronic diseases and their risk factors. (June 9, 2004). Retrieved June 28, 2004, 2002, from http://www.cdc.gov/nccdphp/about.htm

Davies, M., & Sque, M. (2002). Living on the outside looking in: A theory of living with advanced breast cancer. *International Journal of Palliative Nursing, 8,* 583–584, 586–590.

Eberhardt, M. S., Ingram, D. D., Makuc, D. M., Pamuk, E. R., Freid, V. M., Harper, S. B., et al. (2001). *Urban and rural health chartbook. Health, United States, 2001 with rural and urban chartbook* (NCHS Publication No. PHS 01–1232). Hyattsville, MD: National Center for Health Statistics.

Eysenbach, G., Powell, J., Englesakis, M., Rizo, C., & Stern, A. (2004). Health related virtual communities and electronic support groups: Systematic review of the effects of online peer to peer interactions. *British Medical Journal, 328*(7449), 1166–1170.

FitzGerald, M., Pearson, A., & McCutcheon, H. (2001). Impact of rural living on the experience of chronic illness. *Australian Journal of Rural Health, 9,* 235–240.

Gesler, W., Hartwell, S., Ricketts, T., & Rosenberg, M. (1992). Introduction. In W. Gesler & T. Ricketts (Eds.), *Health in rural North America* (pp. 1–22). New Brunswick, NJ: Rutgers University Press.

Husaine, B., & Moore, S. (1990). Arthritis disability, depression, and life satisfaction among black elderly people. *Health and Social Work, 15,* 253–259.

Hwu, Y. J. (1995). The impact of chronic illness on patients. *Rehabilitation Nursing, 20,* 221–225.

Jensen, A. (1991). Psychosocial factors in breast cancer and their possible impact upon prognosis. *Cancer Treatment Reviews, 18,* 191–210.

Long, K. A., & Weinert, C. (1989). Rural nursing: Developing the theory base. *Scholarly Inquiry for Nursing Practice, 3,* 113–127.

Marks, J. S. (2003, *The burden of chronic disease and the future of public health.* Retrieved June 28, 2004, from http://www.cdc.gov/nccdphp/burden_pres/

Mast, M. E. (1995). Adult uncertainty in illness: A critical review of research. *Scholarly Inquiry for Nursing Practice, 9,* 3–24; discussion 25–29.

Meit, M. (2004). *Bridging the health divide: The rural public health research agenda.* Pittsburgh, PA: University of Pittsburgh Center for Rural Health Practice.

Miles, M. B., & Huberman, A. M. (1994). *Qualitative data analysis* (2nd ed.). Thousand Oaks, CA: Sage.

Mishel, M. H. (1984). Perceived uncertainty and stress in illness. *Research in Nursing & Health, 7,* 163–171.

Mishel, M. H. (1988). Uncertainty in illness. *Image: Journal of Nursing Scholarship, 20,* 225–232.

Mishel, M. H. (1993). Living with chronic illness: Living with uncertainty. In S. Funk, E. Tornquist, M. Champagne, & R. Wiese (Eds.), *Key aspects of caring for the chronically ill: Hospital and home* (pp. 46–58). New York: Springer Publishing.

Mishel, M. H., & Braden, C. J. (1988). Finding meaning: Antecedents of uncertainty in illness. *Nursing Research, 37,* 98–103, 127.

QSR NUDIST. (1998). Version 4. OSR International Pty Ltd., Melbourne, Australia.

Robinson, C. A. (1993). Managing life with a chronic condition: The story of normalization. *Qualitative Health Research, 3*(1), 6–28.

Scott, J. (2000). A nursing leadership challenge: Managing the chronically ill in rural settings. *Nursing Administration Quarterly, 24*(3), 21–32.

Strauss, A., Corbin, J., Fagererhaugh, S., Glaser, B., Maines, D., Suczek, B., et al. (1984). *Chronic illness and the quality of life* (2nd ed.). St. Louis: Mosby.

Stuifbergen, A. (1995). Health-promoting behaviors and quality of life among individuals with multiple sclerosis. *Scholarly Inquiry for Nursing Practice, 9,* 31–50.

Sullivan, T., Weinert, C., & Cudney, S. (2003). Management of chronic illness: Voices of rural women. *Journal of Advanced Nursing, 44,* 566–574.

Weiner, C. (1975). The burden of rheumatoid arthritis: Tolerating the uncertainty. *Social Science and Medicine, 9,* 97–104.

Weinert, C. (2000). Social support in cyberspace for women with chronic illness. *Rehabilitation Nursing, 25,* 129–135.

Winters, C. A. (1997). *Living with chronic heart disease: A pilot study.* Retrieved March 31, 2004, from http://www.nova.edu/ssss/QR/QR3–4/winters.html

Winters, C. A. (1999). Heart failure: Living with uncertainty. *Progress in Cardiovascular Nursing, 14,* 85–91.

CHAPTER THIRTEEN

Acceptability: One Component in Choice of Health Care Provider

Jean Shreffler-Grant

Access to health care has deteriorated in many rural areas in the United States as a result of the closure of rural hospitals and the associated loss of local providers and services that often accompany hospital closure. Historically, much of the blame for closures has been attributed to factors external to rural communities, such as limited Medicare reimbursement, the declining rural economy, and provider shortages. More recent evidence has accumulated that suggests that underutilization of the local hospital by rural residents who bypass it to seek care in larger towns is a contributing factor (Amundson, 1993; Bauer, 1992; DeFriese, Wilson, Ricketts, & Whitener, 1992; Reinert, 1991).

Since the early 1990s, variations of Critical Access Hospitals (CAH) have been implemented as alternatives to hospitals that are at risk for closure. CAHs must be located in remote rural areas and are limited to short-stay lower-acuity services and are allowed more flexibility in staffing

This research was funded by Health Care Financing Administration Dissertation Grant 30-P-90510/0-01, Hester McLaws Award, Sigma Theta Tau Zeta Upsilon Resarch Award, and Montana State University–Bozeman, College of Nursing.

and other licensure requirements. They are also reimbursed by Medicare on the basis of reasonable cost instead of prospective payment as compared with traditional rural hospitals. Cost-based Medicare reimbursement is considered advantageous for small hospitals that often serve a high proportion of elderly patients and are less likely to be able to average risk across large numbers of admissions as may be necessary under prospective payment (Christianson, Moscovice, Wellever, & Wingert, 1990). Following implementation of the Rural Hospital Flexibility Program, passed into law in 1997, CAHs became a national model and have gained broad support in rural areas across the nation (Shreffler, Capalbo, Flaherty, & Heggam, 1999). As of 2003, there were over 600 CAHs nationwide (Hagopian, Johnson, Fordcyce, Blades, & Hart, 2003). Whether these new CAH models will be any more viable than traditional rural hospitals will likely be tied to how they are viewed and used by the rural residents they are intended to serve.

Improving equity in access to care has been an ongoing concern throughout most of the past half century (Aday, Bagley, Lairson, & Slater, 1993; Patrick & Erickson, 1993), and rural access to care has been a particularly persistent problem. Although equitable access to care in and of itself may be intuitively desirable, it is through presumed links between access, appropriate use, and resulting positive health outcomes that access becomes important (Millman, 1993). I conducted a study (1996) to examine rural residents' perspectives on access to health care in six communities in Montana with CAHs. The concept of "acceptability" is one dimension of access to care that can be used to explain why people do or do not use local rural health care services. As part of the larger study, a scale to measure acceptability was developed and validated. In this chapter I will focus on the Acceptability Scale (Appendix A).

CONCEPTUAL FRAMEWORK

Access to care was the conceptual framework guiding this study. I conceptualized access to care as having two dimensions. *Potential access to care* includes properties of the population and health care system that affect opportunities to enter into the health care system. *Actual or realized access to care* includes utilization and willingness to use the health care system and satisfaction with the care received (Aday & Andersen, 1975; Andersen, McCutcheon, Aday, Chiu, & Bell, 1993).

In several studies published in the 1980s on the relationship between access to care and utilization of care, Penchansky and Thomas (1981; Thomas & Penchansky, 1984) defined access as the fit between clients and the health care system—an adequate degree of fit was measured by objective utilization and subjective satisfaction. They identified five components of potential access:

1. Availability—an adequate supply of providers and services relative to clients' needs;
2. Accessibility—where services are located relative to where clients are;
3. Accommodation—how services are organized to accept clients;
4. Affordability—costs of services relative to resources of clients; and finally,
5. Acceptability—the clients' attitudes and opinions about the characteristics of providers and services.

Discriminant validity of Penchansky and Thomas' (1981; Thomas & Penchansky, 1984) components of access to care was supported in their studies and subsets of clients were found to differ significantly in utilization of health care based on how satisfied they were with the components that were salient for them. Although these investigators measured acceptability chiefly by consumers' attitudes and opinions about the physical environment in which care was delivered, they proposed that attitudes about personal and technical practice characteristics of providers and services were also relevant.

METHODS

In the larger study to examine rural residents' perspectives on access to health care, I (Shreffler, 1996) employed a descriptive survey design. I sent surveys to a random sample of 100 households in each of 6 communities with CAHs, and I interviewed a subset of respondents by telephone. I obtained a 63.5% response rate on the mail survey (n = 381).

My principal aims in this study were to identify the predictors of use and willingness to use local health care and satisfaction with care. In interpreting the term *predictors,* it should be noted that I sought significant statistical relationships rather than cause and effect relationships. It was not possible to determine from the data whether people used local health care because they thought it was acceptable or whether they thought it was acceptable because they had used it.

There were four dependent variables in the analyses to address this aim: (a) use of the local CAH, (b) use of the local primary care provider, (c) willingness to use the local CAH, and (d) willingness to use the local provider. These *use* variables were dichotomous yes or no indicators of whether or not the respondents reported actual use of the CAH and the local provider in the recent past. The willingness to use variables were dichotomous yes/no indicators constructed from responses to a question about where respondents would first seek care for a variety of future health concerns. The future health concerns counted as *yes, willing to use* were concerns for which the local CAH and provider(s) offered health care services rather than other services included in the question that were not available locally and for which patients needed to be referred elsewhere.

The major independent variables, or potential predictors, included potential access to care factors. All were measured by respondents' self-report and from their perspectives (versus from the perspectives of the hospitals or providers). These included characteristics of the population, such as age, income, health insurance, and health status, and character-istics of the health care system that I operationalized according to the 5 a's from Penchansky and Thomas's work (1981; Thomas & Penchansky, 1984); (i.e., availability, accessibility, accommodation, affordability, and finally, acceptability).

The Acceptability Scale comprised the summed values of responses to twelve 5–point Likert-type rating questions related to the concept of acceptability included on the mail survey. I based my selection of the ques-tions for inclusion in the scale on Penchansky and Thomas' work (1981; Thomas & Penchansky, 1984). I then validated the questions in telephone interviews from responses to the question: "When you and your household members choose a medical care provider and a hospital to use, can you tell me what factors are important to you?" Responses were related to the technical quality of care, "art" of care, and appearance of the facility or office as are the questions included in the scale.

The Acceptability Scale items were components of two questions that asked respondents to rate a wide variety of aspects of health care in their local communities (See Appendix 13). Response options included 1 = *excellent,* 2 = *good,* 3 = *average,* 4 = *fair,* 5 = *poor,* and 6 = *don't know.* The scale had a possible point range of 12–60. The reliability coef-ficients for the Acceptability Scale were Cronbach's alpha = .97 and the Standardized item alpha = .97; the interitem correlations analysis ranged from 0.54 to 0.88.

To identify the predictors of use and willingness to use local health care, I built four separate multivariate logistic regression models (one for each dependent variable) in which I first regressed the dependent variable regressed on a set of 6 community (dummy) variables to control for confounding by community. Then I added independent variables to the model together as a group (not stepwise). Next, I calculated 95% confidence intervals (for β and odds ratios) for the independent variables with $p \leq .05$.

I analyzed qualitative comments on several short answer questions on the mail survey and open-ended questions in the telephone interview regarding access to care by using content analysis methods. I read all qualitative data multiple times and sorted them into similar categories based on the words used in the comments (manifest content) and the apparent meaning of the words (latent content; Catanzaro, 1988). I sought patterns and categories that might add to the understanding of rural residents' views on access to health care in their local communities. I then summarized these themes and categories and identified relevant themes using the actual phrases of the respondents.

RESULTS

Table 13.1 shows the descriptive results of the use and willingness to use dependent variables I examined. As can be seen on the table, relatively few respondents ($n = 37$, 9.7%) reported that anyone in their household had used the local CAH for inpatient care in the prior 2 years whereas roughly two thirds of the respondents ($n = 260$, 68%) reported use of the local provider in the past year. Less that half of the respondents indicated willingness to use the CAH ($n = 162$, 43%) and local providers ($n = 182$, 48%) for future health concerns.

I computed Acceptability Scale scores for 261 of the total 381 households; I excluded the remaining because of missing values or *don't knows*. The mean Acceptability Scale score was 46.48 (SD = 9.87 range = 18–60 points [possible range = 12–60 points]).

Based on the logistic regression analysis (summarized on Table 13.2), respondents for households most likely to use the CAH for inpatient care were those who rated their knowledge of local health care highly, were older in age, and reported lower incomes. The odds ratio indicates the factor by which the odds of use or willing to use change when the corresponding variable is changed by one unit. Because in this chapter I focus on the Acceptability Scale, I do not discuss the other results at length, but just as illustration, for every unit increase in the knowledge rating category with

Table 13.1. Frequencies of Dependent Variables "Use" and "Willingness to Use" Local Health Care ($N = 381$)

Variable	n	%
"Used the CAHs" for inpatient care in prior 2 years	37	9.7
"Used local provider(s)" in the past year	260	68
"Willing to use the CAH" in the future	162	43
"Willing to use the local provider(s)" in the future	182	48

Note. CAHs = critical access hospitals.

Table 13.2. Results of Multivariate Logistic Regression Models to Identify Predictors of Use and Willingness to Use Local Health Care

	β	SE	OR	95% CI
Use CAH and				
Knowledge of local health care	.8362	.400	2.308	(5.05, 1.06)
Respondent age	.035*	.017	1.036	(1.07, 1.01)
Household income	-.533*	.221	.587	(0.61, 0.56)
Use local provider and-				
Acceptability Scale score	.096**	.024	1.100	(1.15, 1.05)
Willing to use CAH and				
Acceptability Scale score	.065**	.021	1.067	(1.11, 1.02)
Use of local provider	.936*	.452	2.549	(6.18, 1.05)
Willing to use local provider and				
Acceptability Scale score	.088**	.023	1.092	(1.14, 1.04)
Use of provider (in the past)	1.88**	.504	6.546	(17.58, 2.44)
Community affiliation	1.54**	.549	4.664	(13.69, 1.59)

Note. OR = odds ratio; 95% CI = 95% confidence interval of the odds ratio. Data includes significant independent variables only.

*p < or = .05. **p < or = .01

an odds ratio of 2.308, the odds of use of the CAH increased by 130%. An odds ratio of 1 is equal odds, so anything significantly over or under 1 is considered. The Acceptability Scale as well as other variables in this model (distance from CAH, use of local provider, ease of transportation, and community affiliation) were not significant predictors of use of the CAH. I anticipated that few if any covariates would be significant in this model, with only 37 households who had reported use of the CAH.

Households most likely to use the local provider(s) were those that had higher Acceptability Scale scores. For each additional point on the scale, the odds of use of the provider increased by 10%. Other variables in this model (knowledge of local health care, distance from CAH, respondent age, income, transportation, and community affiliation) were not significant predictors of use of the local provider.

Households most likely to be willing to use the CAH for future health problems were those with higher Acceptability Scale scores and those that used the local provider(s) in the past year. Based on the odds ratios for each additional point on the Acceptability Scale, the odds of indicating willingness to use the CAH increased by 7%. Other variables in this model (knowledge, distance from CAH, age, income, transportation, and community affiliation) were not significant predictors of willingness to use the CAH.

Residents most likely to be willing to use the local provider(s) in the future were also those with higher acceptability scores, who used the local provider(s) in the past year, and reported that they were affiliated with the local community. Each point on the Acceptability Scale increased the odds of willingness to use the provider by 9%. Other variables in this model (knowledge, distance from CAH, age, income, and transportation) were not significant predictors of willingness to use the local provider.

Among those who used local health care, the Acceptability Scale score was also a significant predictor of satisfaction with care. Because I included only those households that had used both the CAH and local provider(s) in the recent past ($N = 36$) in this analysis, I used Mantel-Haenszel chi-square tests to examine relationships between satisfaction and selected covariates. There was insufficient power to analyze this relationship using multivariate logistic regression models. The Acceptability Scale score was significantly associated with satisfaction with the local CAH, emergency care, local primary care provider(s), and the availability of night or weekend care ($p \leq .01$). Other variables examined were not significantly associated with satisfaction with care.

In the qualitative comments, the rural respondents offered many perspectives related to the relationship between acceptability and use of local health care. "He knows what he's doing. He knows my son and my son knows him and that's comforting." "He's a country type doctor. I like that." "The way a hospital is equipped. I want a doctor who is top of the line." "For the doctor—that you have rapport with him, that he gives you accurate information, that you're comfortable that he knows what he's doing." "For the hospital—the nursing care, cleanliness. The doctor—personality. I go to see him the first time—did the medicines help, did the care help the problem?" "They don't have the services, the doctor's not as good, and it's not as good a hospital."

DISCUSSION AND CONCLUSIONS

In this study, the Acceptability Scale was the most consistent predictor of use and willingness to use local rural health care as well as satisfaction with care. Acceptability is that component of access to care that reflects potential clients' attitudes and opinions about the characteristics of providers and services. Unlike other aspects of access, acceptability reflects an opinion, a judgment, and personal preferences on the part of consumers. The current rural reality for obtaining most goods and services including health care is that with access to vehicles, modern highways, and health insurance, rural residents are not as affected by distance in choosing health care as they once were. And this study suggests that those who do not find local health care acceptable go elsewhere.

It is interesting to note that a large majority (95%) of the respondents in this study indicated that having local health care was very or somewhat important to their household members and "keeping" or maintaining the health services and providers they had was the predominant theme in the qualitative comments—yet only 9.7% of the households had a family member hospitalized in the CAH in the prior 2 years, and only 68.2% had used the local provider(s) in the prior year. A clarification of this discrepancy may be found by considering a second theme that emerged from the data, "just in case." "You always have certain people who are doubters ... but they still want emergency care available in case they need it, even though they don't support it for everyday things." "I know that it's not paying its way in taxes but we need it. It's like having an insurance policy. Insurance policies don't pay for themselves either but you need it just in case." Clearly there was support in these 6 communities for keeping their local health care, but acceptability was associated with use of local health care whereas support or indicating its importance were not.

By improving researchers'understanding of what rural consumers deem acceptable in terms of services and providers, the Acceptability Scale can be used to improve health care access for rural residents. In the practice arena, attending to community residents' perceptions of competence, quality, the art of care, and appearance of facilities as well as developing strategies to strengthen and improve these perceptions may reduce out-migration for health care that is available locally. In the policy arena, as new models of care are developed or refined, paying substantial attention to features or characteristics that influence acceptability to consumers can make the difference between services that will be used and valued and services that will be bypassed by the residents they are intended to serve. When it comes to rural health care, Kinsella's (1982) old baseball adage, "If you build it, [they] will come" does not necessarily hold, unless what is built is acceptable to rural residents.

REFERENCES

Aday, L. A., & Andersen, R. (1975). A framework for the study of access to medical care. In L. A. Aday & R. Andersen, *Development of indices of access to medical care* (pp. 1–14). Ann Arbor, MI: Health Administration Press.

Aday, L. A., Bagley, C. E., Lairson, D. R., & Slater, C. H. (1993). *Evaluating the medical care system: Effectiveness, efficiency, and equity.* Ann Arbor, MI: Health Administration Press.

Amundson, B. (1993). Myth and reality in the rural health service crisis: Facing up to community responsibilities. *The Journal of Rural Health, 9,* 176–187.

Andersen, R. M., McCutcheon, A., Aday, L. A., Chiu, G. Y., & Bell, R. (1993). Exploring dimensions of access to medical care. *Health Services Research, 18*(1), 49–74.

Bauer, J. C. (1992). The primary care hospital: More and better health care without closure. In L. A. Straub & N. Walzer (Eds.), *Rural health care: Innovation in a changing environment* (pp. 65–74). Westport, CT: Praeger.

Catanzaro, M. (1988). Using qualitative analytical techniques. In N. F. Woods & M. Catanzaro, *Nursing research: Theory and practice* (pp. 437–456). St. Louis: C. V. Mosby Co.

Christianson, J. B., Moscovice, I. S., Wellever, A. L., & Wingert, T. D. (1990). Institutional alternatives to the rural hospital. *Health Care Financing Review, 11*(3), 87–97.

DeFriese, G. H., Wilson, G., Ricketts, T. C., & Whitener, L. (1992). Consumer choice and the national rural hospital crisis. In W. M. Gesler & T. C. Ricketts (Eds.), *Health in rural North America* (pp. 206–225). New Brunswick, NJ: Rutgers University Press.

Hagopian, A., Johnson, K., Fordcyce, M., Blades, S., & Hart, L. G. (2003). *Health workforce recruitment and retention in critical access hospitals.* In CAH/FLEX National Tracking Project, 3(5). Retrieved April 9, 2004, from http://rupi. org/rhph-track/results/vol3num5.pdf

Kinsella, W. P. (1982). *Shoeless Joe Jackson comes to Iowa.* New York: Ballantine Books.

Millman, M. (Ed.). (1993). *Access to care in America.* Washington, DC: National Academy Press.

Patrick, D. L., & Erickson, P. (1993). *Health status and health policy: Quality of life in health evaluation and resource allocation.* New York: Oxford University Press.

Penchansky, R., & Thomas, J. W. (1981). The concept of access: Definition and relationship to consumer satisfaction. *Medical Care, 19,* 127–140.

Reinert, B. R. (1991). The impact of hospital closures on rural Texas residents: A nursing perspective. *Dissertation Abstracts International, 52,* 1958. (No. 9128345)

Shreffler, M. J. (1996). Rural residents views on access to care in frontier communities with medical assistance facilities. *Dissertation Abstracts International, 57,* 3131. (No. 9630109)

Shreffler, M. J., Capalbo, S. M., Flaherty, R. J., & Heggam, C. (1999). Community decision-making about critical access hospitals: Lessons learned from Montana's medical assistance facility program. *The Journal of Rural Health, 15,* 180–188.

Thomas, J. W., & Penchansky, R. (1984). Relating satisfaction with access and utilization of services. *Medical Care, 22,* 553–568.

Appendix A. Individual Items Included in the "Acceptability Scale"

1. How would you rate [*facility name*] in each of the following categories?

Circle one answer for each category.

	Excellent	Good	Average	Fair	Poor	
a.) Overall quality of care	5	4	3	2	1	Don't know
b.) Medical care	5	4	3	2	1	Don't know
c.) Nursing care	5	4	3	2	1	Don't know
d.) Staff concern/compassion	5	4	3	2	1	Don't know
e.) "Personal" aspects of care	5	4	3	2	1	Don't know
f.) Building cleanliness and condition	5	4	3	2	1	Don't know
g.) Acceptability as source of care	5	4	3	2	1	Don't know

2. How would you rate each of the following aspects of overall medical care provided in your community? (Care provided by physicians, physician assistants, or other primary care providers at their office or local hospital).

Circle one answer for each category.

	Excellent	Good	Average	Fair	Poor	
a.) Competence of primary care providers	5	4	3	2	1	Don't know
b.) Concern/compassion for patient	5	4	3	2	1	Don't know
c.) "Personal" aspects of care	5	4	3	2	1	Don't know
d.) Competence of support staff	5	4	3	2	1	Don't know
e.) Acceptability of provider as source of care	5	4	3	2	1	Don't know

PART IV

Rural Nursing Practice

Scharff's (1998) seminal work about the role of the rural nurse generalist published in the first edition of this book is the first chapter of this part. It is followed by a study by Raph and Buehler in which they examine another rural nursing theory key concept—health professionals' perception of lack of anonymity. Then, Troyer and Lee build on Scharff's work in their description of the rural generalist in the community health setting. Rosenthal uses the narrative method in her exploration of acute care nursing in two rural hospitals. O'Lynn reports on a study conducted with male nurses in rural settings. In the last chapter of this part, Hendrickx addresses the continuing educational needs of rural nurses.

CHAPTER FOURTEEN

The Distinctive Nature and Scope of Rural Nursing Practice: Philosophical Bases

Jane Ellis Scharff

LOOKING BACK

Plenty and little have changed in 10 years. Rural nursing practice seemed a dichotomous set of the routine and the extraordinary to me back then, as it does now. I was an insider, if not an old-timer, and my findings, although remarkable to some, seemed simply confirmatory to me. Already a budding pragmatist and not yet fully a scientist, I thought, at the time, it was enough to have empiric validation for the practice that I had known and in which my former workplace colleagues continued. For that reason and so many others, I did not publish the findings of my master's thesis in 1987. Subsequently, I have been cited frequently, misrepresented occasionally, and poached a time or two when it comes to references about the world of rural nursing. It is time to uphold my responsibility to nursing science and to set the record straight. The nature and scope of rural nursing IS distinctive. I am now willing to be quoted on that. Furthermore, rural nursing can now be given a definition based on that distinctiveness.

Rural nursing practice, be it hospital practice, private practice, or community health practice, is distinctive in its nature and scope from the practice of nursing in urban settings. It is distinctive in its boundaries, intersections, dimensions, and even in its core. Ten years ago I was loath to claim distinctiveness within rural nursing's core. It seemed too bold to proclaim that at the very level of essence, and not attributable to setting alone, rural nursing could be so different. Today, I am determined to claim it: The core of all nursing is care, and care is the substance of the relationship between nurse and patient; consequently, what happens at the core of rural nursing is something apart from what happens at the core of nursing anywhere else.

Still a pragmatist, my job is to get readers as close to the experience as I can. Thankfully, my growth as a scientist makes the job easier than it was some years back. Although no longer in the practice, I understand rural nursing better today than I did then. The importance of rural nursing has not decreased as my worldview has expanded. On the contrary, the more I dissect and reconstruct my thoughts about life and truth and nursing science, the more clearly I see the beauty emanating from the nature and scope of rural nursing, and the more clearly I appreciate its relevance to all of nursing science.

From an ontological viewpoint, I will share some information about what it means to "be" a rural nurse, and from an epistemological viewpoint, I will express a little of what it means to "know" rural nursing practice. What came as primary expression to me, because I lived it, breathed it, and studied it, is secondary expression as I write it, and I will do my best to translate the experience through common language. However, the story I tell will require imagination to transcend time and space and to gain a sense of the reality of rural nursing practice. The information for this chapter comes from my ethnographic study of rural hospital nurses in the Inland Northwest completed in 1987, from dialogue with key informants before then and up until today, and from my personal experiences within rural health care systems over the past 20 years.

In the last 10 or 15 years, I have made some presentations about portions of this work to nurse clinicians, nurse researchers, and non-nurse health care audiences. Inevitably, following such presentations, I am approached by one or two individuals who have been rural nurses who want to tell me that the presentation struck a chord. I understand their need, which stems from the human desire to be recognized and understood. It stems from the frequent, albeit unintended, distortion of truth about rural nursing communicated by those who do not fully understand what it means to walk a mile in a rural nurse's duty shoes. I may not be able to change that, but I offer my perspective nonetheless.

CONCEPTUALIZING RURAL NURSING PRACTICE

Being Rural

There was a wonderful line in the 1984 science fiction film, *The Adventures of Buckaroo Banzai: Across the Eighth Dimension* (Rausch). The line was delivered by the main character, Buckaroo, a multiskilled neurosurgeon, particle physicist, rock musician, and Zen warrior who, in the midst of chaos matter-of-factly declared, "No matter where you go, there you are." If this sounds simple, I would caution that it is hardly simple. Buckaroo was talking about being in the moment, so imagine for a moment what it means to have *gone* rural. What of rural nursing identity? While the imagery may seem silly or surreal, the truth is real, authentic, important, credible, respectable, and as serious as any nursing practice anywhere. However, as indicated earlier, rural nursing practice is also distinctive from nursing anywhere else. Although I use the analogy of Buckaroo Banzai hoping it will bring a smile, rural nurses will recognize the script of playing a cool and noble professional, simultaneously enacting multiple roles, and managing the continual transition from one part to another with the frankness of Buckaroo.

Being rural means being a long way from anywhere and pretty close to nowhere. Being rural means being independent or perhaps just being alone. Being a rural nurse means that when a nurse saves a life, everyone in town recognizes that she or he was there, and when a nurse loses a life, everyone in town recognizes that she or he was there. Being rural means turning inward for answers, because there may be nobody to turn to outward. Being rural means that when a nurse walks into the emergency room, it may be her or his spouse or child who needs a nurse, and at that moment, being a nurse takes priority over being anyone else. Being a rural nurse means being able to deal with what she or he has got, where she or he is, and being able to live with the consequences.

Knowing Rural

Certainly every reader has heard that a little knowledge can be a dangerous thing. The adage was probably modified from what Alexander Pope said in the 17th century: "A little learning is a dangerous thing." I dispute it now and say that a little knowledge can be a lifesaving thing. The demarcation between danger and safety is the difference between *having* knowledge and *using* knowledge. From time to time, I have had conversations with academic colleagues about dangerous nurses. In these conversations, we have agreed that dangerous nurses are not those who know they do not know what they are doing—although there is certainly an element of danger in that scenario, which ultimately must be addressed. The greater danger, however, emerges with those nurses who think they do know, but actually do not know, what they are doing. Although I have no statistics on the prevalence of such nurses, it is my belief that they hide more easily in urban settings than they do in rural settings.

Knowing rural means knowing that what one knows may be all one has. Knowing rural means personally knowing everyone with whom one works and having knowledge about nearly everyone for whom one cares. As a rural nurse, knowing means sharing knowledge in an informal, yet crucially important exchange, with other professionals, where the addition of one mind can mean expanding the knowledge base by 100%. Although *who* one knows can be important in any setting, the distinction between rural and urban dynamics of whom one knows, is that in the urban setting who one knows is more likely to be related to competitive advantage, whereas in the rural setting who one knows is more likely to be related to cooperative advantage. Knowing rural means that knowledge can mean the difference between perishing, surviving, and thriving, and therefore, knowing is inextricably connected to being when one is rural.

THE NATURE AND SCOPE OF NURSING

For practicality, a framework for the study of the nature and scope of rural nursing practice was sought to identify and describe the distinctive characteristics of practice in rural settings. The American Nurses' Association (ANA) Social Policy Statement (1980) provided the framework for a logical sequence of investigation into details of rural nursing practice. The policy statement includes an organized and systematic approach to studying nursing nature and scope.

1. *Nursing's Nature.* Within the policy statement, the nature of nursing is characterized as a relationship between the nursing profession and society that is mutually beneficial, and nursing itself is deemed an essential outgrowth of the society that it serves. Nursing is described as existing in response to society's needs. From that standpoint, my study of rural nursing was based on assumptions that rural nursing emerges from and is essential to rural society, and distinctions of rural nursing are due, in part, to distinctive interests and needs of rural society.

2. *Nursing's Scope.* The scope of nursing includes four definitive characteristics that are intersections, dimensions, core, and boundary (ANA, 1980). These four characteristics became conceptual foundation blocks for my study of rural nursing.

    a. *Intersections.* Nursing intersects with other professions involved in health care. These intersections are points at which nursing meets and interfaces with other professions as well as expands its practice into the domain of other professions as necessary.

    b. *Dimensions.* Characteristics such as philosophy, ethics, roles, responsibilities, skills, and authority are examples of nursing dimensions. These are qualities that add depth to nursing practice. They are characteristics underscored and influenced by interpersonal relationships and intimacy as well as the intrapersonal quality of nursing.

c. *Core.* The concept of the core of nursing is complex and somewhat more difficult to discuss than are the other concepts. It is oversimplification to say that the needs of people are the core of nursing, although such is true. Nursing exists to deal with human response to health issues, and human response can be equated to human need with respect to health. The patients' *needs* and their *responses* are outgrowths of whom they are as human *beings*. The nursing care we provide is an outgrowth of whom we are as human beings. The core of nursing is the dynamic of nursing care juxtaposed with human response.

d. *Boundaries.* Nursing's boundaries change and expand in direct reflection of the intersections, dimensions, and core of practice. Boundaries are nebulous, unseen, intangible lines of demarcation between what is clearly within the nature and scope of nursing and what is questionably within nursing's scope. Unlike physical boundaries, nursing's boundaries are metaphysical, relationally and contextually based, and sometimes have origins outside the control of nursing.

METHODS

In an effort to describe the nature and scope of rural nursing, it was determined that an ethnographic method, using participant observation and interviewing techniques, would yield the most pertinent data for analysis. Data were gathered throughout several stages of conceptualization concerning rural nursing phenomena. Field notations, printed news media, and taped interviews were employed. The study of rural hospital nurses included an exploratory phase in which 8 rural nurses from northwest Montana were interviewed. These interviews were audiotape recorded, and from initial open-ended questions, a more refined interview guide was developed that contained both closed-and open-ended questions. Twenty-six rural hospital nurses in one of four rural towns in eastern Washington, northern Idaho, or western Montana were interviewed. All interviews were audiotaped and then transcribed verbatim. The findings reported in this chapter are related to many aspects of rural nursing practice and are based on the responses of all 34 rural nurses, as well as several other key rural informants and my own observations. All samples were convenience, and all informants elected to be included in the studies.

FINDINGS

Informant Demographics

All of the informants were women ranging in age from 25–61 years with an average age of 40 years. The number of years actively employed as a registered nurse was 3–35 years. The mean number of years spent working in rural hospitals was 8 years and, for most informants, was roughly half the total active nursing years. Most informants were originally diploma-prepared, 7 were baccalaureate graduates, and 4 were associate graduates. Two informants had achieved a master's degree in nursing. Although informants were not asked about marital or parental status, nearly all said during the interview that they were married and were parents.

Most of the informants worked full-time, and those who worked part-time averaged 23 hours per week. In addition, many were placed on call if they were not working. On call status could be attributed to low census, high census, operating room call, cardiac care call, or emergency department call. Most informants reported one or two days of overtime per month. In almost every case, informants indicated a need to be flexible about their working schedules with regard to the events of the rural practice setting. Turnover rates were low at all facilities, and the most senior nurses had been on staff from 16–25 years.

Hospital Demographics

Information about the hospitals was obtained through interviews with nursing, fiscal, administrative, or other personnel, as well as from public records and the participant observation process. The hospital organizations were between 20 and 60 years in existence, the present structures were between 3 and 35 years old, and all had undergone some renovation over time. Ownership of the hospitals was stated as nonproprietary, public district, or community. Each hospital was governed by a board of directors of three to ten individuals who held fiduciary responsibility, decision-making authority, and to whom the administration was accountable. Board membership was either self-perpetuating or community elected. One facility was accredited by what was then the Joint Commission on Accreditation of Hospitals (JCAH). Administrative personnel said that there was little to be gained by small rural hospitals having JCAH accreditation, especially in light of what the JCAH charged for the process.

The hospitals had licensure ranging from 20 to 44 acute care beds, 0 to 3 intensive or cardiac beds, 5 to 7 newborn bassinets, and 3 to 5 swing beds for extended care. In every case, occupancy was at a fraction of licensure, and occupancy figures averaged to be about 20%–40% for acute care beds. There was some variability in the use of the other services at each facility. Two had fairly active use of the cardiac or intensive care beds. Two had fairly active obstetrical departments. Three had active surgical departments. Emergency cases at these hospitals ranged from 3 to 13 per 24 hour day during the previous fiscal year. One relied on the constant occupancy of swing beds to maintain financial solvency. The number of physicians on medical staff ranged from a low of 3 to a high of 17. Typically, physicians who held admitting privilege at a given facility did not necessarily live within the community. Undoubtedly, the variety of medical practitioners on staff impacted the occupancy of each facility. Usually, nurses were expected to be able to float from medical–surgical areas to emergency, obstetrical, and intensive care areas but not to the operating room, which seemed to be the one sacrosanct specialty area.

The Rural Communities

At the time of the study, I spent several weeks traveling to and about four separate communities in western Montana, northern Idaho, and eastern Washington to gather information regarding the nature and scope of rural nursing. Each of these towns fit the operational definition of being geographically isolated and of having less than 5,000 residents. Upon arrival in each community, time was taken to drive about, observe the local terrain, look for indicators of economy, walk around town to observe the pace and lifestyle, note the casual conversations taking place in public areas, and read each community's local weekly newspaper.

There were many similarities and few differences between the communities in terms of how they appeared to the outsider. Each town was located near railroad tracks, all of which were currently used. Three of the towns were on a river in forested mountain terrain and were logging or lumbermill towns. The fourth town was on an expansive plain and was an agricultural community. Each town was inhabited mostly by Caucasian people and each was laid out in typical western fashion with one main street and several auxiliary streets at which the center of the business district was found. Each town boasted the typical hardware stores, grocery stores, restaurants, farm or logging machinery shops, tool shops, post office, drug store, employment office, beauty shops, ice cream stands, feed stores, junk shops, small motels, bars, and churches. Each town had a well-kept appearance, although each had a few empty buildings or storefronts in the business district.

Residents in these communities were friendly and helpful. They recognized me as an outsider, and although willing to answer my questions, were curious and wanted to know the purpose of my presence in their town. When I explained myself, the residents registered sincere interest and pleasure that their community had been targeted for this study. They acted like they felt privileged and eagerly conveyed their high regard for nurses in general and *their* nurses specifically. Never did these residents express animosity toward the community of nurses. Most of them had a story to tell about how a friend's or relative's life was saved at the local hospital.

Rural Hospital Nurses

The rural nurses I observed and interviewed were a dynamic group of women who could certainly be called expert generalists. They moved quickly, and for the most part easily from one role to another as circumstances required. They explained that most rural nurses have a great deal of knowledge regarding a variety of nursing practice areas. When beginning work in a rural hospital, many nurses suffer reality shock due to the variety of demands placed on them. One seasoned nurse told me, "Although you might start out and you don't have that wide knowledge, you better get it quickly." A relative newcomer nurse expressed admiration about the knowledge level of her rural colleagues, calling them "impressive." The nurses I interviewed routinely worked in three or four different specialty areas of nursing practice every week and, sometimes, every day. When talking with one respondent about this phenomenon and how easy certain nurses made it look, she said, "The ones who are experienced in rural nursing seem to be very comfortable in switching back and forth between specialties."

Nursing Staff Tenure and Group Acceptance

At all facilities nurses were heard to use the terms "new" or "newcomer" and "old" or "old-timer" in reference to a given nurse's tenure on the staff. There was no particular time limit identified when a nurse makes the transition from new to old, nor how one arrives at a level of acceptance. However, tenure of less than 2 years was apparently definitely considered new, and tenure of 3–5 years in combination with competence generally constituted acceptance. Tenure beyond 10 years was considered seasoned, and in special cases of achieving high proficiency or social acceptance, one of these nurses might be called an old-timer, but usually this term was reserved for someone who had been around for 20 or more years. What I discerned was some gray area depending on a nurse's tenure, level of proficiency, and sociability related to group fit. It seemed that a nurse who was very skillful, flexible, and likeable might reach old-timer status sooner than a nurse who was lacking one of those characteristics.

Although I cannot pinpoint a "typical" rural nurse, certain characteristics were confirmed as traits of distinctive advantage for a rural nurse's success. For example, good common sense, good judgment ability, the ability to set priorities, good physical assessment skills, and physical and emotional strengths were considered of survival significance to these nurses, due, in part, to the aloneness of their practices. They made comments such as, "You have to make all your own decisions. There's no one to do that for you." "You have to be able to be autonomous." "You can't go to somebody for concurrence with decision making." "At any time during your shift, your assignment may change drastically." "You can make the difference between life or death—the judgement calls are yours." All informants were adamant that the prevalent feeling of aloneness and serious responsibility were distinctive to the rural setting. None would concede that the feeling was anything like that experienced in an urban setting. These nurses expressed a very real and pervasive sense of responsibility which rural nurses bear for their patients. The nurses who do not have the ability consistently to carry the burden of such decisional responsibility are the ones who do not survive as rural nurses. Old-timers claimed they could often tell right away, or within a few weeks, if a newcomer was going to catch on or not. Old-timers based such predictions on their assessments of a newcomer's characteristics as mentioned above, combined with evidence of adaptation to the new environment.

Education and Professional Development

The burden for self-responsibility of education is greater in the rural setting than in the urban setting, and most rural nurses accept this burden in stride. There are a wide variety of sources from which rural nurses receive their continuing education, such as out-of-town workshops or conferences, in-service education, journals, textbooks, practice sessions, physicians, and other nurses. The greatest educational needs voiced were in cardiac, trauma, maternal-child, and complex medical nursing.

Informants indicated a thirst for knowledge in accredited professional continuing education. Several respondents reported attending more than ten continuing education events in a year. Most attended between three and ten events annually. These events were either developed and held locally, developed elsewhere but held locally, or developed and held in urban settings. Although expenses were a factor, they were not the central factor in respondents' attending continuing education events.

Nearly all informants also relied on journals for new information, read journals regularly, and reported the most popular journals to be *Nursing, American Journal of Nursing, RN, Journal of Nursing Administration,* and *Nursing Management,* in that order. Current journals were visible in each facility, and notations were seen hanging on bulletin boards in nursing report rooms or locker rooms with a suggestion from one nurse to others that everyone review a given recent journal article germane to a given current case.

Rural nurses, in fact, identify one another as their most important single source of information and education. This was often explained as information being imparted from a peer when it was needed most, so that learning occurred while doing, which tended to heighten the memory. Comments that supported these phenomena included, "We try to share everything we can with each other." "New nurses sometimes come in with great new information or real current ideas. It helps a lot." "Sometimes the new girls expect you to know things, and I don't, and it can be embarrassing. So we look it up together." "When you've been around for awhile, you develop a camaraderie. We know what we can expect from each other."

Out of town workshops were identified as the next most important source of continuing education to rural nurses. Informants qualified this by stressing that the topic or presentation needed to be relevant to the rural environment. One informant said, "It's got to be meaningful. You know, you go up to the city and they tell you how to do something, and they don't realize how different the setup is."

Interpersonal Relationships and Nursing Practice

Rural nurses know everyone who works at the hospital, all of the physicians, and most of their patients. Rural nurses say that the interpersonal closeness of knowing everyone with whom they work, and for whom they care, generally has a positive influence on their practice. The intensity of this interpersonal dynamic is unique to the rural setting. Although it is likely that nurses in any setting develop close relationships, rural nurses are in a distinctive situation of being personally acquainted with all of those around them, so that the depth of interaction is potentially greater, and the accountability for interpersonal exchange is a constant that is simply not present in other settings. An informant explained the bond she felt with coworkers by saying, "It's nice to know the people you're working with. You work more together, you try harder, and you work closer." Another nurse shared that among many rewarding qualities of rural nursing, "The cooperation of the other nurses and the cohesiveness of the group is probably the biggest."

An old-timer at one hospital said, "I don't have to explain when I say something. They believe me, and they do it without wasting time." It was easy to verify this through observation. Certain old-timers could communicate a virtual reassignment of responsibilities through the tone of their voices as they disappeared momentarily to deal with arisen crises, such as the admission of trauma victims in the emergency room. On occasions it was like watching a dance, the motions of which were so well understood, each dancer so valued and respected, that without missing a step, workers would change places based on available expertise and would back each other up without visible cues. Even physicians were seen deferring to old-timer nurses at such times. Yet, the choreography depended heavily on the direction of the one in charge, and on other occasions, with an inexperienced newcomer directing, the dance was frantic, and the flow chaotic.

Practicing Medicine

Rural nurses are understandably reluctant to admit that they practice medicine, but they know their boundaries are sometimes stretched by circumstance. "You take it upon yourself and do what has to be done to make sure the patient's stable before you can call the doctor," said one nurse to me. When patient crises occur, calling the physician is considered important, but it simply does not rank at the top of the list. The nurses I interviewed and watched used a standard A-B-C (airway, breathing, circulation) order of setting priorities to respond to patient needs. Thus, they often began written or unwritten medical protocols while the aide would be sent to summon the physician. Physician response times varied from 5–30 minutes at the rural hospitals, resulting in nurses being responsible for considerable decision making during the time lapse. At each site, I heard or saw variations on the themes of nurses stabilizing cardiac or trauma victims and nurses managing precipitous births without benefit of physicians present. In interviews, nurses were adamant that they had a responsibility to patients to do whatever was required during an emergency, and that although it sometimes felt uncomfortable, inaction would have constituted neglect. The words of one nurse summarize the collective opinion, "We do it because we have to, because it would be wrong if we didn't."

There were also circumstances of newcomer physicians relying on seasoned nurses for insight into or even direction regarding a given patient case. Per physician request, the nurse would literally advise what medications and treatments to order in cases where the doctor did not have the familiarity with a patient's history that the nurse did. This was especially true in after-hours situations of physicians covering for another's patients. My assessment of these circumstances is that each party acted within unseen lines of mutual trust and understanding with the dynamic of trust specific to a given relationship.

Another observation I made at these facilities, which struck me then and which I have informally reconfirmed on multiple occasions since, is that rural physicians seem more likely to read and respond to nurses' notes about patients than do urban physicians. Doubtless there is great individual variability, yet it is tempting to hypothesize that rural professionals have a better grasp than do their urban counterparts of pertinent information that is necessary to communicate to the health care team. Certainly, further study would be required to confirm the probability.

Rural Expertise: Aces, and Pinch Hitters

Rural nurses generally believe that no one can be an expert in every area of rural nursing practice. However, a few nurses are extremely proficient in all clinical areas, and these nurses become role models and mentors to the other nurses with whom they work. At two study sites many informants identified a colleague or two who fit this category. Interestingly, those who were identified by others as *aces* did not identify themselves as such. Each nurse was very modest about her own capability, but the pride toward aces among the staff was obvious. I was aware that talking to or watching these aces in action was as much an honor for the locals as it was for me as an investigating outsider.

All rural nurses interviewed agreed that they must be competent in more than one clinical area to be considered an acceptable staff member. The top four clinical areas deemed to be most important for competency were emergency nursing, obstetrical nursing, intensive or coronary nursing, and medical-surgical nursing. A supervisory nurse told me, "There's a difference between competent and expert. I think everybody who works in this hospital should be able to walk into any specialty area and function." But there was an expectation held by all informants that they be clinically strong, if not expert, in at least two of the above-named areas and be able to float to any other department and still function well in a pinch.

With regard to functioning in a pinch, in the early 1980s two rural Montana nurse executives who are admitted baseball fans coined the *Pinch Hitter Theory of Rural Nursing*. One of those persons, Jean Shreffler, now an academic, is author of other chapters in this text. The second person, Maura Fields, was then and remains today the nurse executive at a rural hospital in Montana and is arguably one of the most innovative and masterful nurse leaders I have ever had the good fortune to know. Her rendition of the theory went like this:

> In rural nursing, you have to be like a pinch hitter. You may not perform a task or procedure or work on a very specialized case but once a year. But when you go to do it, you have to do it like you do it every day. In baseball, a batting average of 300 is good. But the pinch hitter, well, you want them to be better than that, really, you want them to bat a thousand. That's what it's like for a rural nurse, when they go to

work, you want them to bat a thousand. (Personal conversation, Maura Fields, 1983.)

For those readers who are doubting that there can be that many instances in which the above theory becomes important, rest assured that it happens all the time. Industrial and recreational traumas are frequent in these communities. Rural citizens experience their share of severe burns, drug overdoses, cardiac arrests, head injuries, freak accidents, and critical illness. Although transfer to larger medical centers is sometimes preferred, stabilization is first necessary, and transfer is sometimes not possible. One hospital in this study is 90 road miles from the nearest medical center of any size and 150 road miles from a trauma center. Rotary blade or fixed wing aircraft are often used to transport cases that require more care than can be delivered locally, but northwest mountain weather conditions can be a significant factor in keeping aircraft grounded.

Although rural nurses do not expect an easy routine, frustration is common surrounding the conflict of trying to achieve expertise in such a complex practice. Boredom is rare as they face the constant variety of demands. One informant related the example of the prior day's evening shift. The informant was one of two RNs on duty at the time, assisted by one aide. The scenario she described began after change of shift report and went like this:

> Just yesterday evening there were seven patients in the house with nothing going on. Within an hour, there was one admitted with a depression state, an OB came in, and there were four or five cases in the ER, one being a child with rectal bleeding, which makes you wonder about child abuse.

Although two nurses and an aide would have no difficulty caring for seven stable medical surgical patients, the admission of the depressed patient was a wrench in the works. Mental health diagnoses are among those which rural nurses feel least appropriately prepared for, and they lack confidence in rural physicians' ability to treat mental health patients appropriately, as well. The depressed patient required suicide precautions for a period of time which meant that the aide was assigned to remain with the patient at all times. The pediatric patient in the emergency room required careful documentation, delicate interaction, and a social services consultation. The obstetrical patient admission required nurse assessment and individual care until it was determined that the patient was in early labor. One nurse moved back and forth between the emergency room and the general care unit; the other moved back and forth between the labor room, the depressed patient, and the general care unit.

Here is an account from another informant about another evening shift where three RNs were on duty but without assistance from an aide:

> Not long ago we had an OB with a bad baby, small for gestational age, and at the same time we got two ambulances five minutes apart, and they were both cardiacs with chest pain. While that was happening, there was surgery going on, and there was somebody in the unit. I don't know if God is watching you or what, but, for the most part, things seem to come out okay in the end.

In this case, one nurse was already assigned to the intensive care unit, and one was required to remain with the obstetrical patient to do monitoring and other procedures. When the first ambulance arrived, the third nurse was dispatched to the emergency room. Fortunately, some ambulance crew members were emergency medical technicians and could help with continued patient monitoring and calling in the physician, laboratory, and respiratory personnel. Also fortunately, the physician arrived within 10 minutes and was designated to care for both patients. The final good fortune is that nothing went wrong on the general care unit while hell was breaking loose elsewhere.

Knowing Patients Personally

Most rural nurses subscribe to the belief that when they know patients personally, they can give better care. The possibility of experiencing fear when caring for family members or best friends notwithstanding, the rewards are considered rich. A gradual loss of anonymity occurs to rural nurses as they become immersed in and assimilated into rural society, making anonymity nonexistent for old-timers. "I can be more supportive emotionally when I know them," one said, and another elaborated, "Let's say in the ER, with chronic lungers, you know them, and they feel secure because they know we remember them." I saw instances of rural nurses informally calling to check on patients after discharge. As far as I know, patients were always glad to have these calls. The loss of anonymity is generally considered reassuring for those professionals who are comfortable with rural life, but it can be constricting as well. It should not be assumed, however, that negative aspects of anonymity loss are necessarily related to poor patient outcomes. On the contrary, one informant told me,

> I know of several situations where knowing my OB patients who had poor outcomes made a difference to them, where I was really able to help them get through the experience. It's a real emotional drain, but you're ahead of the game, because the trust is there.

The argument could be made that patients perceive their care to be better based on the close personal contact that is often made in the rural setting. A nurse who believes that her relationship to a patient made a difference in the patient's outcome said,

> I recovered my little neighbor girl after her surgery. Most little kids are scared when they wake up, but when she woke up she knew me and wasn't afraid and recovered really fast. Because fear generates pain, but she wasn't afraid, she recovered faster than usual.

It is a cultural expectation of many rural people to be taken care of by someone they know. This differs from the expectation in urban settings. For the most part, informants agreed that rural people do expect to have their medical needs met, even though they live far from a major medical center. However, one informant said that rural patients often wait until they are "half dead" before they seek intervention and are "grateful for what they get." Another nurse said, "People have told me they were glad I was on when they were here, that if I said it was going to be okay, then it was going to be okay."

Nearly all rural nurses could confirm that sometimes they had patients from out of town who had previously experienced urban hospital admissions. These patients, whether vacationing in the rural setting or passing through the rural area, ended up in rural hospitals for reasons not important to this story. Their comments about the care they received in rural hospitals are important. The nurses were told by these patients that the care was of better quality, that they felt more cared for, that the rural nurses took more time to listen, that care was accomplished more quickly and smoothly, and that they felt more like people and less like numbers in the rural hospital than they did in any urban hospital. The outsider patients often expressed surprise at the high level of competence they encountered in the rural setting.

DISCUSSION

Rural Nursing's Distinctive Nature and Scope

Analyses of the reports of rural nurses show that the nature and scope of rural nursing are clearly distinctive. Using a framework to focus the discussion, the distinctions can apparently be categorized as those pertaining to rural nursing's nature, as well as the four components of rural nursing's scope, those being intersections, dimensions, core, and boundary.

The Nature of Rural Nursing

Most rural nurses have difficulty defining their practice, although they can describe it. Their descriptions are a variety of rich, thoughtful, colorful, and articulate responses. Rural nursing is generalist nursing, not to be mistaken for mundane, and includes an intensity of purpose which makes it distinctive. Rural nurses may feel misunderstood and poorly recognized by the larger nursing community, but they are nonetheless a proud lot.

The Scope of Rural Nursing

The intersections of rural nursing are distinctively marked and fluid. Rural nurses consistently and necessarily practice well within the realm of other health care disciplines, the most notable being respiratory therapy, pharmacy, and medicine. The intersection between nursing and medicine has the most extensive implications. It is a gray area that hinges on circumstances and relationships, and the most complex intersections occur during emergent situations; "until the doctor gets there." Some rural nurses embrace this intersection more willingly than others, but none do it casually. Reflective concern is apparent in comments related to this intersection. One informant said, "It means putting your neck out there on the line, but you have to make the judgment and go on." Another told me, "It sometimes feels uncomfortable, but it's part of my responsibility to the patient."

It is evident that the practice of rural nursing is dimensionally distinctive. Rural nurses embrace an ethic of openness and honesty that is pervasive. The dimension of interpersonal knowing is viewed as a positive feature of rural practice, and it exists between nurses and patients as well as among coworkers. A nurse administrator shared with me that, "in terms of practice outcomes, your accountability is right in front of your face." Rural nurses talked about being able to accomplish goals more quickly with their patients and said that guidance, teaching, and counseling behaviors are automatic to their practice in the rural environment. Communication patterns in the rural setting are more direct and suffer less obfuscation than do those in urban settings. There are fewer barriers to go through when imparting messages from one to another. As a result, there are probably fewer errors of omission and commission related to practice in the rural setting than there are in the urban setting. Confronting and managing conflict is more common in the rural setting, avoidance being an unacceptable dynamic for group cohesiveness that stems from mutual concern and regard for one another. Independent decision making is a given in rural practice, but rural nurses are aware of their limitations. One said, "You have to know when you don't know, and you have to know where to go to find out." Rural nurses are mindful, if not fully informed, about the legal dimensions of their practice. However, with respect to questions of patient safety and survival, rural nurses sometimes decide their ethical obligation to do what is right for their patients carries more weight than their legal responsibility to uphold the law. These cases generally become lessons of learning, are scrutinized and discussed by the group, and are entered into memory for future reference.

Human responses, which nurses diagnose and treat, are the core of nursing. Some sources have suggested, and informants in this study agreed, that rural dwellers are known to delay health seeking, and tend to define health as the ability to get out of bed and go to work. Thinking in terms of nursing diagnosis, one might call this behavior "dysfunctional perceptual orientation to health" which requires distinctive intervention at nursing's core. Rural nurses are faced with determining an appropriate line of demarcation between a rural dweller's rugged individualism and stubborn disregard for health. Inextricable from rural nursing's core are the relational issues of what it means to be rural. As introduced earlier in this chapter, from an ontological standpoint, rural nursing is distinctive at its very core.

Boundary being dependent on the intersections, dimensions, and core of nursing, there can be no question as to rural nursing's distinctive boundary. Rural nursing is constantly changing in response to complex intersections and dimensional intricacies distinctive to rural society. The boundary is, therefore, neither smooth nor even static. When nurses come to a rural setting from an urban setting they are very aware that the boundary of their practice changes. The transitional period for these nurses is not always easy, and boundary expansion can be accompanied by ambivalence, anxiety, and frustration. Newcomers must become adjusted to the rural culture to function effectively, and not all survive. Rural experts can play a key role in the success of newcomer transition, and those "aces" who invest themselves in the orientation and mentoring of newcomers know the importance of the payoff.

Defining Rural Nursing

Rural nursing is a special variety of nursing in which the nurse must have a wide range of advanced knowledge and ability, in combination with commitment, to practice proficiently in multiple clinical areas simultaneously along the career trajectory. The practice requires constant and continual personal and professional adaptation in developing identity. A rural nurse has both an ontological sense of being and an epistemological sense of knowing that connect the nurse with the surrounding community and through which the rural nurse creates a reality of rural professional nursing practice. In no other setting is a nurse's practice so thoroughly and integrally a constant factor in a nurse's life. In a society where separating one's private life from one's professional life is considered obligatory, rural nurses are singularly challenged, stripped of their own anonymity while simultaneously charged with protecting their patients' privacy.

Closing Thought

The newcomer practices nursing in a rural setting, unlike the old-timer, who practices *rural nursing*. Somewhere between these spectral extremes lies the transitional period of events and conditions through which each nurse passes at her or his own pace. It is within this temporal zone that nurses experience rural reality and move toward becoming professionals who understand that having gone rural, they are not less than they were, but rather, they are more than they expected to be. Some may be conscious of the transition, and others may not, but in the end, a few will say, "I am a rural nurse."

REFERENCES

American Nurses' Association (ANA). (1980). *Nursing: A social policy statement* (Publication No. NP-63 20M 9/82R). Kansas City, MO: Author.

Pope, Alexander. (1711). Essay on criticism. Cited in B. Evans (Ed.), *Dictionary on quotations* (1978). New York: Avenel Books, Delecort Press.

Rausch, E. M. (Screenplay Author). (1984). *The adventures of Buckaroo Banzai: Across the eighth dimension.* [Film]. (Available through Vestron Video.)

CHAPTER FIFTEEN

Rural Health Professionals' Perceptions of Lack of Anonymity

Susan J. Raph and Janice A. Buehler

The development of a separate and distinct theory of rural nursing has led to several germane concepts. One such concept is "lack of anonymity." Shellian (2002) notes that a strong sense of accountability occurs for the nurse who cares for people she knows. Long and Weinert (1998) assert that rural health care providers must deal with a lack of anonymity and greater role diffusion than urban providers. Lee (1998, p. 76) defines lack of anonymity as "taking care of clients who are known through associations other than the nurse/client relationship," and proposes three characteristics that illustrate the concept. For lack of anonymity to occur, the nurse must be visible and identifiable, and experience diminishes personal and professional boundaries. Alterations in the personal or professional boundaries of a nurse would suggest that both positive and negative experiences might occur in the relationship between a nurse and a client. Although there may be many factors associated with diminished personal and professional boundaries, Fazzone, Barloon, McConnell, and Chitty (2000) suggest that complacency toward the actual risks involved in providing care to patients may increase the public health nurse's risk for threat or injury. In her summary, Lee suggests that lack of anonymity has varying impact for rural health professionals and suggests this is an area in need of further study. Our purpose in this qualitative study conducted by the first author (S. Raph) was to explore the perceptions of a small group of rural health professionals and identify the variables affecting their lack of anonymity.

OVERVIEW OF COMMUNITY, SETTING, AND METHODOLOGY

I (S. Raph) chose a rural county health department in northern Montana as the setting for this pilot study. The county has a population density of 2.6 persons per square mile, classifying it as "frontier" (Montana Department of Health and Human Services, 1998). There is one full-time public health nurse and several part-time health department staff. The health department informants used in the study are representative of the multidisciplinary approach common to rural Montana health departments.

I conducted formal, semistructured interviews with four informants, three professional health care providers and one support staff member. I recorded the interviews on audiotape for accuracy. I used theoretical sampling, a component of grounded theory (Chenitz & Swanson, 1986), in data collection and analysis. After the second interview, I open-coded data to identify emerging categories and their properties, and I developed questions for the remaining interviews that reflected the identified emerging theory. I repeated the process of constant data comparison to identify relationships among categories and use of theoretical sampling throughout the analysis to allow for the grouping, collapsing, and renaming of categories, and for the emergence of some relationships. I used theoretical coding and memo writing to identify the emerging concepts, properties, and relationships (Chenitz & Swanson).

FINDINGS

The phenomenon of lack of anonymity was the focus and context of this study. A perception of "lack of anonymity" is experienced on two levels: personal and professional. The analytic paradigm that emerged appears in Figure 15.1 and serves as the basis for the discussion of the findings.

The antecedent condition "professional relationship" emerged from the data, as this was the basis of all interactions identified by the informants. Given the varying professional disciplines of the study group, we defined this condition as a caregiver–patient relationship. There were four responses to lack of anonymity identified in the analysis: (a) personally affirming, (b) professionally affirming, (c) professionally threatening, and (d) personally threatening. The "increasing negative perception of lack of anonymity" continuum at the bottom of the figure illustrates the varying

Antecedent Condition:
Professional relationship: caregiver–patient

Perceptions:

Personally affirming   Professionally threatening

       Professionally affirming   Personally threatening

Positive   Increasing negative perception of Lack of Anonymity   Negative

Figure 15.1. Rural health professionals' perceptions of lack of anonymity.

impact this phenomenon has on the rural health professional. An analysis of the antecedent condition and the responses associated with the variable of "increasing negative perception" revealed the following relationship: The more personally threatening the encounter becomes, the more negative the perception of lack of anonymity becomes. As a result, we suggested a tentative hypothesis that a negative perception of lack of anonymity is related to the degree to which the interaction invades or threatens one's personal life.

Personally Affirming

The most positive of interactions identified by the informants is the perception of *personally affirming,* and thus begins the continuum of positive to an increasingly negative perception of lack of anonymity. Personally affirming interactions were friendly encounters that did not place the informant in a professional role. Primarily, these were family and friends of the informant who were aware of unwritten rules regarding "shop talk" and knew to separate the informant's personal and professional lives. These encounters were brief and usually included general health-seeking behavior, such as "Do you think I should get a flu shot this year?" The setting for these encounters was typically the informant's home, a place of safety. Strategies to avoid these types of encounters were not identified by the informants as they did not see them as intrusive or negative.

Professionally Affirming

The perception of *professionally affirming* extends across the continuum of increasing negative perception of lack of anonymity. These interactions were generally regarded as positive for the informants. However, the frequency with which they occurred modified this positive perception. The encounters associated with this perception were impersonal interactions with participants of the health department, who often sought clarification on general information about vaccines, appointments, or needed after-hour services. The settings of these interactions were usually public places in the community, such as the grocery store, the post office, or a restaurant. The informants viewed the encounters as "no big deal," and were often "glad to help." One informant spoke of the effect this had on her professional role. "It makes you feel good that people think you're knowledgeable about what you do. And once people approach you about questions, you want to know more about your work, so that you can answer those people properly."

The informants emphasized the use of nonjudgmental attitudes during the interactions with these patients. "You just need to see them as individuals … as people. I guess you can separate the client when you're at work from the person in the community." Strategies for coping with the varied effects of these incidents included networking to enhance the professional's knowledge base and lateral or peer support. Although the encounters were primarily positive and often enhanced the professional relationship, the informants noted the frequency with which they occurred and the valuable time they took in some instances. An increase in the frequency and length of the interaction were mitigating factors in how the primarily positive encounter was perceived by the informant.

Professionally Threatening

The perception of *professionally threatening* is placed further along the continuum of negative perception for the informants. The informants expressed concern over encounters that placed them in a position of potentially doing harm if not handled correctly. They feared giving wrong advice during these interactions or felt inhibited enough by the setting so as not to be able to offer any therapeutic advice. The frequency and length of these interactions, the inappropriateness of the setting, and the confidential nature of the conversation all played a key role in how negatively the informant perceived the interaction More often than not, the informant felt more embarrassed for the client than intruded upon.

Other encounters focused on the internal struggles of professional obligations. One informant spoke of the internal conflict she experienced knowing a patient's medical history of substance abuse and the professional obligations of maintaining confidentiality, despite the fact that the patient was a school bus driver.

> The same person that I was taking to [name] for an alcohol-induced heart dysrhythmia, was the bus driver for the community schools. When you know that this person has an alcohol problem but they're also the bus driver for the children in your community and you're a parent also and so, things do get kind of weird sometimes.

The informants also highlighted issues of professional obligations surrounding their employment. Encounters of being "constantly at work" illustrated greater negativism for the informant. One informant spoke of the professional obligations she had felt from a former employer. Another informant related similar feelings that she was "always at work" and always aware of how her actions would be perceived. She noted that many of her patients have an expectation that health care professionals are "helping people and good listeners," and that they are always going to seek her out for an opportunity for storytelling or advice. As a result of this, she expressed concern over losing the patient's business if the interaction was not helpful.

> I feel that I have to stop and listen to somebody's story of their blood sugars, and I have to be that way if I want to continue that good relationship. Because also in the small towns, people talk to other people. So if they see me outside the facility, whether it's WIC [Special Supplemental Nutrition Program for Women, Infants, and Children], or the hospital, and I'm not helpful, then they may not come back. In our small businesses, we can't afford to lose even a few. They're just lonely people who want someone to talk to.

The setting of these encounters varied as noted, but also occurred while out with family or friends. Strategies to counter the negative feelings associated with these incidents included participation in outside interests, limiting the interaction time, changing the setting to allow for confidentiality and therapeutic intervention, or deferment to another time.

Personally Threatening

The perception of *personally threatening* illustrated the most negative perceptions of lack of anonymity and is at the end of the continuum. Two informants spoke of personally intrusive encounters that provoked fear and anger. These interactions included some degree of personal threat from the patient that ultimately forced the informant to protect herself or her family. One informant spoke of her frustration over "feeling as though I must practice what I preach ... if I want to eat a Ding-Dong I have to go to Canada!" This frustration stems from frequent interactions in the grocery store or while out to eat, where patients watch everything she purchases or consumes.

> They watch what I buy in the grocery store, and they make comments about it too. They screen my shopping cart! ... Sometimes I just want [my husband] to take me some place far away where I won't run into anybody that I know ... I can go to Canada or I just stay home.

While this Montana county borders Canada, having to leave the country illustrates the degree of frustration and intrusiveness of the interactions that warrant fleeing from home. The act of isolation further speaks to the degree of invasion this informant experienced.

Another encounter illustrates the potentially dangerous avenue patients can take when expectations are not met by the health care professional. In this encounter, a family who was involved with child protective services had requested the staff member to write a letter to the district judge on their behalf. When she refused, the family informed her they were coming over to her house.

> They were calling me from a pay phone and said they were on their way over to my house and they were irritated with me for refusing to write this letter. I was home with my daughter at the time and I told her, "grab your coat; we're going to grandma's." And so we sneaked out of town the back way to my grandmother's ... I felt like I should have faced this head on, but I wanted to get my daughter out of there ... This same family later stalked our social worker. It was really frightening.

This frightening encounter prompted the informant to flee her home to protect her child.

Although the informant denied any consideration of leaving her position because of this interaction, she did take steps to preclude any further invasion into her personal life by getting an unlisted phone number and setting limits with the family. The degree to which these interactions posed a threat to the personal well-being of the informant illustrates a direct relationship to negative perceptions of lack of anonymity in the rural setting.

RELEVANCE TO RURAL NURSING THEORY

Nurses in the rural setting felt reassured and constricted by the lack of anonymity experienced in the community (Scharff, 1987). This perception, though more extreme than what was seen by Scharff, was also evident in this study group and was illustrated through the detail of interactions that ranged from positive and helpful to threatening. Weinert and Long (1991) noted that nurses in rural communities reported a sense of always "being on duty." The authors pointed to the fact that rural nurses find themselves as sources of health information for neighbors and friends in a variety of settings. Results of this study are consistent with Weinert and Long's finding in the perception labeled as *personally affirming* and *professionally affirming*. Although these interactions were viewed as positive and helpful, they reflect a lack of anonymity. The informants were visible, identifiable, and experienced diminished personal and professional boundaries as identified by Lee (1998).

IMPLICATIONS FOR RURAL NURSING PRACTICE

The findings of this study identify a range of perceptions associated with lack of anonymity for the rural health professional. This range of positive or "no big deal" to negative or "frightening" demonstrates the equally wide implications for rural nursing practice. As an administrator of a rural health department it is important to be aware of the stresses affecting the staff. Support, whether it is peer or administrative, is essential in maintaining healthy working relationships and the overall function of the department. Assisting the staff to recognize this range of possible perceptions of lack of anonymity may enhance staff morale, job satisfaction, staff safety, and ultimately patient care. Specific actions or strategies identified in this study that helped to mitigate the negative perceptions associated with lack of anonymity were nonjudgmental attitudes, professional networking, peer support, outside interests, and being able to limit inappropriate interactions by changing the setting or deferring to another time. The benefits of the positive interactions offered the staff a sense of professional growth, personal satisfaction, and the reassurance of consistent caseloads and funding. And although isolation and fleeing home may be strategies used in highly threatening situations, the basis of coping is being aware of the potentially frightening encounters that can occur. An increased awareness of the range of perceptions associated with lack of anonymity will assist the staff to balance their private and professional lives.

REFERENCES

Chenitz, W. C., & Swanson, J. A. (1986). *From practice to grounded theory: Qualitative research in nursing.* Menlo Park, CA: Addison-Wesley.

Fazzone, P. A., Barloon, L. F., McConnell, S. J., & Chitty, J. A. (2000). Personal safety, violence, and home health. *Public Health Nursing, 17,* 43–52.

Lee, H. J. (1998). Lack of anonymity. In H. J. Lee (Ed.), *Conceptual basis for rural nursing* (pp. 76–88). New York: Springer Publishing.

Long, K. A., & Weinert, C. (1998). Rural nursing: Developing the theory base. In H. J. Lee (Ed.), *Conceptual basis for rural nursing* (pp. 3–18). New York: Springer Publishing.

Montana Department of Public Health and Human Services. (1998, June). *Montana County Health Profiles.* Helena, MT: Department of Public Health and Human Services Health Policy and Services Division.

Scharff, J. (1987). *The nature and scope of rural nursing: Distinctive characteristics.* Unpublished master's thesis, Montana State University, Bozeman, MT.

Shellian, B. (2002). A primer on rural nursing. *Alberta RN, 58*(2), 5.

Weinert, C., & Long, K. A. (1991). The theory and research base for rural nursing practice. In A. Bushy (Ed.), *Rural nursing* (Vol. 1, pp. 21–38). Newbury Park, CA: Sage Publications.

CHAPTER SIXTEEN

The Rural Nursing Generalist in Community Health

Linda E. Troyer and Helen J. Lee

Fewer nurses live and work in rural settings as compared with urban settings. According to Stratton, Dunkin, Juhl, and Geller, in 1995, the mean registered nurse (RN)-to-population ratio was twice as large in metropolitan areas compared with nonmetropolitan areas. And yet a higher percentage of rural nurses work in community-based nursing, 11.8% compared with 7% of the overall RN population (Dunkin, Stratton, Movassaghi, & Kindig, 1994). Rural nurses are described as generalists (Bigbee, 1993; Scharff, 1987). Although literature on rural nursing has increased since the late 1980s, the majority of literature describing the characteristics of rural nurses is based on descriptions of hospital-based nurses. Our purpose in this chapter is to describe a study conducted by the first author (L. Troyer) to explore whether the concept of rural nurse generalist could be extended to the practice of community health nurses.

In my study I used the four characteristics of the scope of nursing used by Scharff in a previous chapter: intersections, dimensions, core, and boundaries. The most distinctive finding of Scharff's (1989) study was that rural hospital nurses do not specialize but rather expand the scope of their practice.

METHODS

My study was qualitative descriptive in design; I collected data using interviews of a convenience sample of rural community-based nurses. *Rural* was defined as a nonmetropolitan county not having a city of 50,000 population within its boundaries.

Sample

I recruited a convenience sample of 7 rural community-based nurses in central and eastern Montana through networking with Montana State University-Bozeman community health faculty. Three participants were exclusively public health nurses (PHN), three were home health nurses (HHN), and one nurse was a tribal nurse with both PHN and HHN responsibilities. All participants were female, ranging in age from 27–56 years. Three nurses had a bachelor of science degree in nursing whereas the remaining four held associate degrees in nursing. Reported nursing years of experience varied from 3–24 years, and experience in rural community-based nursing ranged from 2–14 years. The sample included nurses with and without previous urban work experience. Four nurses worked full-time; three were part-time, working 20–32 hours per week. Nurses who worked full-time were on call up to 20 nights of the month. All full-time nurses reported working overtime, varying from a few hours a month to 20 hours per week.

Procedures

Following approval by the Human Subjects Review Committee of the College of Nursing, Montana State University-Bozeman, I collected data using focused semi-structured interviews. After I collected demographic information from the study participants, I asked broad general questions followed by prompts pertaining to the scope of their practice and experience. Examples of the questions included: "Tell me what you do," "Describe a typical work day," "Tell me about the people you care for," "To whom are you responsible?" and "If you had complete control of your job, what would you change?" The interview ended by quoting Scharff's (1998) definition of rural nursing: "a special variety of nursing in which the nurse must have a wide range of advanced knowledge and ability, in combination with commitment, to practice proficiently in multiple clinical areas simultaneously along the career trajectory" (p. 37). I then asked the participants whether they saw themselves fitting the definition. I audiotaped and transcribed interviews for analysis.

Data Analysis

I summarized and categorized demographic information by the community-based practice represented—home health, public health, and tribal nurse. I categorized and organized into tables the percentage of time spent and the job responsibilities verbalized by the participants. Then, I performed content analysis of the data (Mayring, 2000) in two stages. In the first stage, I coded all data systematically for emergent categories (inductive coding). I used open coding to find tentative categories and their properties. In the second stage (deductive coding), I used the codes (intersections, dimension, core, and boundary) derived by Scharff (1987) from the 1980 American Nurses' Association (ANA) Social Policy Statement to categorize the data pertaining to the interviewed nurses' practice. As the deductive coding progressed, particularly for the dimension of nursing, the similarities and differences between the three categories of nursing represented in the sample became evident.

RESULTS

I present the study findings in three sections. First, I report the percentage of time nurses spent in general job responsibilities. Then, I describe community-based nursing using Scharff's (1998) scope of nursing codes derived from the 1980 ANA Social Policy Statement. That description includes a comparison of the community-based nursing responsibilities between and among the three types of community-based nurses represented in the sample. Finally, I present the continuum of autonomy, job variety, and job satisfaction that emerged from the inductive content analysis process.

Nursing Job Responsibilities

Table 16.1 shows the percentage of time spent in general nursing job responsibilities. The majority of the nurses' time was spent with client contact (range = 15%–50%) and paperwork (range = 8%–50%). The nurses, whether home health, tribal, or public health, had unique ways of dividing their time; no clear-cut differences in their use of time could be seen between the three categories of nurses. Driving took up a considerable amount of work time for most of the nurses in the sample (range = 2%–30%).

Intersections

The intersections of nursing are points where nursing meets, interfaces, and extends its practice into other areas of other professions. The interview data revealed that rural community-based nursing practice intersects or

Table 16.1. Percentage of Time Spent on General Job Responsibilities

Job responsibility	HHN#1	HHN#2	HHN#3	Tribal RN	PHN#1	PHN#2	PHN#3
Client contact	50	30	15	50	35	50	45
Paperwork	10–20	50	33	8	15	15	40
Driving	10–20	10	6	30	25	2	5
Meetings	<5	2	15	10	10	5	5
Phone calls	10	10	12	2	10	5	2
Computer	10	2	0	0	5	5	0
Other							
Public relations	5						
Inservices,							
public relations			19				
Continuing nurse							
education							3

Note. HHN = home health nurse; PHN = public health nurse; RN = registered nurse.

subsumes the practice of several other professions. One nurse said, "You get so used to doing different things that you may do more in the scope of another discipline than you realize."

In home health nursing the greatest overlap was with mental health and the social work issues of finances and insurance coverage. In public health nursing the greatest overlap with other allied health areas was with nutrition and social work.

Dimensions

The dimensions of nursing are the roles, responsibilities, and skills that nurses use in practice. The dimensions of nursing provided further description of the scope of nursing. The nurses' philosophy, ethics, and authority influenced these dimensions.

The practice of the rural community-based nursing distinguished itself in terms of the wide variety of roles within each practice and between types of practice as shown in Table 16.2. Most of the listed nursing responsibilities are self-explanatory except for "gap-filling." Reported by the PHNs and the tribal nurse, gap-filling adding services based on the needs of individuals and agencies in the community. For example, if the local hospital stopped teaching prenatal classes, the PHNs would start childbirth classes.

In analyzing the interview data, the similarities and differences between and among the study participants became evident. The following paragraphs describe the contrast.

Table 16.2. Responsibilities of Community-Based Nurses

Responsibilities	HHN ($n = 3$)	PHN ($n = 3$)	Tribal Nurse
Administration	(3/3)	3/3	yes
Allied health tasks	3/3	3/3	yes
Assessment	3/3	3/3	yes
Continuing education	3/3	3/3	yes
Coordination of care	3/3	3/3	yes
Family planning	0/3	2/3	yes
Gap-filling	0/3	3/3	yes
Head start[a]	0/3	3/3	yes
Home visits	3/3	2/3	yes
Hospice	3/3	0/3	yes
Immunizations	0/3	3/3	yes
Maternal-child health	0/3	3/3	yes
On call	3/3	0/3	yes
Patient education	3/3	3/3	yes
Prison	0/3	1/3	yes
Reimbursement[b]	3/3	1/3	no
Satellite clinics	0/3	2/3	yes
School nursing	0/3	3/3	yes
Staff supervision	3/3	1/3	yes
Travel to > 1 county	3/3	3/3	no
Well-child care	0/3	3/3	no
WIC nutrition program	0/3	3/3	no

Note. HHN = home health nurse; PHN = public health nurse; WIC = Women-Infant-Children. Data for HHN and PHN represent ratio of nurses with responsibility to the total number of nurses.

[a] Head Start Developmental and Health Screening. [b] Reimbursement responsibilities included (1) ensuring services and supplies were covered by insurance and (2) grant paperwork.

Similarities among HHNs. As the HHN served mostly elderly clients, all were concerned with cuts in Medicare reimbursement for home health care especially for clients who lived long driving distances from the home health office. They reported spending long hours completing Outcome and Assessment Information Set (OASIS) forms (Center for Health Services and Policy Research, 1998) and other paperwork.

Differences among HHNs. Two HHNs were in combined administrative and staff positions. One HHN did not have a hospice program in the counties where she worked. She thought her cancer patients did not get the number of visits they required because of Medicare reimbursement issues. She reported making unpaid visits to these clients; she ultimately quit her home health job because of this issue.

Similarities among PHNs. The three PHNs conducted similar mandated programs, such as the Women-Infant-Children Nutrition Program (WIC), well-child clinics, immunizations, maternal-child health programs, and Head Start developmental and health screening. They were responsible for the nursing administration tasks of their offices. They kept records of the services provided to justify funding of programs. Often the paperwork required to justify a program took more time than the actual program itself.

Differences among PHNs. One PHN primarily provided school nursing for her county, did not deliver elder programs, and did very little maternal–child health. The other two PHNs completed home visits for clients who did not meet home health agency guidelines and traveled to satellite clinics. One PHN set up medications for the prison inmates in her county.

Tribal nurse—both a PHN and HHN. The tribal nurse carried out PHN programs, such as immunizations and maternal-child health, but did not do well-child clinics or WIC. In addition, she undertook school nurse responsibilities for an outlying school on the reservation. In conjunction with the county home health office, the tribal nurse participated in home visits and hospice nursing.

Core

The core of nursing dealt with human responses to health or illness issues. Based on the rural nursing theory work, nurses in the rural setting keep in mind that often the clients' view of health is the ability to work, to be productive, and to do usual tasks (Long & Weinert, 1989). HHNs reported that typically clients waited too long before getting hospice or home care, whereas, PHNs frequently encountered clients too proud to use public health services.

Boundary

The boundary of rural community-based nursing is a combination of the intersections, dimensions, and core of nursing. As with rural hospital nursing, rural community-based nurses' boundaries of practice changed continually as the nurses moved between nursing activities as the following excerpts from two different nurses portray.

> I walked in the office at 7 a.m. and the phone was ringing off the hook. My client 50 miles away pulled out his central intravenous line. The

closest ambulance couldn't make it to his place because it was broken down. I called the ambulance here but I beat them out there and applied pressure until they got there. When I got back, a client 30 miles away in another direction was having cardiac problems. I went out there and had to call the ambulance because he was in third degree heart block. And cell phones don't work out here so I can't get things done while I'm driving.

On my way to work, I was flagged down and informed that someone had been sick all night. I haven't got a telephone in the car because cell phones don't work out here. That client needed to go to the emergency room. I always follow up and go to the emergency room with a client. You're always breaking rules. So you have to have good common sense on when to break the rules. Then there was a sick baby somewhere where the child had a positive blood culture and they want me to find the baby so the parents can bring the child in. Then I got a report on children somebody was neglecting. I got an anonymous call to check on them because they were left alone. So I had to go out and check if they were left alone and then call social services. Our social service department is overwhelmed. If there is medical neglect, the public health nurses deal with that too. Then a school called to say that five kids have head lice. They're brought to my office and we treat the head lice and contact the parents and educate the parents on the treatment of head lice. Then the clinic called me to say there's a lady in labor and she's 17 and she's scared, can you come over and give her a crash course on some breathing exercises? How can you say no? So you throw down all your paperwork and run over to the clinic and start demonstrating the blowing and puffing. It's just too wild sometimes. You have to be very flexible.

Fit of Rural Nurse Generalist Definition

When asked whether they fit the rural generalist definition provided by Scharff (1998), these community health nurses all agreed they did. Two responses are shared below:

Yes, I fit this definition but I don't consider myself to have advanced knowledge, I mean, I'm learning every day. But you have to know something of everything in order to work in a rural setting. Like peds, maternity, geriatrics, med-surg, orthopedics, dermatology. There's always something to learn.

As a new graduate I am working towards this knowledge and ability but I have a long ways to go. I see that I need a wide range of knowledge in different areas. Being aware of other resources that are available to get the knowledge I need, I'm gradually getting to that point. I don't have all that knowledge in myself but I'm learning who I can go to. Like social work, physical therapy, occupational therapy, speech therapy. Knowing who your resources are and being aware that I don't have to be totally knowledgeable in all those areas, although it would be good to have a greater knowledge in those areas. Definitively a lot of the knowledge falls into nursing. But if someone is available with greater knowledge, I feel it is my job to refer to those people. Nursing is cool in that we have a little bit of knowledge in a lot of areas and we can do a lot of things. Sometimes a specialist can only work so many hours or only get reimbursed so much, so then it is our place to go back in and work with them and make sure they are getting followed up on adequately.

Summary

The content analysis of the interview data using Scharff's (1998) constructs demonstrated that the rural community-based nurses in the sample were generalists and did not specialize. The roles they included in their practice were flexible and expanded to meet the needs of their rural communities. Because the majority of their clients were elderly with acute health care needs, HHNs experienced the most similarity in tasks performed. The practice of HHNs was also more similar to rural hospital nurses than other community-based nurses. The practice of PHNs included more variety in the ages of clients served and the many different programs with which they were involved. While PHNs did home visits, HHNs reported that they were not responsible for public health programs. The tribal nurse experienced the greatest amount of variety in her practice as it included both home health and public health nursing.

CONTINUUM OF AUTONOMY AND JOB VARIETY AND SATISFACTION

The content analysis of the responsibilities of the community-based nurses and the comparison of the three differing levels of nurses resulted in a continuum based on (a) autonomy, (b) job variety, and (c) job satisfaction. *Autonomy* referred to being able to function alone and make independent decisions (Davis, 1991). *Variety* in the job was defined as the ability to be flexible in adapting to the needs of the individual and the community; not being tied to one area of nursing (Troyer, 2000, p. 37, 47). *Job satisfaction* referred to being happy while fulfilling the job requirements (Mish, 1989, p. 646)

The seven nurses were placed on the continuum starting from left to right, from less to more job autonomy, job variety, and job satisfaction, which covaried among the participants. The continuum is depicted in Figure 16.1.

← Less   AUTONOMY   More →
                          JOB VARIETY
                       JOB SATISFACTION
HHNs, PHN (new graduate), PHN (newcomer), PHN (old-timer), tribal nurse

Figure 16.1. A continuum of autonomy and job variety and satisfaction.

HHN = home health nurse; PHN = public health nurse.

HHNs

The three HHNs experienced the least autonomy, job variety, and job satisfaction because of constraints of home health regulations and concerns regarding insurance coverage and Medicare reimbursement. Homebound status regulations limited their flexibility in providing care. A vast amount of paperwork took time away from patient care and resulted in decreased job satisfaction. An example is depicted in the following HHN interview excerpt:

> Admissions were lengthy with paperwork taking two-and-one-half hours and now it takes 4 hours to do with the OASIS form. If you transfer a patient to the hospital there's more paperwork. If they go home you have to do the OASIS all over again even if you haven't had them off services for a week yet. There's another form to do when a patient gets discharged. There's just a lot of paperwork. And starting July 1, 1999 they passed a 15 minute increment billing deal, where now you have to track all the time in the home. You don't start counting until you've been in the home 8 minutes. If there's any interruption greater than 3 minutes, you're supposed to subtract time if they're in the bathroom or on the phone or whatever. It's an asinine regulation. I think all the staff feels bogged down with paperwork requirements.

PHNs

The PHN who was a new graduate thought she had a lot of autonomy but felt uncomfortable with the lack of set priorities in her job description. She mainly focused on school nursing, immunizations, and well-child clinic work. As time progressed, she stated she was becoming more comfortable in starting new programs in the community.

A second PHN was labeled a newcomer because she was new to her community and had only recently started her public health position. Previously, she worked for a home health agency in an adjacent county and felt comfortable in seeing clients in their homes as a PHN. She and her co-PHN were developing policies and procedures for their office and had the freedom to develop programs based on the needs of the community. As a newcomer to public health nursing she felt she was still growing in the role. She stated she was very pleased with the variety and flexibility of the job and her ability to do what is needed to promote positive health outcomes in her county.

The third PHN had worked for a long time in public health and lived most of her life in her community. She reported that a few years ago, county officials tried to combine the public health and home health nursing offices. Because she did not want to learn all of the home health regulations and paperwork guidelines, she restructured her position so that it would not be combined with home health. Her restructuring plan focused on meeting the public health needs of the community. She reported feeling highly satisfied in seeing the effect of her practice on all age levels in the community. However, because she lives a long distance from a major health center, she fills gaps and serves as a safety net, providing care to clients who otherwise would not qualify for home health or other programs.

Tribal Nurse

The widest variety in roles and tasks was seen with the tribal public health and home health nurse. She structured her job to best meet the needs of the tribe she serves. She performed classic public health activities as well as coordination of home health or hospice care for tribal members. Because of the isolation, poverty, lack of home phones, and lack of cell phone coverage on the reservation, she made decisions independently, often dealing with acutely ill patients in the home. She expressed great satisfaction with nursing; she thought using flexibility and ingenuity worked to improve the lives of clients.

DISCUSSION

The community-based nurses' descriptions reflected similarities and differences to Scharff's (1998) definition of rural nurse generalist. The nurses incorporated different roles and worked in different areas of nursing within the same work day, a key characteristic of the rural generalist reported in the literature (Bigbee, 1993; Weinert & Long, 1991).

In comparing the findings for the first ANA code *intersection,* both hospital and community-based nurses met, interfaced, and extended their practice into other professional areas of practice. However, differences existed in intersection between the two groups. Hospital-based nurses overlapped with pharmacy and medicine, particularly in emergency situations, whereas the community-based nurses' overlap occurred with mental health and social work. With regard to dimension, the rural hospital nurses performed roles, responsibilities, and skills specific for individual patients within the hospital setting. The community-based nurses were more likely to perform a variety of roles, responsibilities, and skills that focused on the needs of individuals and groups within the community. The core of nursing, dealing with human responses to health or illness, was the same for rural hospital and community-based nurses. The boundary (combination of intersection, dimension, and core) was similar for the rural hospital and community-based nurses in that both changed their boundaries in response to the variety of clinical or health care situations experienced. The differences between the two groups were the environments in which the boundaries were changed, the hospital or the community.

The findings of this study validated those from the single community-based nurse in Davis' (1991) study of rural nursing. Davis explored the rural nurses' domains of practice; the community nurse described a broader scope of practice within the community as compared with the practice of the rural hospital nurses in Davis' sample.

The continuum of autonomy, job variety, and job satisfaction was supported by the findings of a study of job satisfaction between PHNs and HHNs in a rural midwestern state (Juhl, Dunkin, Stratton, Getler, & Ludtke, 1993). The study findings demonstrated that PHNs were more satisfied than HHNs with their task requirements. The PHNs reported more diverse role expectations, and the HHNs indicated they had considerable more documentation of tasks for reimbursement purposes.

Rural community-based nurse novices need to attain a wide variety of knowledge, to learn what resources are available, and to learn how to access these resources. Personal traits, such as enjoying variety, may lead to experiencing more satisfaction as a rural community-based nurse. Flexibility is required when alternating between working with individuals and then with groups, particularly for PHNs.

Holistic nursing practice was exemplified in the study by the numerous insights related about their clients' environmental and social situations. The holistic view was fostered by the increased opportunities for social interaction with the client and their family and friends at their home and in the rural community. Often, these community-based nurses had taken care of the family or friends of the client and had a nearly complete picture of their health situation.

NURSING IMPLICATIONS

Based on the findings of this study, the ability to work as a generalist is required in the practice of the rural community-based nurses. More needs to be done to facilitate meeting the educational needs of rural community-based nurses. The importance of the work of rural community-based nurses should be recognized and efforts made at local, state, and national levels to improve their staffing conditions. The burden of the large amount of paperwork in home health nursing needs to be addressed. Nurses need to keep aware of changes occurring in the health care system and participate in designing policy and other changes that promote adequate care for clients in the rural setting in and out of the hospital.

Rural community health nurse novices need to develop a network of resources to assist them when starting their practice. Because a baccalaureate education is considered the entry level education for community nurses, associate degree prepared nurses would benefit from continuing their academic education; spending time as a student in a rural community-based setting with an experienced community-based nurse would be beneficial (Ide, 1992).

Limitations of this study were its small sample size and the possibility of regional bias. These findings cannot be generalized to other rural community-based nurses; however, the implications may be applicable if community nurses are employed in similar working circumstances in sparsely populated areas.

RECOMMENDATIONS

Replication of this study in other areas of Montana and similar sparsely populated areas is recommended. Replication is needed that compares larger samples of home health, public health, and tribal nurses. Further research is needed to verify or refute the concepts presented in the continuum of autonomy, job variety, and job satisfaction.

Further research needs to be done on the financial and regulatory constraints on the delivery of home health services in rural settings and how these affect job satisfaction of HHNs in other regions. Many home health agencies are closing in the region of Montana where this sample of nurses was employed largely because of changes in Medicare reimbursement occurring since 1997. The consequences of this decrease in services to clients and their community needs to be examined. The practice of PHNs filling the gap when home health offices close in these areas and other locations warrants further study.

REFERENCES

American Nurses' Association. (1980). *Nursing: A social policy statement* (No. NP-63 20M 9/82R). Kansas City, MO: Author.

Center for Health Services and Policy Research. (1998). *Outcome and Assessment Information Set (OASIS)*. Denver, CO: Author. Retrieved August 14, 2004, from http://www.hcfa.gov

Bigbee, J. L. (1993). The uniqueness of rural nursing. *Nursing Clinics of North America, 28*(1), 131–144.

Davis, D. J. (1991). *A study of rural nursing: Domains of practice-characteristics of excellence.* Unpublished master's thesis, University of Nevada, Reno.

Dunkin, J., Stratton, T., Movassaghi, H., & Kindig, D. (1994). Characteristics of metropolitan and non-metropolitan community health nurses. *Texas Journal of Rural Health, 7,* 18–27.

Ide, B. A. (1992). A process model of rural nursing practice. *Texas Journal of Rural Health, 9,* 18–27.

Juhl, N., Dunkin, J. W., Stratton, T., Getler, J., & Ludtke, R. (1993). Job satisfaction of rural public and home health nurses. *Public Health Nursing, 10,* 42–47.

Long, K. A., & Weinert, C. (1989). Rural nursing: Developing the theory base. *Scholarly Inquiry for Nursing Practice, 3,* 113–127.

Mayring, P. (2000, June). Qualitative content analysis. Forum: *Qualitative Social Research, 2.* Retrieved October 7, 2004, from http://www.qualitative-research.net/fqs-texte/2–00/200mayring-e.htm

Mish, F. C. (Ed. (1989). *The New Merriam-Webster Dictionary.* Springfield, MA: Merriam-Webster.

Scharff, J. (1987). *The nature and scope of rural nursing: Distinctive characteristics.* Unpublished master's thesis, Montana State University, Bozeman.

Scharff, J. (1998). The distinctive nature and scope of rural nursing practice: Philosophical bases. In H. J. Lee (Ed), *Conceptual basis for rural nursing* (pp. 19–38). New York: Springer Publishing.

Troyer, L. E. (2000). *Rural generalist: Community-based nursing.* Unpublished master's thesis, Montana State University, Bozeman.

Stratton, T. D., Dunkin, J. W., Juhl, N., & Geller, J. M. (1995). Retainment incentives in three rural practice settings: Variations in job satisfaction among staff registered nurses. *Applied Nursing Research, 8,* (3), 73–80.

Weinert, C., & Long, K. A. (1991). The theory and research base for rural nursing practice. In A. Bushy (Ed.), *Rural nursing* (Vol. 1, pp. 21–38). Newbury Park, CA: Sage.

CHAPTER SEVENTEEN

The Rural Nursing Generalist in the Acute Care Setting: Flowing Like a River

Kathryn (Kay) Ayres Rosenthal

Nurses working in rural hospitals are characterized as expert generalists, often caring during single shifts for a diverse group of patients who would have been admitted to a specialty unit had the care occurred in an urban setting. As a generalist, however, the nurse is held to the same standards of care established by specialty nursing (e.g., operating room [OR], intensive care [ICU], obstetrics [OB], postanesthesia [PACU]). This can create struggles, opportunities, and threats to generalist nurses specific to the practice of rural nursing. In this chapter I illuminate the issues and concerns, and rewards and challenges faced by rural nurses by presenting an overview of my research (Rosenthal, 1996). I present subthemes, themes and the metatheme as well as one example of a story cocreated by me on the basis of the data I obtained. I describe implications for nursing practice, administration, education, and research.

DESIGN

I chose exploratory descriptive as the design for the study. I encouraged nurses to tell stories of their experiences working in a rural acute care hospital to illustrate the lived experience of the rural nurse generalist. The assumptions of the design include: a) the topic has not previously been studied or explored or has not been studied from the point of view of the participant or informant, and b) the participants had personal experience in, or knowledge about, the topic (Brink & Wood, 1989, p. 145).

I use narrative to present the findings. Polkinghorne (1988) defined *narrative* as the equivalent of story, the primary form by which human experience is understood and made meaningful. Narrative processes organize human experiences into meaningful episodes providing a means of increased understanding of life's events and a mechanism to verbalize unspoken aspects of life.

Research Question

What are the stories told of the lived experience of rural generalist nurses who work in an acute care hospital with fewer than twenty-five beds located in a mountain setting?

Agency Access and Setting

Two rural hospitals with fewer than 25 beds were the settings for this study. These hospitals were located in western mountain communities in the United States. Hospital A was approximately 90 minutes and Hospital B was approximately 3 hours from urban hospitals. Neither hospital selected for this study provided high technological care (e.g., cardiac catheterization, angioplasty, neurosurgery). Hospital A had computer axial taxonomy (CAT or CT) scanning capabilities. Hospital B had magnetic resonance imagery (MRI) and CT scanning.

Referrals to larger hospitals were made when technological support services were needed. Patients were sent to larger hospitals for continued treatment transported by personal car in nonacute situations, by ambulance when ground transport was appropriate, or by helicopter when time was critical. Helicopter transports took less than 30 minutes from Hospital A to reach metropolitan hospitals north or south of their location. Hospital B had fixed wing transportation that arrived in a metropolitan area within 40 minutes. Transferring patients within the "golden hour" of emergency medicine, the hour that predicts mortality and morbidity, success or failure, was easily met in normal weather situations. In typical mountain weather conditions, such as lightening storms in May and June, low cloud covering common in the winter and spring months, and intermittent wind storms throughout the year, the uncertainty of helicopter support was an ever-present issue at Hospital A. Hospital B was less affected by weather because of fixed wing navigational capabilities.

Sample

The Director of Nursing (DON) at each hospital obtained facility permission to conduct the study, identified generalist nurses who worked in multiple subspecialties within the hospital (e.g., OR, emergency department [ED], OB, medical-surgical, and gastrointestinal lab [GI]), and scheduled interviews with them. The study sample comprised 7 registered nurses (RN) and one licensed practical nurse (LPN) who agreed to participate in the study (see Table 17.1). Three nurses worked entirely in a rural setting. The other 5 nurses in the study had multiple years of experience in rural and urban settings. One of the eight nurses had rural nursing practicum as part of her nursing education. Ethical approval was obtained for the study from the University of Colorado, Denver, Review Board.

Interviews

Interviews were conversational in style and manner. Each interview began with an introduction to the lens under which I conducted the study, the research question, and a list of probing questions, which facilitated but did not prescribe the interview direction. I conducted interviews after assuring the nurses that I would maintain their confidentiality and anonymity. In these interviews, I encouraged the nurses to share their stories. I tape recorded and transcribed the interviews. I disguised specifics in the story that would aid the reader in identifying the person or place. For example, a motorcycle accident became a car accident; I changed the nurses' name

Table 17.1 Demographics

Characteristic	Hospital A nurses				Hospital B nurses			
	1	2	3	4	5	6	7	8
Age	44	66	52	39	44	51	36	56
Gender	F	F	F	F	F	F	M	F
Ethnic	C	C	C	C	C	C	C	C
Education	DIPL	DIPL	ASSOC	LPN	BSN	DIPL	ASSOC	DIPL
Rural/Clinical	N/N	N/N	N/N	Y/Y	N/N	N/N	N/N	N/N
Work status	FT	FT	FT	FT	FT	FT	FT	FT
Total years in nursing	23	40	4.5	19	22	26	3	34
Rural nursing, years	20	28	4.5	19	18	20	2	34
Career in rural nursing, %	86	70	100	100	81	86	66	100

Note: Female=F; Male=M; Caucasian=C; Education=Educ; Diploma=DIPL; Associate Degree=ASSOC; Baccalaureate=BSN; licensed practical nurse=LPN; No=N; Yes=Y; Full Time=FT); Part Time=PT; Rural nursing clinical offered in nursing program/Participated in Rural clinical=Rural/Clinical.

to a pseudonym, and ommited the highway number. I verified interviews in writing with each nurse. I collected stories until redundancy occurred and no new themes emerged.

Data Analysis

According to Brink and Wood (1989), the analysis of data for an exploratory study "requires a fluid, flexible, somewhat intuitive interaction" between the data and researcher (p. 151). Living with the data, explained as reading and rereading the transcripts, looking for what is present, absent, what fits, and what does not fit, is recommended. Data analysis for the present study had two distinct aspects. One was the identification of themes with supporting subthemes and exemplar transcripts. I sent transcripts, themes, subthemes and stories to the participants as well as faculty members for confirmation. The second aspect of data analysis was the creation of narratives, stories rewritten by me on the basis of the interviews with rural generalist nurses.

FINDINGS

Four themes emerged from the data: (a) Going With the Flow: Fluid Role; (b) Fish Out of Water: Expert to Novice; (c) Still Waters Run Deep: Self Reliance; and (d) Life in a Fish Bowl: Contextual Knowledge of Patients. I explicate briefly each of the themes here. See Rosenthal (1996) for a full description of the themes and subthemes with supporting transcript excerpts.

Going With the Flow: Fluid Role

The first theme, Fluid Role, emerged from several subthemes: (a) Flexibility was needed by the rural nurse as the workload and area of nursing care to be delivered varied based on the patients' age and diagnoses; (b) Shifting Priorities occurred throughout the rural nurse's day (e.g., the nurse in the middle of one procedure may be required to move immediately to another more urgent priority); (c) Continuity of Care was demonstrated by nurses caring for patients from ED to OR and PACU all in the same shift; (d) the Lack of 24–hour Ancillary Support forced the rural nurses to fill these roles e.g., cook, dispatcher, phone operator, laboratory and x-ray personnel on the off-shifts and weekends; (e) the Anticipatory Generosity to Limited Availability of Nursing Staff was described as off-duty RNs hearing sirens and coming to the hospital to see if help was needed; (f) the feelings of Team Support, interdisciplinary Rapport, the Give and Take of the team, and Implicit Trust were illuminated; instances of Role

Transcendence were described in which nurses may act in the role of physician until the physician arrived and the physician acted as RN in the absence of another nurse.

Fish Out of Water: Expert to Novice

The second theme, Expert to Novice, represented the dualism within the nurse's knowledge base. Although rural nurses could be experts in surgical nursing, they were concomitantly novices in other areas of nursing. Many nursing skills were transferable from one specialty to another, but some skills were specific to a certain branch of nursing. Nurses came to the rural nursing setting feeling confident of their previous knowledge base. Their confidence is challenged almost immediately because of the breadth of knowledge needed in the rural setting. The theme Expert to Novice was a compilation of the subthemes discussed by the nurses in their interviews. The rural nurses who were former urban nurses described how Urban Nurses Are in for a Big Surprise when they decide to "go rural." The nurses felt they Never Have Enough Knowledge and sometimes had to learn in the midst of actions, which they termed *Trial by Fire*. They frequently were alone in situations where they realized they were the Most Qualified; in situations where they were caught not knowing a particular skill or theory, they would Know That Next Time. Their Confidence Increased Through Certification.

Still Waters Run Deep: Self-Reliance

The third theme, Self-Reliance, emerged from subthemes of the rural nurse's ability to Thrive on Variety. One nurse commented, "I stay sane by changing my job within the facility, clinically too. I learned OB, ED, then ICU ..." instead of being threatened by it. The nurse's ability to Stay Calm in the middle of chaotic situations was described by one nurse who stated, "And I can stay very calm ... I do get flustered by things but they happen inside." Self Reliance addresses the rural nurses' realization that One is Alone; You're It in many situations, when one would like to have had another professional's guidance or support, as well as Humor and Confidence while dealing with one's own humanness. One nurse described having been taught to start intravenous lines (IVs) but not having done any. When a patient needed an IV, the DON said, "Go in and start it." And she did.

Life in a Fish Bowl: Contextual Knowledge of Patients

The final theme, Contextual Knowledge of Patients, illustrated the unique position of the rural nurses in that the majority of the patients would be personally connected to themselves, their family, or friends in the context of the community. In the urban setting, nurses working across town would rarely care for patients that they knew personally. In the rural setting, all employees were known; if they or their children came to the hospital for service, the rural nurses provided the care. Because the community was small, the odds of caring for an acquaintance or family member are greatly increased. That can be terrifying for rural nurses. Even the tourists could be connected to the rural nurse because they were often visitors of friends of the nurse.

Subthemes of Contextual Knowledge include: (a) caring for a Known Person, (b) the Discomfort of Caring for a Friend, (c) the Positive Aspects of Knowing the Patient, (d) and how knowing the patient Touches Your Heart and Soul. One nurse described dealing with rape cases and how upsetting that was. "Almost everything that goes on in a rural hospital this size, it touches one's heart and soul really, because you know everybody or almost everybody."

Metatheme

The metatheme, Flowing Like a River, emerged from reviewing the transcripts, the four themes, and their subthemes. The metatheme is an image that united all the findings of the study and provided an overall impression of the lived experience of rural nurses.

STORIES OF RURAL NURSING

The creative outcomes of the interviews of rural nurses were a compilation of six stories explicating the lived experience of rural nurses. I wrote the stories in the first person so that emotions could be expressed. They were based on the data but certain aspects of the stories were fictionalized, (i.e., names of participants, date, time, and place.) However, the substance of the stories' situations and events were true to the transcribed interviews. "Injured? Dying? This Can't be Happening!" reflected the nurses' stories of caring for patients who are family members or acquaintances. "Man, Am I a Good Metro Nurse! I'll Show Those Rural Nurses a Thing or Two" reflected interview content from former urban nurses who moved to rural areas thinking it would be easy because they know more than their rural colleagues but find they have a lot to learn. "Code Blue Boots" reflected the training scenarios practiced to help prepare staff for "what-if" situations that will eventually occur while they were on duty. "We're All in This Together" reflected the community collegiality between the school and the hospital in the rural setting. "Orientation. You Call This Orientation?" described how despite orientation or lack thereof rural nurses became oriented to the variety of roles. I present here excerpts from one story, "Western Slant."

Western Slant

It was Labor Day. The town was hosting multiple events. The parade of horses, antique cars, motorcycles always left us short staffed. We had three nurses scheduled and a fourth on call for the Emergency Department (ED). The day started out quiet enough. Then we heard a vehicle in the ambulance bay.

It was Rancher Bob, former board member of the hospital, very prominent business man in the community, director of the city planning committee. He had his horse trailer blocking the ambulance bay and wanted our help. Of all things, he wanted his horse's leg x-rayed. Bring out the portable x-ray machines, work quickly we need to keep the bay open for "real" emergencies! I couldn't believe my eyes and ears. I've worked in the rural setting for three years now and knew the local vet sometimes borrowed operating room (OR) lights, some drugs from the pharmacy but this really caught me off guard. As we were finishing up, the ambulance pagers blared.

"Multiple motor vehicle accident (MVA) on the pass, two vans with multiple passengers involved in a head on." Primary and secondary crews were being dispatched. They asked, "Could we please coordinate the staffing of the third vehicle?"

"No." I respond. "They are staffing the parade in the event of injuries."

A flurry of thoughts enter my head. We need to get that horse out of the ambulance bay. Start calling the disaster roster list. As I think of staffing, it hits me what a mess this is going to be. We'll need help and most of the employees are either at the parade, at work already or out of town for the holiday. Well, just start calling.

Admitting tells us that there is a husband and wife in the lobby, the wife has an ankle injury. "Tell them we are setting up the ER for a major car accident and they are going to have to wait." Tossing her an ice pack and pillow, I add, "Here, put an ice pack on the ankle, take this pillow to elevate her leg." Calling out after her I ask her to, "Ask how much discomfort or pain she is in and let me know if it's a lot. We'll come out and check her as soon as we can." I say somewhat tersely.

"Is that horse out of the ambulance bay?" I speak into the room.

"Yes," comes a reply. Hearing Cindy in the corner of the room and seeing her setting things up I delegate: "Cindy, can you go look at this ankle in the lobby ... ? I'll finish opening the trauma tray and I'll pull the chest tube trays while you're gone ..."

Report is called in, one Black (Dead on Arrival, DOA), one Red (Critical), permission to chopper from the site received. Six Yellow (Unstable), and two Green (Stable, "Walking Wounded"). Two nurses from Home

Health Care have arrived. I assign one to the morgue. I assign the other to the two patients triaged as "greens" telling her, "Take them to the ... chemotherapy room, that way if you need to lay them down, the chemo chairs stretch out."

A nursing home aide comes to command center, how can she help? "Go to the Med Surg floor and ask for a census and status report from one of the nurses." I recognize I am not using please or thank you, I'm just barking out commands.... OK. I've got six nurses in the ED. Next person that comes in can cover the floor or switch places with one of the floor nurses in the ED. Patients one and two arrive. Ten minutes later patient three arrives. We're starting IVs, hanging blood and IV fluid, inserting chest tubes, foleys, nasogastric tubes, recording assessments, doing EKG's, x-rays, running labs.

The patient in the lobby is what?! Complaining about the what?! The wait! Tell them we're sorry but we have to take care of the critical patients in this accident first and they are just going to have to wait.

Patients four and five arrive. Another nurse, who just happened to hear the ambulance sirens by her house came in to see what was going on. Great!

"Go assess the patients on the floor and see where they are at with meds, treatments, are they doing OK? There's an aide there that can help you."

"Wait," one of the floor nurses says, "You start this IV, I can't get it and I'll go check the patients on the floor, I know them already."

"Good idea. Let's go." Patient six arrives and is no longer a yellow, they are retriaged a red and we need a chopper now.

There are no more carts, I thought maintenance was bringing one from the basement? Where is it? ...

The x-ray technologist asks, "Are we done with all the x-rays? Can we do the lady in the lobby? Hey, who are all those people in the lobby anyway?"

"What do you mean?" I go to the lobby and there are at least twenty people there. I quietly tell the admitting clerk "Let's get some traffic control here." ...

... Seeing a housekeeper walk in I send him to command center and tell them to assign him as Security. ...

Finally the chopper arrives and after assessing the patient themselves, listening to report, they are out of the building. One down, five to go.

"Let's see if we can transport the two patients in room four in the same ambulance. Patient #4–1 needs to be transported to Metro OR and patient #4–2 needs to get a CT scan." I say ..."

I'll go see them (the greens in chemo) when we get the yellow's taken care of," says ED doc number two.

The ambulance bay doors open and it's one of the local family practitioners walking in, "Need any help? I was at the parade and heard a lot of commotion, what's going on?"

"Here," Jane calls out, "we've had a major MVA, go see the patient in five, possible head injury and rib fracture." She tells him, "x-rays have been done and are in the room. Let us know if they need to go to Metro for a CT or MRI."

He comes out after assessing the patient and says, "Let's admit to our hospital and just watch closely." he announces calmly.

"OK," I say, "But you're taxing my staffing. Almost everyone is here right now and nights will only have three nurses on. How close are we going to have to watch him?" We decide if he's the only ... yellow ... that we keep we'll have adequate staffing.

"Come see the patient in bay one, he might have abdominal injuries from his seat belt." calls Cindy. We decide to send him to Metro Trauma ED for abdominal CT and surgical consult. We'll send bay three with him for a surgical consult unless Orthopedics can come up and do surgery here. Then we reconsider, a C-arm (specialized x-ray equipment) will probably be needed so we better send him down.

"Let's send the two kids to Children's Metro, their injuries aren't too bad but they can watch them closer." ED doc one yells to the unit secretary.

She starts dialing Children's Metro. "ER or ICU?" she clarifies.

"ER, and pull some antidumping law (COBRA) forms and start copying the chart as soon as you can. Did anyone fax those labs to Metro OR when they came back?" No one knows. Lab is paged to fax the results and copy the charts of the kids so they can go down by ambulance. It's interesting how all departmental lines, minimal as they are, disappear in an emergency, x-ray is copying charts, getting maps for friends in the lobby so they can meet them at Children's Metro, cleaning the cart when bay two leaves by chopper. The paramedics and EMTs are all helping with vitals, writing the nurses' notes as dictated by the RN's assessment; helping hold legs while foleys are inserted, and helping cut off clothes so we can really see the extent of injuries.

Now, back to deal with the greens, ED doc number one goes to evaluate and hopefully discharge to home. ED doc number two is debriefing with the ED staff.

"Hey," I call out, "let's do this later, get this ankle out of the lobby before the prima donna or her husband strokes from waiting, her x-rays are over there."

Finally, the ED is cleaned out but the husband of the woman with the hurt ankle has come unglued. We've called the police department back in to remove him from the ED. The officer approaches the doctor and the husband who are yelling at each other at the top of their lungs. The doctor pulls the officer's pistol, aims it at the husband and says, "You can just get out of my ER." We all stand there flabbergasted! In Metro ED it's the patients or visitors who draw the guns, here's it's the doc!

"CALM DOWN EVERYONE" yells the police officer. He takes his gun from the doctor and secures it in his holster. I grab the arm of the ED doc and kind of push/pull him into room five, closing the door behind us and tell him to "Stay." By now I'm visibly shaking. It's been enough to deal with the accident to now have to deal with this. The police officer has taken the husband outside and has threatened to take him to jail if he doesn't calm down.

Cindy has called the debriefing team, but since it's a holiday she had to leave a message, they'll get back to us Tuesday. ED doc number one has discharged the greens downstairs and has agreed to put a splint on the lady with the broken ankle and discharge her.

In the meanwhile, we are cleaning the ER and getting ready for the next round just in case. Happy Holiday! NOT. The safety director/Certified Registered Nurse Anesthetist (CRNA) says, "Let's write this one up so we don't have to have a fake disaster drill." We all agree! This one was enough for the whole year.

"But YOU write it up," calls ED doc number two from room five. He is shaking his head and says he's "Off to the showers." He's cooled off and embarrassed, we nickname him "Quick Draw McGraw" ... behind his back and all start laughing when he is out of hearing range. We hope he was out of hearing range!

DISCUSSION

In the story, "Western Slant," written with actual interview data, I incorporate the reality of rural nursing on a holiday shift. In the story I demonstrated several of the themes and components of the metatheme. Going With the Flow: Fluid Role was evidenced by the nurses' flexibility, changing priorities, limited staff, and the team support during the emergency. Fish Out of Water: Expert to Novice was demonstrated by the nurse on the floor, possibly an expert in OB, coming to ED to help where she may be a novice. Still Waters Run Deep: Self Reliance is demonstrated by the variety of the situation, the need to stay calm during the emergency, and the sense of humor exhibited by the staff to survive the stress of the situation. Life in a Fish Bowl: Contextual Knowledge of Patients was not clearly illuminated in this story as victims were not identified as family members or visitors of any of the employees.

Implications for Nursing Practice

The nurses described characteristics of successful rural nurses during the interviews. These characteristics included "flexibility," "emotional strength," and "being able to ask for help from a coworker or knowing when advice is needed from a Metro ED, ICU, or burn unit." The successful rural nurse "cannot be afraid to ask questions." The rural nurse needs personal accountability to "learn from the situation because there are times when she must go ahead and do something, carry out a new procedure, or administer a medication for the first time, when there is no one else to ask or to help." The nurse who "looks up the information before or after the situation" will be prepared for the next time. The rural nurse who is able to "recognize skills and knowledge of others" and "tap into their strengths without feeling that she is less proficient or less of a nurse for not knowing" will be more successful in the rural setting. Furthermore, the nurse who is determined to succeed in the setting and "desires to live in a rural community" will have a greater rate of success. Nurses are bound to be "self-critical" and constantly assess their work. The nurse should be "confident but not overly so."

Rural nurses need to love the challenge of learning, the thrill of doing it all, and being a "jack-of-all-trades." Nurses who "thrive on variety" and do not like the comfort and security of established routines may excel in rural nursing. Rural nurses need to know how to get along with people because the ability to build relationships and establish community rapport is crucial. Tact and assertiveness and being a team player are skills needed by rural nurses. Being able to read instructions and policies and procedures in front of patients during a crisis may be required. Rural nurses must be practical, "have common sense," "know how to triage, set priorities, delegate, and use good judgment." Having the ability to implement theory and be able to turn knowledge into action even if they have never done the procedure before will enhance the nurses' confidence.

Nurses may act as physicians in the absence of physicians, starting the resuscitation procedures, administering medications per Advance Cardiac Life Care protocol, and determining what IV solution to hang before the physician arrives. Nurses may begin appropriate diagnostic tests, laboratory and x-ray, so that when physicians arrive they will have the information needed to immediately begin treating the patient.

The nurses spoke of rewards and benefits of rural nursing. One reward identified was "having time to do the little things for patients. To be able to sit with the patient and talk about what is really going on in their life. To give back rubs and offer foot soaks." Because there is less hierarchy in the rural setting, nurses' voices are more easily heard. Nurses can make a difference and feel ownership for the rural hospital. Although there are few positions for promotion, nurses who want to learn will identify many opportunities for lateral promotion into different clinical and nonclinical opportunities.

Implications for Nursing Administration

Cross training rural nurses so they feel prepared for any situation is a critical aspect of nursing administration. Financial support for training as well as providing multiple support systems is essential. The nurses recommended support systems that enable the rural nurse to function with limited resources. Systems were also recommended to relieve nurses during traumatic events when the situation involves a family member. A system to cover extreme fluctuations in census during popular community events (e.g., a rodeo) or sick calls and holidays is needed. With no ability to "divert" the patient to a different unit, to a different floor, or to a different hospital within town, systems are needed to support the nurses on duty.

The stories (Rosenthal, 1996) can be used as orientation scenarios to help decrease fear of "what if," who might come in the ED doors or be admitted to the floor. New nurses will need assistance with planning, identifying personnel to be called in, appropriate supplies to be pulled for use in an emergency, and determining division of tasks. These scenarios will assist to prepare rural nurses for multiple possibilities and to preplan what their responses could be.

The nurses in this study identified a need for assertiveness training and conflict resolution skills so they could confront coworkers and physicians while maintaining a collegial relationship. Professional and practice organizations, such as the Emergency Nurses' Association, the state's nurses' association, American Association of Critical Care Nurses, and Sigma Theta Tau International, can link rural nurses with other nurses for information exchange and support (Long & Weinert, 1992).

Implications for Nursing Education

Several implications for nursing education arose from this study. They include increasing faculty and students' sensitivity to the unique and challenging aspects of rural nursing and providing insight into the lives of rural nurses, particularly the diversity, ambiguity, and uncertainty of rural practice. Further implications for nursing education encompass exchange programs between rural and urban hospitals and universities. For example, university faculty could provide in-services to rural nurses and urban nursing students could be assigned to rural clinical rotations. Urban nurses might provide educational outreach (e.g., trauma courses offered on site at the rural setting). Contracts between urban and rural facilities enable rural nurses to practice in specialized urban settings to strengthen skills.

The stories (Rosenthal, 1996) composed by me from the interviews can be used by nursing faculty to ask nursing students how they would respond to the situations. Or the stories could be used as exemplar cases in ethics discussions. Benner (1991) calls for an increase in storytelling in both practice and in ethical discussions. There are no right or wrong answers to be determined from the stories, only multiple possibilities, multiple realities, and multiple choices that could be discussed between faculty and students.

Implication for Nursing Research

Implications of this study for future research include further narrative inquiries and expansion of the stories to develop rural nursing theory. Gadow (1990) suggested "The cultivation of personal knowing as a form of inquiry may be the most important contribution of nursing to the human sciences" (p.167). Perhaps this study will encourage others to expand their inquiry into personal knowing and further ask, "What is it like?" regarding other aspects of nursing.

Future research may focus on what sociologists would call deviant case analysis. Strauss and Corbin (1990) discussed negative cases and stated, "the negative or alternative cases tell us that something about this instance is different. Following through on these differences adds density and variation to our theory" (p.109). Research questions might include: What are the stories of unsuccessful rural generalist nurses? What are the stories of rural generalist nurses who remain in the setting but are not comfortable in the generalist role, who stay in the setting not by choice but because of family obligations? In this study, the DON recruited successful rural nurses. Altering the sample selection method may reveal totally different perceptions of the lived experience of rural nurses. Repeating this study with nurses from other rural settings would provide additional insight into the lived experience of the rural nurse generalist.

In future studies, another style of interview or research methodology could be used. I did not share my personal stories with the participants. It would be an interesting comparison to repeat the study with the researcher engaging in the interviews instead of staying passive. Being more openly empathic might encourage nurses to share more threatening stories, to further expand on stories or offer insight into why treating a known patient was so difficult. Another possibility would be a focus group of rural nurses. This technique might reveal other stories that are stimulated by participation of other group members.

SUMMARY

Conducting this study generated a rich data source. It examined a setting rarely studied that encompasses a focus on patient care and nursing services. It adds to the knowledge base of rural nursing practice and of nursing administrators and sensitizes nursing educators and others to the needs of rural leaders.

REFERENCES

Benner, P. (1991). The role of experience, narrative, and community in skilled ethical comportment. *ANS, 14*(2), 1–21.

Brink, P., & Wood, M. (1989). *Advanced design in nursing research*. Newbury Park, CA: Sage.

Gadow, S. (1990). Response to "Personal knowing: Evolving research and practice." *Scholarly Inquiry for Nursing Practice: An International Journal, 4,* 167–170.

Jager, B. (1975). Theorizing journeying, dwelling. *Phenomenological Psychology, 11,* 235–260.

Long, K. A., & Weinert, C. (1992). Rural nursing: Developing the theory base. In Winstead-Fry, P., Tiffany, J., & Shippee-Rice, R. (Eds), *Rural health nursing* (pp. 389–406). New York: NLN.

Polkinghorne, D. (1988). *Narrative knowing and the human sciences*. Albany: State University of New York Press.

Rosenthal, K. (1996). *Rural nursing: An exploratory narrative description*. Unpublished doctoral dissertation, University of Colorado, Denver, CO.

Strauss, A., & Corbin, J. (1990). *Basics of qualitative research*. Newbury Park: Sage.

CHAPTER EIGHTEEN

Men Working as Rural Nurses: Land of Opportunity

Chad O'Lynn

A growing body of literature suggests that rural residency is associated with poorer health outcomes than urban residence (Center on an Aging Society, 2003; Goins & Mitchell, 1999; Kumar, Acanfora, Hennessy, & Kalache, 2001; National Institute of Nursing Research, 1995). The suggested reasons for this disparity generally relate to barriers of access to health services because of distance and lack of available providers in rural areas. One strategy to address the health disparities in rural settings is to recruit and retain and then to support health care providers, including nurses. However, amidst the rural health literature, relatively little has been published describing the experiences of nurses who care for rural dwellers.

This gap in the literature is significant, in that recruitment and retention of nurses in rural practice is challenging and more difficult than in urban practice because of rural wages, paucity of jobs for spouses, and the negative perceptions of rural nursing (Bushy, 2002; Hopkins & Domrose, 2001; Long, 2000; Trossman, 2001; Vukic & Keddy, 2002). This challenge serves as an overlay for an already well-documented nationwide

This research was funded by Montana State University-Bozeman College of Nursing, Block Grant Program. The author acknowledges Helen J. Lee and Charlene A. Winters for their assistance with this study.

nursing shortage. To meet projected vacancies, the profession has begun to implement general recruitment strategies targeting groups such as ethnic minorities and men (Buerhaus, Staiger, & Auerbach, 2000; Gordon, 2002). Increasing the number of men in the nursing profession will assist in meeting the demands for future nurses and in improving the diversity of the nursing workforce (American Association of Colleges of Nursing, 1997, 2001; Anders, 1993; Davis & Bartfay, 2001; Sullivan, 2000; Villeneuve, 1994). However, virtually nothing is known about the experiences of men in rural nursing and what recruitment strategies might be appropriate to attract men to practice in rural settings.

Because men only comprised 5.4% of the U.S. RN workforce in 2000, one may assume that there is opportunity for increased recruitment (Spratley, Johnson, Sochalski, Fritz, & Spencer, 2001). However, there is some suspicion that men leave nursing shortly after entering the profession at higher rates than do women (Davis & Bartfay, 2001). The reason for this is unclear. O'Lynn (2004) noted that men in nursing felt that their basic nursing education program did not prepare them well for working with primarily female coworkers.

To recruit and retain men into rural nursing practice, a better understanding of rural nursing from the masculine perspective is needed. This understanding will assist in the development of gender-appropriate strategies to recruit men to critical shortage areas, as well as assist in the development of gender-appropriate supports to retain men in rural nursing. My purpose in this study was to examine the experiences and perspectives of men working as rural nurses. I asked two research questions: What are the experiences of men working as rural nurses? What would be appropriate strategies to recruit and retain men in rural nursing practice?

BACKGROUND AND SIGNIFIGANCE

Limitations of the Literature on Rural Male Nurses

Houde (2002) and Thompson (2002) report that invisibility of men occurs when researchers do not include men in study samples or when data generated from men is folded into the data generated by a majority of women. Most studies noted in this book do not include men. As such, the findings from these studies have questionable generalizability to men working or considering working in rural nursing. No study located for review described rural nursing practice from a male perspective. In the current study, I addressed this gap by providing an initial understanding of the experiences of men in rural nursing practice and how men may be recruited and retained to work in rural communities.

Significance

The implications of the invisibility of men in the nursing literature are profound. A review of literature by O'Lynn (2004) showed that men experience nursing education and nursing practice differently than women do. These differences stem from a variety of reasons, including historical discrimination of men in nursing, differing gender roles, and different approaches to caregiving. If men are to be recruited and retained in rural practice settings, strategies developed from the current understanding of rural nursing practice may not be gender appropriate.

METHODS

I used the hermeneutic phenomenology in the Heideggerian tradition for this study. According to Koch (1995) and Benner (1999), hermeneutic phenomenology assumes a constructivist reality, in which people encounter phenomena with uniquely individualized preunderstanding and historical knowledge that cannot be stripped away. Phenomena are experienced and understood in a highly contextualized and interpreted world. Consequently, reality is not absolute and cannot be reduced to essential truths, although individuals may have many similar experiences (Koch, 1995; Lincoln & Guba, 2000). From an epistemological perspective, hermeneutic phenomenology assumes that knowledge is cocreated among individuals. The researcher cannot be an objective observer, but rather serves as a vehicle through which understanding occurs from transactions with others and existing world contexts can only be corrected and modified (Benner). Hermeneutic phenomenology is a research approach appropriate for exploration of poorly understood phenomena and the meaning they hold for persons.

Procedure

I used open-ended interviews with six men working as RNs in frontier communities in Montana. Inclusion criteria for participation were (a) RN licensure in Montana, (b) employment in a frontier county and a community of less than 5,000 residents, and (c) the ability to speak English. I obtained informed consent from all participants. The Human Subjects Committee of Montana State University-Bozeman and the Institutional Review Board of Oregon Health & Science University approved this study. I completed the study as partial requirement for a research practicum credit at Oregon Health & Science University.

I recruited a purposive sample of participants from a list of all RNs licensed in Montana supplied by the State Board of Nursing. This list provided only the names and residential addresses of the nurses. It provided no indication of the nurse's sex or ethnicity or race. I examined the list for names of nurses believed to be male residing in frontier counties. If more than one nurse resided in a community, one name was highlighted for enrollment. The rationale for this procedure was to ensure maximum representation of rural communities in the sample. From the screening of the list, I identified 30 potential participants and sent letters in the spring of 2004 inviting them to participate. Seven letters were returned stamped "No longer at this address/No forwarding address." Of the 21 remaining potential participants, seven agreed to participate. However, one withdrew from the study prior to his interview.

The 6 men in the sample were Caucasian. The men's age range was from 34–58 years ($M = 40.7$ years). Their years of experience as a nurse was less than 1–30 years ($M = 11.4$ years). All had some nursing experience in an urban setting at some point during their careers. The range of time spent working as rural nurses was less than 1–20 years ($M = 7.7$ years). Five worked in rural hospitals as staff nurses. The 6th worked as a pediatric nurse practitioner in a primary care clinic. Nursing was a second career for all of the participants.

The size range of communities in which the men worked was 940–2,874 residents ($M = 1,668$; U.S. Bureau of the Census, 2002). Two of the six communities were located on or near Indian reservations. The major economic activity of five of the communities were ranching and farming. One community relied on tourism as it was located near Yellowstone National Park.

Two participants lived in the communities in which they worked. The other 4 participants commuted 340, 129, 53, and 35 miles one-way to the agencies where they worked. The participants working in hospitals not in their communities grouped their shifts, staying in town either at the hospital or in a motel and returning home during their off days. One participant had been doing this for 20 years.

The hospitals in which five participants worked were designated CAHs (range-e.g. 4–15 beds). All had long-term care facilities either attached to the hospital or located next door. None of the participants worked as staff in these long-term care facilities at the time of the interviews. All hospitals were served by volunteer ambulance services. As such, local ambulance availability was not guaranteed on a 24–hour basis. Participants noted that it was not uncommon for patients to present to the emergency department who had transported themselves or were transported by family or friends or by the local sheriff. The nearest emergency services from these hospitals were located 23–65 miles away (*M* = 37 miles). However, the hospital located 23 miles from another emergency facility was accessible only by secondary roads, with a usual driving time of 45 minutes in the best of weather. All hospitals had access to helicopter transport to a regional medical center. Although some had improved heliport pads nearby, one helicopter service was 7 miles away. However, if needed, there was a grassy area next to the hospital upon which a helicopter could land in good weather. For the helicopter to land safely, the participant needed to ensure that the area was clear of debris and turn on the outdoor lights if it was dark.

Data Collection and Data Analysis

I conducted interviews over the telephone at a time and date selected by the participants that lasted 45–100 minutes in length. Consistent with phenomenological methods, I used loosely structured interviews, which allowed for free discussion of topics in which the participant or I deemed relevant. I asked some general (grand-tour) questions of all the participants to obtain information on rural nursing, gender, and recruitment. These questions included (a) What is rural nursing? (b) What is your typical work day like? (c) What is it like being a man working in rural nursing? (d) Why do you work in a rural area? and (e) What would attract men to work as rural nurses?

I tape-recorded all interviews, then transcribed them. I analyzed transcripts sequentially as each interview occurred. I read transcripts in-total to gain a general perspective. I then analyzed each transcript section-by-section for codes. I used direct quotes when possible for codes to best represent the participants' responses. I then organized codes into categories that represented emerging themes. I compared categories and themes from each transcript to each other to determine similarities and differences among the transcripts.

After I completed and analyzed interviews with 4 participants, I noted a redundancy in themes. However, the transcript of 1 participant, the pediatric nurse practitioner, included details of his duties and work day that were very different from the other transcripts. These differences were most likely reflective of the fundamental differences between the nurse practitioner and the staff nurse role. On the other hand, his discussion of other aspects of rural living and his rural clientele generated findings similar to the transcripts of the rural staff nurse participants. Because of this, I decided to include the transcript but did not pursue further exploration of the practice characteristics of rural advanced practice nurses.

After I conducted the first four interviews, I gave copies of the uncoded transcripts to two experienced rural nurse researchers and a graduate student who resided in a rural community. These peer auditors, working independently, examined these interviews for categories. They contrasted categories with the categories from the original data analysis. Although there were slight differences in the wording of the categories, the meaning of the categories were similar.

With redundancy in the transcripts and similarity in the categories derived from the peer auditors, I enrolled two additional rural hospital staff nurses and interviewed them to seek saturation of the themes. The findings were consistent with the previous findings and I did not conduct any more interviews.

RESULTS

Generally, the participants painted a very positive view of rural nursing and the rural environments in which they worked. For the men who were seasoned nurses, all were happy with rural nursing and had no plans for relocation. The men who were relatively new to rural nursing demonstrated a general excitement and enthusiasm with the characteristics and challenges of rural nursing practice. Although opportunities did not appear in the transcripts, it was an overarching theme. The term reflected the positive accounts provided by the participants and may reflect the desired perspective of a potential nurse recruiter looking to fill vacant nursing positions in rural communities. The specific themes of opportunities include (a) expanded practice, (b) autonomy, (c) meaningful relationships, (d) challenge, (e) rural rewards, and (f) recruitment.

Opportunity for Expanded Practice

All men described rural nursing as generalist practice that extended beyond the typical generalist practice employed by float or resource pool nurses in larger facilities. Typically, in larger hospitals, nurses who work on multiple units develop generalist skills for select patient populations. Rarely do nurses working in larger hospital care for all the types of patients seen in that hospital. In rural nursing, the men stated that they take care of pediatrics to geriatrics, emergency care to long-term care, all within the same shift, every shift. The term *jack-of-all-trades* was used by several of the participants. One participant described his typical shift this way:

> Well, I guess a good example would be not too long ago, we had a serious motor vehicle accident involving a motorcyclist that we were stabilizing and trying to transport elsewhere. At the same time, we had a mom and a newborn baby ... postpartum patient, and then with all

that, we had an ambulance call with an 89–year old patient who had
respiratory distress who died on us that night … In the meantime, we
had two or three patients down the hall, one was on a cardiac monitor,
while another was just … I don't remember what the other one was, but
you know, it's every night, you can see everything all in one night.

Four participants stated they were the only RN on duty, accompanied
by a nurse's aide. As such, all skilled procedures and care coordination
were completed by them for all of the patients present during their shift.

In addition to the expanded patient population of the rural nurse, all
participants described the expanded role of the rural nurse. The specific
duties of each of the participants varied depending upon his workplace,
but all discussed the completion of roles typically done by ancillary staff
in larger hospitals. These roles included emergency department assistant,
respiratory therapist, ward clerk, billing clerk, phlebotomist, electrocar-
diograph technician, security officer, central supply clerk, pharmacy technician, community educator, social worker, and ambulance personnel. The
men noted that as the nurse on duty, they were the "only game in town."
One participant described the time-consuming task of taking inventory of
all medications and treatments provided to a patient during the previous
24–hour period for billing purposes. Another participant indicated that
the RN also served as the hospital's security officer. Another participant
provided the following description.

> Of course, in that facility, we do all the paperwork. We do the patient
> charts, we write out the lab slips. Sometimes if lab's not there, we go
> ahead and do the blood draw … We basically do all the ward clerk du-
> ties. We do all the transfer paperwork. We dispense medications from
> what we call the pharmacy. We don't have a pharmacy … Well, actu-
> ally, we have the hospital pharmacy, but we're it as far as dispensing
> and keeping track of what we have and what needs ordering and that
> kind of stuff. Of course, there's a lot of paperwork there involved in
> tracking, you know, what medication is going to what patient and that
> kind of thing … We copy paperwork. We make sure we have insurance
> information. We do all the HIPPA privacy paperwork, you know, I
> mean we'll cook the meals if need be. We pretty much are there to do
> whatever needs doing.

The men discussed a blending of the roles noted earlier, but in particular, the blending of roles between medicine and nursing. This blending
occurred most frequently in the emergency room and involved tasks such
as initiating treatments and diagnostic work while waiting for the physician to arrive. However, all participants noted that they were practicing
within their scope of practice as defined by the State of Montana.

Despite the seemingly overwhelming burden patient diversity and expanded roles might create, participants noted the benefits (and hence, opportunities) of these characteristics of rural nursing. One participant stated that working in a rural hospital was "less frustrating" than a larger hospital because he did not have to wait on other health care personnel to come and do their task for a patient before he could move forward with nursing care. "Instead," stated another participant, "you just do it yourself." Several participants described the expanded roles as a way to become more involved with their patients, and thus, become more knowledgeable about their individual care needs. They indicated that nurses may treat a patient in the emergency room, admit that patient to a hospital bed, take comprehensive and holistic care of that patient for several days, then work with that patient as they transition to a swing bed or are discharged to the community. The participants criticized the care received by patients in larger hospitals as being disjointed and poorly coordinated, because patients receive care by numerous providers and disciplines as they progress through a hospital stay. As such, the participants felt that the patients in rural hospitals receive more personalized care.

Opportunity for Autonomy

All participants described the increased level of autonomy enjoyed by rural nurses compared with their nonrural colleagues. Several of the men specifically used the term *autonomy,* whereas others used the terms *independence, having more leeway,* or *freer to make decisions.* One participant noted that rural nursing is a "self-driven practice." All described increased autonomy as a benefit of rural nursing practice.

Autonomy was categorized in two ways: (a) greater freedom to make decisions impacting patient care and (b) greater freedom to use one's own work routines. The participants described using nursing judgment in making revisions to an individual patient's plan of care more freely than they had experienced while working in larger hospitals. Several noted that rural nurses are able to request needed supplies, initiate protocols, or deliver necessary treatments that were once commonplace in nursing practice, but are now becoming increasingly dependent upon the decisions of other professionals (e.g., respiratory therapist required to initiate incentive spirometry). The greater autonomy described by the participants suggests greater integrity of the domains of collaborative and independent nursing practice, whereas the trend in larger hospitals may be increasing the domain of dependent nursing practice.

Some participants described the freedom to set one's own schedule and routines on any given shift as a positive experience. Because they usually worked with only one other individual, how and when specific tasks were to be accomplished during a shift was negotiated. The freedom to set work routines was not only desirable, but necessary to provide the flexibility for unpredicted emergency room visits and patient admissions. On hospital units with more staff, an individual nurse has much less freedom for establishing routines, as these types of decisions will impact a larger group of workers and may conflict with preestablished unit routines and cultures. It is interesting that with a perceived increased level of autonomy, none of the participants noted autonomy-based conflicts with coworkers. Instead, the participants described how staff worked together better than in larger hospitals, hence, described more meaningful relationships with coworkers.

Opportunity for Meaningful Relationships

All participants described at length the improved ability to develop and maintain positive and meaningful relationships in rural practice settings with coworkers, clients, and the community. With coworkers, the men described the higher level of teamwork than they had experienced in urban settings. One participant noted,

> Basically, the biggest thing I found with rural nursing is the teamwork. When I worked in [urban setting] for so many doctors, you never really got to know any of them. I mean, there were some that were easier to work with than others, but you didn't get to know them very well. And in a rural community, your doctors and nurses really work together as a team. They have to because there are only so many of you.

This teamwork not only included nurses and physicians, but all health care workers. Several participants praised the nurse's aides with whom they worked. Because they were sometimes busy in the emergency room, participants relied upon their aides to "keep an eye on the other patients" for them. They noted the skill and dedication of their aides. The reliance upon and admiration for their aides led to a higher level of trust than they had experienced with the aides with whom they had worked in larger hospitals.

Because there were fewer employees and more frequent contact with other employees, participants stated that they really "got to know" the people with whom they worked. Teamwork was demonstrated by everyone "pitching in and helping out" and doing whatever it takes to "get the job done." As one participant noted,

> If we have something major going on, generally the ambulance crew is there to help. They can do CPR, help start IV's. Usually if it's something major, when the ambulance crew brings them in, they will stay and help.

All participants had access to an on-call nurse or nurse at the nursing home that they could call for assistance. Also, physicians and physician assistants were able to get to the hospital in a very short period of time when needed. This readiness to help each other was such that none of the participants felt isolated when working at the hospital.

Participants commented on how patient the staff and physicians were when asked questions and how willing they were to teach. This milieu facilitated teamwork and collaboration, maintained trust among the staff, created a climate of mutual respect, and enhanced camaraderie. And although two participants noted there were occasional conflicts ("everyone is human"), none reported troubled relationships with coworkers that eroded teamwork.

Another benefit of working in a rural practice is direct access to management. Small numbers of staff in the hospitals meant few, if any, layers of middle management that separated frontline workers from hospital administration. One participant sat on the hospital's foundation board; he stated he was able to bring representation directly from the patient care staff to hospital decision makers. Such access can translate into beneficial power that directly affects the nurses' work environments.

All participants talked about meaningful relationships with their patients and with the communities in which they worked. Relationships with patients and communities have been described as inherently different than those in urban settings because of the lack of anonymity many rural health care providers experience (Lee, 1998). Lack of anonymity makes it difficult for rural health care providers to maintain professional role boundaries (Lee; Scharff, 1998). However, all participants in this study described familiarity with their patients as a benefit and improved their ability to provide quality care. One participant stated,

> Generally, patients coming in . . . if they recognize somebody, if they know somebody, then they are more confident. They feel more comfortable, you know, and more confident in the care. I don't know how many times that I've had people say that. They come into the ER or they're patients in the hospital and they go, "Oh, it's so nice to see someone I recognize." You know, but it's actually a real benefit for the patients.

Rural nurses "treat generations of families." For example, a woman may be admitted to the hospital. One month later, her son may come to the ER with an injury. Several months later, a grandmother is admitted, and so on. Because of the small population, each rural nurse can impact a relatively large percentage of the community, and unlike urban settings where nurses may never see their patients again, in rural areas a nurse may encounter former patients several times a week at the store, a high school sporting event, etc. Participants did not seem burdened by off-duty contacts from the community.

Several participants remarked how supportive the community was of the hospital. Examples of the support included voluntarily raising taxes to support the local hospital, holding fundraisers to purchase an up-to-date ambulance, stopping by to visit patients and cheer them up, and volunteering a few hours to "do anything that we might need help getting done."

Opportunities for Challenge

All participants remarked that rural nursing was challenging. One stated, "The first eight months were tough.... REALLY tough." Most challenges stemmed from the realities of working with an expanded patient population and in an expanded practice role. In addition, the increased accountability required by working in multiple roles created additional challenges that the men felt were not as pronounced in nonrural practice settings. Such challenges require that rural nurses be flexible, have excellent triage and prioritization skills, and have broad-based nursing knowledge supplemented by emergency, critical care, and trauma certifications. Preparation for the unexpected was seen as crucial by the participants. One noted, "You don't see a lot of everything, but you see a little bit of everything a lot."

However, despite the challenges of rural nursing, all participants expressed a sense of pride in their accomplishments and their skills. One noted that when urban nurses come to a rural setting, they are amazed at the talent and versatility of rural nurses. Another who was new to nursing commented on how much better trained and skilled he was than his former classmates who were working in highly specialized urban practices. Another noted that because of his skill set and experience, he could go "just about anywhere" and be an asset to a potential employer.

Another challenge mentioned by the participants was maintaining confidentiality. As stated previously, some community members are actively involved in hospital activities. In addition, one participant commented that the stereotypes of small towns as "everyone knowing everyone's business" and "there are no secrets in a small town" are true. However, maintaining patient confidentiality was not particularly difficult, as long as nurses stayed vigilant. One participant stated, "You just know that you don't talk about certain things. If someone is persistent in finding out information, you just say 'I'm sorry, I can't share that information.'"

Opportunities for Rural Rewards

I asked each participant why they chose to work in a rural practice. Some commented on the ability to gain diverse nursing experiences, and two reported financial incentives. The pediatric nurse practitioner reported receiving a higher salary from the Public Health Service for working in an underserved rural area. The participant just out of nursing school discussed a federally funded loan repayment program available to him for agreeing to work in a critical (rural) shortage area. In addition, all commented on the beneficial aspects of a rural lifestyle. These aspects included picturesque surroundings, less stressful lifestyle, lower crime rate, and friendly people in the rural communities. However, most important were the close proximity to outdoor activities such as hunting and fishing, and the family-friendly environments of the rural communities. One participant commented,

> Basically, the lifestyle in the small community is more conducive to family. Schools are closer. You have more involvement with the children in school. You can take the kids to the park, or they can go out on their own to the park and play.... So you don't have as much concern in a small town. The kids have much more freedom ... a better way to grow up.

Gender and the Opportunities for Recruitment

Participants did not feel that nursing practice differed between male and female rural nurses. In addition, all felt well-received and respected by their employers and their local communities. One participant said, "They told me they were excited to have a male nurse." Men provide physical strength and were able to balance out an all-female nursing staff. One participant felt he was able to confront belligerent males in the ER better than his female coworkers. He stated,

> I think that in the emergency room ... sometimes just seeing a male quiets them down a little bit. They don't act quite as offensive ... [Although] some of the [female] nurses are pretty tough, some of them will get a little intimidated and walk out and ask me to take care of the patient or ask me to help settle them down.

Other participants stated that their experience with team sports provided a sound foundation for the teamwork necessary for effective rural practice.

All participants felt that rural nursing would be attractive for men. When I asked them about recruitment strategies, the participants stated that autonomy and diversity of experiences are particularly attractive for men. Two noted that, in their experience, men tend to like emergency and trauma nursing and believed that rural nursing would routinely provide these experiences. However, a number of participants pointed out that salaries are lower in rural areas than in urban areas and believed that rural hospitals need to be competitive with larger hospitals to attract men to rural practice.

DISCUSSIONS AND IMPLICATIONS

The findings from the current study support those of other studies describing rural nursing practice that primarily used the perspectives of female samples. In particular, the current study found similar descriptions of increased autonomy, collaboration, role expansion, patient diversity, challenges, and lack of anonymity as characteristics of rural nursing practice. Consistent with other studies, the men in this study also reported the need for flexibility, extensive generalist knowledge, emergency and trauma certifications, and a "can-do" attitude to be effective in rural nursing. Not found in the current study was the theme insider or outsider. Generally, the men were well received as they came to work in their rural communities.

The study provides new insight on the positive aspects of rural nursing practice (Hegney, McCartey, Rogers, Clark, &Gorman, 2002; Rosenthal, 1996; Scharff, 1998). The men described potentially negative aspects of rural nursing, such as lack of anonymity and the diversity of patients as benefits and attractions to rural nursing. The positive depiction of rural nursing provided by the men supports the term *opportunity* as a connecting theme. The participants in the current study took pride in their accomplishments at meeting the challenges of rural nursing and felt that their experiences in rural nursing made them better nurses overall.

In terms of recruitment, the findings are somewhat different from those noted by Australian researchers (Hegney et al., 2002). In both studies, factors that attracted and retained nurses to rural practice focused on the positive aspects of a rural lifestyle (Hegney et al. did not include outdoor recreation) and on positive relationships rural nurses have with coworkers and members of the community. However, the Australian study did not include the diversity of experiences offered in rural nursing, the increased autonomy available to rural nurses, the challenges of rural nursing practice, or the pride felt in meeting those challenges as attractions to rural nursing. Also, the Australian study identified that the emotional and physical demands of rural nursing as key factors in causing nurses to leave rural nursing. The men in the current study did not mention emotional or physical demands as part of their practice. In fact, several indicated their physical strength was of benefit in the practice setting. The only negative aspect of rural nursing mentioned by the current study participants that might dissuade someone from rural nursing practice are the lower wages offered by most employers.

According to participants in the current study, nurse recruiters hoping to fill vacancies in rural settings by accessing the undertapped male nurse labor pool should highlight the following in their marketing strategies: (a) increased autonomy; (b) increased opportunity for diverse patient experiences including emergency and trauma nursing; (c) more meaningful relationships with coworkers, patients, and the community, and (d) the outdoor recreation and family-friendly environments.

LIMITATIONS AND RECOMMENDATIONS
FOR FURTHER RESEARCH

The sample size of the study was small. However, consistent with phenom-enology, sample sizes are generally small, but data are rich from lengthy interviews (Creswell, 1998; Patton, 2002). Because I obtained saturation of the themes in the study, expanding the sample size may not have contrib-uted additional themes. Consistent with qualitative studies, findings from this study cannot be generalized to rural nursing populations (Creswell; Patton). Yet, because the findings of this study are consistent with the find-ings of other qualitative studies of rural nursing practice, the findings may have high transferability to other nurses working in rural hospitals.

Another limitation is self-selection of the participants. It is possible that men working as rural nurses who had very different perspectives chose not to participate in the study. In addition, all of the participants are Cau-casian. It is unclear how many male nurses of ethnic minority background are working in rural Montana communities because the State Board of Nursing did not provide this information with its list of RNs. However, there was some diversity within the sample in terms of years of nursing and rural nursing experience and of the types of communities in which they worked. Further research is needed to understand the experiences of men in other rural locations and practice settings, particularly in long-term care and in advanced practice, and men of other ethnic backgrounds.

CONCLUSION

My purpose in the current study was to examine the experiences and perspectives of men working as rural nurses. The findings indicate that men find rural nursing practice a very positive experience that can be described as a land of opportunities. These include the opportunities for expanded practice, autonomy, meaningful relationships, challenges, and rural rewards. Nurse recruiters trying to attract men to rural nursing should emphasize the positive aspects of rural nursing, the opportunities for outdoor recreation, and the family-friendly environments offered by rural communities.

REFERENCES

American Association of Colleges of Nursing. (1997). *Diversity and equality of opportunity*. Retrieved March 12, 2002, from http://www.aacn.nche.edu/Publications/positions/diverse.htm

American Association of Colleges of Nursing. (2001, December Issue Bulletin). *Effective strategies for increasing diversity in nursing programs* (AACN). Washington, DC: American Association of Colleges of Nursing.

Anders, R. L. (1993). Targeting male students. *Nurse Educator, 18*(2), 4.

Benner, P. (1999). Quality of life: A phenomenological perspective on explanation, prediction, and understanding in nursing science. In E. C. Polifroni & M. Welch (Eds.), *Perspectives on philosophy of science in nursing: An historical and contemporary anthology* (pp. 303–314). Philadelphia: Lippincott.

Buerhaus, P. I., Staiger, D. O., & Auerbach, D. I. (2000). Implications of an aging registered nurse workforce. *JAMA, 283,* 2948–2954.

Bushy, A. (2002). International perspectives on rural nursing: Australia, Canada, USA. *Australian Journal of Rural Health, 10,* 104–111.

Center on an Aging Society. (2003, January). Data profile: Rural and urban health. *Challenges for the 21st century: Chronic and disabling conditions* 1–6 Georgetown University: Institute for Health Care Research and Policy.

Creswell, J. (1998). *Qualitative inquiry and research design: Choosing among five traditions.* Thousand Oaks, CA: Sage.

Davis, M. T., & Bartfay, W. J. (2001). Men in nursing: An untapped resource. *Canadian Nurse, 97*(5), 14–18.

Goins, R. T., & Mitchell, J. (1999). Health-related quality of life: Does rurality matter? *Journal of Rural Health, 15,* 147–6.

Gordon, S. (2002). *A hemorrhage in the hospitals.* Retrieved June 4, 2002, from http://www.latimes.com/la-000038996jun03.story

Hegney, D., McCarthy, A., Rogers-Clark, C., & Gorman, D. (2002). Why nurses are attracted to rural and remote practice? *Australian Journal of Rural Health, 10,* 178–6.

Hopkins, M., & Domrose, C. (2001). *Remote control.* Retrieved January 11, 2004, from http://www.nurseweek.com/news/features/01–04/rural.asp

Houde, S. C. (2002). Methodological issues in male caregiver research: An integrative review of the literature. *Journal of Advanced Nursing, 40* 626–40.

Koch, T. (1995). Interpretive approaches in nursing research: The influence of Husserl and Heidegger. *Journal of Advanced Nursing, 21,* 827–36.

Kumar, V., Acanfora, M., Hennessy, C. H., & Kalache, A. (2001). Health status of the rural elderly. *Journal of Rural Health, 17,* 328–31.

Lee, H. (1998). Lack of anonymity. In H. Lee (Ed.), *Conceptual basis for rural nursing* (pp. 76–88). New York: Springer Publishing.

Lincoln, Y. S., & Guba, E. (2000). Paradigmatic controversies, contradictions, and emerging confluences. In N. K. Denzin & Y. S. Lincoln (Eds.), *Handbook of qualitative research* (2nd ed., pp. 163–188). Thousand Oaks, CA: Sage.

Long, C. (2000, October 9). *Rural communities feel sting of nursing shortage.* Retrieved November 28, 2004, from http://community.bouldernews.com/news/statewest/091nurs.html

National Institute of Nursing Research. (1995). *Chapter 2: Rural America: Challenges and opportunities.* Retrieved April 9, 2003, from http://ninr.nih.gov/ninr/research/volq/chapter2.htm

O'Lynn, C. E. (2004). Gender-based barriers for male students in nursing education programs: Prevalence and perceived importance. *Journal of Nursing Education, 43,* 229–236.

Patton, M. Q. (2002). *Qualitative research & evaluation methods* (3rd ed.). Thousand Oaks, CA: Sage.

Rosenthal, K. (1996). *Rural nursing: An exploratory narrative description.* Unpublished Dissertation, University of Colorado, Denver.

Scharff, J. (1998). The distinctive nature and scope of rural nursing practice: Philosophical bases. In H. J. Lee (Ed.), *Conceptual basis for rural nursing* (pp. 19–38). New York: Springer Publishing.

Spratley, E., Johnson, A., Sochalski, J., Fritz, M., & Spencer, W. (2001). *The registered nurse population March 2000: Findings from the National Sample Survey of Registered Nurses.* Washington, DC: U.S. Department of Health and Human Services, Bureau of Helth Professions, Division of Nursing.

Sullivan, E. J. (2000). Men in nursing: The importance of gender diversity. *Journal of Professional Nursing, 16,* 253–254.

Thompson, E. (2002). What's unique about men's caregiving? In B. J. Kramer & E. Thompson (Eds.), *Men as caregivers: Theory, research, and service implications* (pp. 20–50). New York: Springer Publishing.

Trossman, S. (2001, July/August). Rural nursing anyone? Recruiting nurses is always a challenge. *The American Nurse, 1,* 18–19.

U.S. Bureau of the Census. (2002). *U.S. summary: 2000* (Census profile No. C2KPROF/00–US). Washington, DC: U.S. Department of Commerce.

Villeneuve, M. J. (1994). Recruiting and retaining men in nursing: A review of the literature. *Journal of Professional Nursing, 10,* 217–228.

Vukic, A., & Keddy, B. (2002). Northern nursing practice in a primary health care setting. *Journal of Advanced Nursing, 40,* 542–548.

CHAPTER NINETEEN

Continuing Education and Rural Nurses

Lori Hendrickx

The availability of continuing education (CE) is essential for maintaining skilled, competent nurses in the practice setting. Access to CE programming has been an issue for nurses practicing in rural and frontier areas, yet rural nurses have reported their desire and commitment to remain current through CE (Hendrickx, 1998). Rapidly changing technology, advances in health care and the complexity of patients make it necessary for nurses in general to keep abreast of new information. In rural areas, complex situations may occur less frequently and nurses may often be working alone or with minimal support staff, making it even more imperative that these nurses remain current and have access to CE.

The rural health care environment provides nurses with an opportunity to practice as a generalist. Although the generalist role is ideal for those who appreciate a variety of experiences, some nurses are challenged by the concern that there is too much to know when caring for a diverse population of patients (Trossman, 2001). Bigbee (1993) identified a unique challenge of rural nursing as the multiple functions and generalist orientation. As a generalist, a rural nurse might practice in labor and delivery, medical, surgical, pediatric, or emergency departments, often within the same shift and with limited numbers of other nurses or support staff available. Limitations on nurses' time and the financial constraints facing rural hospitals have contributed to the increasing difficulty of maintaining proficiency for nurses in a generalist practice.

Providing high quality care in rural health care facilities is essential if rural facilities are to remain open. Moscovice and Stensland (2002) stated that rural dwellers often perceived higher quality care existed in more metropolitan hospitals. Although this perception is often based on non-empirical evidence, patients may decide to bypass the local rural provider in favor of a larger facility. A key component in providing quality health care in the rural area is ensuring that rural nurses are up-to-date and have access to current knowledge through continuing education. The lack of CE opportunities or other barriers to obtaining CE have been identified as factors in nurses' decisions to work in nonrural areas (Hendrickx, 2001).

LITERATURE REVIEW

The nursing shortage has been well publicized; however geographic areas experience the shortage in differing ways. Historically, rural areas felt the impact with larger numbers of shortage areas in the United States being in rural counties (Stratton, Dunkin, & Juhl, 1995). In a study examining nursing workforce issues in rural and urban settings, LaSala (2000) found that when major vacancies existed, they were greater in rural areas (19.2%) than urban areas (2.7%). Trossman (2001) stated that rural facilities face enormous challenges when trying to fill a registered nurse vacancy and that the nursing shortage is making recruitment of nurses to rural areas more difficult.

It is not uncommon to find that nurses residing in nonmetropolitan counties travel to metropolitan areas to work, further compounding the problem of recruiting nurses to rural areas. Even though salaries in both urban and rural areas have improved, rural administrators reported that urban areas continue to draw rural nurses by offering higher salaries (LaSala, 2000). In addition to salary differences, other issues related to recruitment and retention of rural nurses have been identified. In studies describing nurse recruitment and retention concerns in rural areas, the lack of CE opportunities has often been identified as problematic related to the ability to recruit or retain nurses (Farmer & Richardson, 1997; Hendrickx, 1998, 2001).

For rural nurses, several deterrents to participation in CE have been identified. The most commonly identified factor has been distance to travel (Hedman & Lazure, 1990; Hegge, Powers, Hendrickx, & Vinson, 2002; Hendrickx, 1998, 2001). Hegge et al., (2002) reported that 39 participants in a study related to competence and CE indicated they traveled greater than 200 miles to obtain CE. In that same study, 75% of the participants had not attended a national conference in the past 2 years;

63% had not attended a regional conference; and 40% had not attended a local conference.

South Dakota is not a state that requires CE credits to renew nursing licensure. However, given the distribution of the respondents in a study across several specialty areas and among different areas within nursing, the need for continued exposure to current practice literature and education is important. In a study (Hendrickx, 2001) of barriers to CE experienced by rural nurses, I asked study participants to identify reasons they did not attend CE activities. Seventy percent ($n = 28$) responded that distance to travel was the major reason they had not attended more CE. Other reasons for not participating in CE were (a) cost, (b) difficulty getting time off from work, (c) topics not of interest, (d) not being able to be away from family, or (e) not knowing about possible CE activities being offered (Hendrickx, 2001). Several respondents also chose to add comments related to their CE activities. Comments often related to distance or cost. One respondent commented, "Many times I would have to travel 6–8 hours to receive 2–4 hours of CE. The cost of that is prohibitive, not to mention the time." Another respondent wrote,

> Usually they (CE) are too far away and if they're more than one day I need motel and food money since it takes another day to drive there and back. There aren't enough nurses at the hospital I work to cover me for that many extra days and I don't want to use my vacation days for that (Hendrickx, 2001).

In the same study, I reported that 12 (26.5%) respondents indicated they had not attended any CE activities during the previous year. Twelve (26.5%) had attended 1–5 hours of CE, 12 (26.5%) had attended 6–10 hours, one had attended 11–15 hours, and 11 (22.4%) had attended more than 15 hours. Nurses were also asked to indicate the distance they had traveled to attend CE. Only 5 (10.2%) nurses indicated they had been able to attend CE activities offered less than 50 miles from their homes. Six (12.2%) traveled 51–100 miles, 12 (24.5%) traveled 101–150 miles and 20 (41%) indicated they traveled greater than 150 miles to attend CE.

In addition to distance issues, nurses have identified the lack of financial resources to support CE attendance, limited transportation opportunities, weather, and inability to get time off from work as deterrents to obtaining CE (Hedman & Lazure, 1990; Hendrickx, 2001). The American Nurses Association also has reported that reduced access to advanced and continuing education was one of several challenges that face rural and frontier nurses (Weinert et al., 1996).

INCREASED OPPORTUNITIES THROUGH
COMPUTER EDUCATION

The use of computers has been proposed as a solution to alleviate the barrier of distance related to CE (Hegge et al., 2002). Bushy (2002), stated that a potential benefit of online courses is the reduction or elimination of commuting time. In addition, technological advances have been purported to be a possible solution to the isolation of rural nurses. Dunkin (2002) stated,

> With the advances in technology that have occurred in the last 10 years, isolation from other nurses is no longer a necessary part of rural nursing. While geography has not changed, there are many resources available to rural and remote nurses, primarily through the Internet (p.1).

Although nurses have identified advantages, such as the convenience of taking courses from home and the increased variety of Internet topics, I reported that rural nurses use computers but not for CE (Hendrickx, 2001). In a study of 559 nurses, Hegge et al. (2002) reported that although 72.5% of respondents had computers at home and 76% of respondents had computers at work, only 100 of the nurses (17.9%) had used computers for CE. Reasons those nurses did not use computers for CE included (a) lack of knowledge about computer continuing education programs, (b) lack of access to a computer, (c) lack of Internet access, (d) lack of time, (e) discomfort using computers, (f) preference for books or other written material, or (e) that continuing education was not required (Hegge et al.).

I conducted a study (Hendrickx, 2003) examining the level of involvement and factors that influence professional development of rural nurses. I also asked these nurses (n = 49) whether or not they use a computer and if they had ever used a computer for CE. Eighty-six per cent (n = 42) reported they had used a computer but only 2 of those had ever used a computer to obtain CE. One of those two reported she was in an online baccalaureate of science in nursing completion program so was taking all her classes over the Internet.

Although the Internet has provided a new method for obtaining CE, there are other methods, such as interactive video conferencing, audio conferencing, and the use of telemedicine networks, that have been developed in rural areas. Telemedicine systems have been used in rural areas for some time to deliver health care services to rural dwellers. Telemedicine has been defined by the Institute of Medicine as "the use of electronic information and communications technologies to provide and support health care, when distance separates the participants" (Geyman, Norris, & Hart, 2001, p. 250).

Nurses in rural areas have used telemedicine systems to deliver CE to other nurses with distance barriers. The American Association of Critical Care Nurses (AACN) recently awarded the 2004 Outstanding Chapter Communication System Award to the Siouxland Chapter of AACN for its use of a telemedicine network to deliver their annual meetings and CE offerings to nurses across the state of South Dakota. In their exemplar submitted for the award, the Siouxland Chapter indicated that South Dakota is a state with only one AACN Chapter, located in the extreme southeast corner of the state and accessible to only a portion of the state's AACN members and critical care nurses. The Siouxland Chapter committed itself to reaching out to AACN members in South Dakota and critical care nurses without physical access to AACN through the use of the Avera McKennan TeleHealth Network. Chapter members established an interactive distance communication method using the TeleHealth network. Monthly meetings and CE then became available through the network to critical care nurses in several towns across South Dakota.

The Siouxland Chapter interactive system allows remote attendees to see and listen to meetings and contribute to discussions, while the local site attendees also see those at remote sites. Microphones stationed throughout the room allow attendees to talk between the sites and ask questions. All of the speaker's materials, such as slides or videos, are sent via the network and available in real time. The Siouxland Chapter communication system has enabled several critical care colleagues to attend meetings and earn CE while in their own communities, reducing travel time and time away from work and families.

The American Nurses Association envisions that telemedicine systems for nursing (termed *telenursing*) are especially relevant for nursing education through distance learning. For rural nurses, this technology has the potential for use "for formal coursework, continuing education, attendance at televised conferences, or participation in clinical teaching rounds" (American Nurses Association, 1997, p. 2).

The increase in distance delivery formats for education will be effective only if the education providers increase awareness and support for the use of distance education among rural nurses. Training programs will have to be developed for use in the professional educational setting as well as in continuing education that assist the learner with the technology.

ACADEMIC EDUCATION

Rural nurses have limited access to advanced academic programs. In rural areas, there tends to be a greater community college presence rather than university presence, making continuing academic education difficult for those nurses interested in completing a baccalaureate or graduate degree (Szigeti, 2000). The emergence of distance learning programs at universities has greatly expanded the availability of academic programming at the baccalaureate level and higher for rural nurses. Many nurses are demanding greater flexibility in educational programming and for some rural nurses, a distance education program is the only type that allows nurses to complete or continue their education (McPeck, 2001). The most prevalent distance programs are the completion programs, which enable registered nurses with an associate degree or diploma in nursing to earn a bachelors or graduate degree in nursing.

A recent Internet search netted 86 online graduate degree programs in nursing in the United States. This number will continue to rise as more colleges of nursing become aware of the advantages of distance learning for nurses. Szigeti (2000) reported that at a Doctoral Conference sponsored by the American Association of Colleges of Nursing, "Faculties in colleges of nursing are aware that it is difficult for many nurses to be on a university campus to earn a doctoral degree. They are developing doctoral programs for these potential students" (p. 2).

At South Dakota State University, since its inception in 2001, the Online Master's Degree Program has admitted the maximum number of students (15) and has had a waiting list each year. For Fall 2004, an additional section of students was added so that two groups of online students could be admitted, accommodating the increased number of applicants. Most applicants have been from South Dakota and neighboring states, such as Minnesota, Iowa, Nebraska, and Montana; however, the Fall 2004 class also had applicants from North Carolina, Missouri, Michigan, Wisconsin, and Texas as well (P. Powers, personal communication, June 7, 2004).

For the registered nurse wishing to obtain a baccalaureate degree, the online RN-to-BSN programs have increased the availability of this option. Programs that used traditional approaches to RN-to-BSN education have moved to online delivery with substantial increases in enrollments. The University of Kansas saw dropping enrollment in its traditional RN-to-BSN program. A change to an online program resulted in a 53% increase in enrollment (McPeck, 2001). Similarly, at South Dakota State University, enrollment numbers in the RN to BSN program were around 8–12 students prior to initiation of online course delivery. The change to online delivery has resulted in increased enrollment, and there are currently 275 students taking either nursing courses or prenursing support courses (S. Rosen, personal communication, June 9, 2004).

Another area that has seen increased growth related to distance delivery of continuing education is RN and LPN refresher courses. These refresher courses have successfully facilitated the return of many retired and inactive nurses to the workforce (Blankenship, Winslow, & Smith, 2003). Rural nurses that are interested in reentering the nursing workforce and need a refresher course for licensing have also taken advantage of online programs. Since 2002, the RN and LPN refresher courses at South Dakota State University have seen a substantial increase in enrollment with the development of online delivery (see Table 19.1; T. Herrold, personal communication, June 9, 2004).

PROFESSIONAL NURSING ORGANIZATIONS

Numerous professional organizations have now added online CE content to their Web sites. For example, the American Nurses Association and Sigma Theta Tau International offer online CE on a variety of topics for a minimal fee while other organizations offer a number of free CE units as a membership benefit. Additionally, complete online educational programs have been made available for purchase, such as the Essentials of Critical Care Orientation (ECCO) program available through the AACN (AACN, 2004). The ECCO program has been beneficial to rural hospitals that do not have the resources to support an education department. This online educational program is useful for hospitals who want to deliver a standardized orientation program to nurses or when a hospital educator's time needs to be "freed up to focus on learning transference, supplemental information development, and learner's educational needs" (Berke & Wiseman, 2004, p. 80). Practicing nurses can then attend the orientation program on their own time or from home, balancing the didactic portion with the hands-on orientation in the practice setting.

The Rural Nurse Organization offers a variety of services for the professional development of nurses specifically interested in rural issues. Its Web site (www.rno.org) provides a newsletter, information about the organization, and access to the *Online Journal of Rural Nursing and Health Care*.

Table 19.1. Enrollment in Refresher Course at South Dakota State University

Year	RN program, *n*	LPN Program, *n*
1999	62	47
2000	65	46
2001	61	53
2002[a]	117	71
2003	168	81

[a]Online delivery began.

SUMMARY

Rural nurses are committed to maintaining quality care in their practice environments but often find that physical distance from programming and other barriers limit their ability to attend CE or academic programs. It is essential that rural health institutions, those responsible for the delivery of CE, and those in academia recognize and address the challenges that rural nurses face with regard to CE. With creative use of technology and commitment by all those involved, rural nurses need not be isolated from activities that will help them maintain current, competent practice.

REFERENCES

American Association of Critical Care Nurses. (2004). *Essentials of critical care orientation.* Retrieved June 9, 2004, from http://www.aacn.org

American Nurses Association. (1997). Telehealth: A tool for nursing practice. *Nursing Trends & Issues, 2*(4), 1–7.

Berke, W., & Wiseman, T. (2004). The e-learning answer. *Critical Care Nurse, 24*(2), 80–84.

Bigbee, J. (1993). The uniqueness of rural nursing. *Nursing Clinics of North America, 28*(1), 131–144.

Blankenship, J. S., Winslow, S. A, & Smith, A. U. (2003). Refresher course for inactive RNs facilitates workforce entry. *Journal for Nurses in Staff Development, 19,* 288–291.

Bushy, A. (2002). Cyber-learning: A primer to get you started. *Online Journal of Rural Nursing and Healthcare, 2*(2). Retrieved March 11, 2004, from http://www.rno.org/journal/issues/Vol-2/issue-2/EdIssues_2_2.htm

Dunkin, J. (2002). Isolation: Real or perceived? *Online Journal of Rural Nursing and Healthcare, 2*(1). Retrieved March 11, 2004, from http://www.rno.org/journal/issues/Vol-2/issue-1/LtrEditor_2_1.htm

Farmer, J., & Richardson, A. (1997). Information for trained nurses in remote areas: Do electronically networked resources provide an answer? *Health Library Review, 14*(2), 97–103.

Geyman, J. P., Norris, T. E., & Hart, L. G. (2001). *Textbook of rural medicine.* New York: McGraw-Hill.

Hedman, L., & Lazure, L. (1990). Extending continuing education to rural nurses. *Journal of Continuing Education in Nursing, 21,* 165–168.

Hegge, M., Powers, P., Hendrickx, L., & Vinson, J. (2002). Competence, continuing education, and computers. *Journal of Continuing Education in Nursing, 33,* 24–32.

Hendrickx, L. (1998). Attitudes of rural nurses toward computers: Implications for continuing education. *Dissertation Abstracts International, 59*(03A), 0690.

Hendrickx, L. (2001, March). *Continuing education needs and perceived barriers of South Dakota nurses in geographically isolated areas.* Paper presented at the Sigma Theta Tau Twelfth Annual Nursing Research Symposium, Brookings, SD.

Hendrickx, L. (2003, March). *Level of involvement and factors that influence professional development of rural nurses.* Paper presented at the Sigma Theta Tau Fourteenth Annual Nursing Research Conference, Brookings, SD.

LaSala, K. (2000). Nursing workforce issues in rural and urban setting: Looking at the difference in recruitment, retention, and distribution. *Online Journal of Rural Nursing and Healthcare, 1*(1). Retrieved March 11, 2004, from http://www.rno.org/journal/issues/Vol-1/issue-1/LaSala.htm

McPeck, P. (2001, July 9). Education evolution: Nursing education models take a tech turn as students demand greater flexibility. *Nurseweek.* Retrieved June 1, 2004, from http://www.nurseweek.com/news/features/01–07/evolution.html

Moscovice, I., & Stensland, J. (2002). Rural hospitals: Trends, challenges, and a future research and policy analysis agenda. *Journal of Rural Health, 18*(Suppl.), 197–210.

Stratton, T., Dunkin, J., & Juhl, N. (1995). Redefining the nursing shortage: A rural perspective. *Nursing Outlook, 43,* 71–77.

Szigeti, E. (2000). Education at a distance. *Online Journal of Rural Nursing and Healthcare, 1*(3). Retrieved March 11, 2004, from http://www.rno.org/journal/issues/Vol-1/issue-3/EdIssues_1_3.htm

Trossman, S. (2001). Rural nursing anyone? Recruiting nurses is always a challenge. *The American Nurse, 33*(4), 1, 18–19.

Weinert, C., Fuszard, B., Wasem, C., Haldane, S., Yocum, D., & Schultz, C. (1996). *Rural/frontier nursing: The challenge to grow.* Washington, DC: American Nurses' Association.

PART V

Rural Public Health

The chapter authors in this part focus on rural public health. In chapter 20, Kuntz and her colleagues describe rural and frontier health nurses' perspective on emergency preparedness. Then, Hill and Butterfield describe the first phase of a 5–year project focusing on the environmental risks in the homes of children living in rural southwestern Montana—environmental tobacco smoke (ETS), radon, carbon monoxide, lead, and impurities in well water. Intrigued by the lack of school nurses in rural Montana, Glover interviewed school secretaries about their role in meeting the health needs of children. Jones and colleagues report on improving the health literacy of rural elders living in Kentucky through the use of an interdisciplinary educational program. In the last chapter of this section, Findholt reports on the culture of rural Oregon communities through an examination of relevant rural nursing concepts—insider or outsider, old-timer or new-comer, lack of anonymity, isolation, and distance.

CHAPTER TWENTY

Public Health Emergency Preparedness in Rural or Frontier Areas

Sandra K. Kuntz, Jane Smilie, and Melanie Reynolds

Preparedness for public health emergencies, including intentional, accidental, or natural disasters, has become a post 9–11 national initiative in small and large communities across the United States. Although one of the six goals of public health includes "response to disasters and assistance to communities in recovery" (Public Health Functions Steering Committee, 1994, p. 1), most local public health agencies prior to the World Trade Center attack and subsequent anthrax events had few resources and limited specific directives for addressing the disaster objective (Department of Justice, 2000; Henderson, 1998; Wetter, Daniell, & Treser, 2001). Early efforts to bolster the sagging public health infrastructure included reprioritizing the critical need for "response" and "assistance" and adding "preparedness" of the public health system and workforce to increase response capacities during significant events (Gebbie, 2002; Koplan, 2001).

Congressional funding and focused local and national efforts have resulted in gradual but significant public health infrastructure improvements since the 2001 incidents. However, despite the positive changes, the American Public Health Association (2002) noted the following unmet service needs in some communities: "coordination at a regional (and local) level is still lacking ... preparation in rural areas falls behind the level of preparedness in major metropolitan areas" (p. 3). To learn more about local preparedness capacities, the Centers for Disease Control and

Prevention (CDC) funded states to conduct an assessment of local public health agencies (counties and Indian tribes) to determine the current preparedness status and needs. Our central aim of this chapter is to examine the qualitative description of challenges and benefits encountered by local public health agencies in Montana when they partner for preparedness with LEPCs, such as local emergency planning committees (LEPCs) and tribal emergency response commissions (TERCs).

BACKGROUND AND SIGNIFICANCE

In 1986, Congress passed the Emergency Planning and Community Right to Know Act, also known as the Superfund Amendments and Reauthorization Act (SARA). The intent of this law was in part to develop community-based local emergency planning committees to protect the public's health, safety, and the environment from chemical hazards (U.S. Code, 1986). Fifteen years after the SARA legislation, Lindell and Perry (2001) questioned the current status of implementation of SARA at the local level including the required LEP. Landesman and Leonard (1993) found that when an LEPC existed in a community, often hospitals and public health agencies were not included or had failed to become active in LEPC meetings and activities.

Public health emergency preparedness requires an all-hazard approach and a wide-range of sustainable public health workforce skills and competencies. Officials of the CDC's 2002 Public Health Practice Program Office stated that "establishing relationships among public health system partners is likely the most critical aspect of emergency (preparedness) and response" (p. 1). Evidence of dynamic, transforming, and often synergistic outcomes related to intersectoral partnerships and complex community problems (substance abuse, teen pregnancy, violence) is documented by researchers (Florin, Mitchell, Stevenson, & Klein, 2000; Lasker, Weiss, & Miller, 2001; Matessich, Murray-Close, & Monsey, 2001; Polivka, Dresbach, Heimlich, & Elliott, 2001). For the Community Tracking Study McHugh, Staiti, and Felland (2004) collected data through telephone and in-person semistructured interviews from 12 metropolitan statistical areas. Results show that readiness was related to (a) previous experience with public health emergencies, (b) adequate funding, (c) successful collaboration, and (d) strong leadership. These themes are projected to help guide policy and funding decisions as federal and state agencies search for the most efficient and effective preparedness tools and methods.

No study to date has described the qualitative aspects of the rural preparedness experience. The categorical differences between frontier spaces and urban places creates a great divide in capacity to mobilize, educate, and sustain workforce; or in some rural areas, volunteer workforces partner for emergency preparedness and other public health concerns (Reynolds & Leahy, 2002). Cowie, Elder, and Leibowitz (2000) made the following observations regarding local emergency response capacity: "Frontier facts are simple. There are probably no or few paid responders, outdated or nonexistent equipment, no tax base, no time to train, and possibly no active local emergency planning committee (LEPC) as required by law" (p. 6).

In Montana, 45 of 56 (80%) counties are classified as frontier with a population density of six or fewer people per square mile and 11 of 56 (20%) counties categorized as rural with more than six but fewer than 50 people per square mile. Three of the eleven rural counties are classified as metropolitan areas with at least one city with 50,000 or more inhabitants (Montana County Profiles, 2000). The public health workforce consists of a variety of professionals employed by counties and tribes including nurses (48%), sanitarians (34%), health educators (11%), and registered dieticians (6%) (Montana County Profiles, 2002). In large and small counties, nurses serve in a range of roles from health officer to public health case worker. In some frontier counties, the nurse is the only part-time or full-time public health employee. According to the Montana Department of Public Health and Human Services (2003) statewide capacity assessment report, 26% of respondent counties reported they had been a member of a LEPC for less than 6 months; 19% had been members for under one year; and 10% were not currently members but were considering joining a committee. Most of the "new member" respondents were from the smallest frontier counties with total populations under 10,000. Most of the respondents who had been members of a LEPC for over 1 year were from large counties with populations over 20,000. With over half of Montana's counties in the early stages of partnering for preparedness, exploring public health perception regarding the collaborative experience is timely and could inform future development and sustainability efforts. Therefore, the question for this study was: How does the rural Montana public health workforce perceive the challenges and benefits of partnering for preparedness?

METHOD

The 2002 Montana Public Health Emergency Preparedness and Response Capacity Assessment (PHEPRCA) conducted by the Montana Department of Health and Human Services (MTDHHS, 2002) provided the data for this study. Lead local public health agency officials, their designee, or a selected team of individuals with expertise from inside and outside the agency completed the assessment. The paper and pencil, 61–page survey came with a projected time commitment of approximately 24 hours. The

University of Montana Technical Assistance Center provided help, answered questions, and supplied local technical assistance to counties and tribes across the state throughout the assessment time period. An initial training session was held in a central location in Montana to explain the purpose, process, and expectations of the PHEPRCA to local officials. At the end of the day-long session, the survey was distributed with full instructions, technical assistance contact information, and a 12–week time period for submitting the completed survey for contract reimbursement. The overall PHEPRCA response rate was 84% with 50 of the 56 counties (89%) and three of seven tribes (43%) participating in the capacity assessment.

The extensive PHEPRCA data set provided opportunity for four types of analyses. First, data were entered into SPSS version 11.5 for Windows, and analyzed by the University of Washington, Northwest Center for Public Health Practice generating descriptive counts, frequencies, and means. These results were reported in regional and statewide summaries. In addition, each local agency received an individual jurisdiction report. Secondly, the data were analyzed by Smilie (2003) and Kuntz (2004) to investigate preparedness levels and establish a matrix for scoring preparedness. Third, Kuntz (2003) investigated the relationship between preparedness and collaboration. The fourth study and the focus of this chapter emerged from two qualitative PHEPRCA questions. The two open-ended questions included in the survey helped to identify key components of the preparedness experience in rural and frontier areas. The first qualitative question asked: What is the greatest challenge your agency has experienced in joining or leading a LEPC? The second question queried: What is the greatest benefit your agency has experienced in joining or leading a LEPC?

Data Analysis

We used textual discourse analysis (Denzin & Lincoln, 1998) to identify "themes, issues and recurring motifs" (p. 43). We entered the data from the two questions into a Microsoft Access database. In the first analysis phase, we identified primary themes. In the second phase, we sorted themes based on county population data. For this study, we stratified counties by population number rather than population density. This designation allowed for greater stratification of the frontier counties. The three population categories included 33 small frontier counties (population < 10,000); 8 medium frontier counties (population between 10,000 and 20,000), and 9 rural counties (population > 20,000). We incorporated reservation data into the county counts to avoid the possibility of identifying specific Native American groups. All seven Indian Nations have population numbers of < 10,000 so we counted them with the small frontier groups for this research (see Table 20.1).

Table 20.1. Respondent Characteristics: Population Density, Agency
Staffing

Characteristic	All jurisdictions reporting ($n = 50$)	Small frontier ($n = 33$)	Medium frontier ($n = 8$)	Rural ($n = 9$)
Population, M	16, 358	4,663	12,840	66,746
Agency staff FTE				
Range	0–90.0	0–13.2	0–10.0	6.0–90.0
M	8.8	2.7	4.4	38.8
SD	18.32	2.81	3.01	31.95

Note. Small frontier < 10,000 in jurisdiction; medium frontier = 10,000–20,000; rural = > 20,000; FTE = (full time equivalent) From *An Assessment of Montana's Capacity to Respond to a Public Health Emergency: Statewide Report,* by Montana Deparment of Health and Human Services, April 2003, University of Washington; Northwest Center for Public Health Practice, Seattle.

FINDINGS

Two primary themes emerged from the thematic analysis. Respondent answers to both open-ended questions could be categorized as either agency-based or partnership-based perceptions related to both challenges and benefits. Agency-based perceptions referenced internal organizational issues. Partnership-based perceptions alluded to the external collaborative formed with other agencies to address preparedness issues. Four themes in each category of "challenges" emerged. Table 20.2 shows the challenges cited by all respondents according to the themed responses made by small frontier (<10,000), medium frontier (10,000–20,000) and rural (>20,000), local public health agencies. Table 20.3 identifies the primary themes related to benefits of partnering for preparedness and differentiates the themed responses made by small frontier (<10,000), medium frontier (10,000–20,000), and rural (>20,000) local public health agencies. Because frontier agencies (both small and medium) outnumber rural agencies by 4:1 and respondent agencies listed different numbers of challenges and benefits, our intent of Tables 20.2 and 20.3 focuses on acknowledging differences rather than serving as a comparison between jurisdiction types.

Perceptions Related to Challenges

Coordinating efforts among partners, time constraints, and the need for fiscal and human resources represented the most commonly cited challenges to partnering for preparedness in Montana (Table 20.2). With so many pressing public health issues, generating interest, overcoming apathy,

Table 20.2. Preparedness Challenge Responses of All Agencies Stratified by Local Public Health Agency

Type of challenge	Jurisdiction Size*		
	SF	MF	R
Agency-Based			
Time constraints (*n* = 11)	7	2	2
Human resources (*n* = 11)	8	3	—
Generating interest or overcoming apathy (*n* = 8)	6	—	2
Fiscal resources (*n* = 11)	10	1	—
Partnership-Based			
Organizational coordination (*n* = 19)	9	5	5
Communication (*n* = 4)	2	1	1
Turf (*n* = 5)	1	3	1
Roles and inclusion (*n* = 8)	8	—	—

Note. SF = small, frontier < 10,000 population in jurisdiction (*n* = 30); MF = medium, frontier 10,000–20,000 population in jurisdiction (*n* = 7); R = Rural > 20,000 population in jurisdiction (*n* = 9).

and establishing a sense of commitment aimed toward preparedness efforts confronts local agencies. Turf, role, and inclusion surfaced as issues with comments indicating some public health representatives search for purpose and identity in previously organized groups. Some comments related to frontier agency status included few employees covering numer-

Table 20.3. Preparedness Benefit Responses of All Agencies Stratified by Local Public Health Jurisdiction Size

Type of Benefit	Jurisdiction Size*		
	SF	MF	R
Agency-Based			
Networking (*n* = 18)	11	3	4
Recognition or respect (*n* = 15)	10	4	1
Increased disaster awareness (*n* = 8)	7	1	
Partnership-Based			
Effort synergy (*n* = 14)	6	35	
Resource sharing (*n* = 12)	9	1	2
Education/Training (*n* = 9)	7	2	

Note. SF = small, frontier < 10,000 population in jurisdiction (*n* = 30); MF = medium, frontier 10,000–20,000 population in jurisdiction (*n* = 7); R = Rural > 20,000 population in jurisdiction (*n* = 9).

ous mandates with limited funding. Respondents from frontier counties most often mentioned agency-based challenges, whereas participants from larger rural counties with normally more fiscal and human resources named partnership-based issues as the primary point of concern. The following comments are representative of the challenges related to partnering for preparedness:

> (It is difficult to) maintain momentum between perceived threats. (Rural)
> Our agency has a kind of "New Kid on the Block" feeling but the LEPC (the local emergency planning committee) seems willing to accept public health (Small, Frontier)
> Difficult communication between public health and the DES (department of emergency services) coordinator. (Rural)
> The RN in the Health Department works part time. All emergency group members work full time and volunteer countless hours as EMTs, firemen, etc. There isn't much time for more group meetings. (Small, Frontier)
> Our involvement is in the early stages—everything is challenging. (Small, Frontier)
> We have been attending these meetings for ten years. We feel like a part of their meetings. No challenges at the moment. (Rural)
> Educating the group about the role public health plays in emergency preparedness is a big challenge. (Small, Frontier)
> Public health has not been recognized as a "player" and I've had difficulty determining my role in the group (i.e., what I can offer). I have progressed but I still need role/responsibility clarification. (Small, Frontier)
> LEPC seems to be a back-burner item in our county. Public health has been sharing bioterrorism information but no LEPC meetings have been held despite requests by this agency for the same. (Small, Frontier)
> The same people are involved in many organizations and everyone is involved in too many things to attend. Also, it is challenging to avoid stepping on someone else's toes. (Small, Frontier)

Perceptions Related to Benefits

The most prevalent theme from the benefits question was the perception that synergy was possible through joining forces to develop preparedness plans—opposed to going it alone (Table 20.3). Several agency respondents mentioned that preparedness partnering seemed to strengthen cooperation and coordination among agencies on other community issues. Although garnering respect for public health contributions was noted as a challenge, the act of participating in partnership activities helped raise recognition of and respect for public health contributions so was listed as a benefit by some agencies. Another important acknowledged benefit is the advantage gained when public health personnel train alongside emergency response personnel and other providers.

Sample comments representative of the benefits question posed to local agency personnel include the following:

> Networking with other agencies strengthens each participating agency in preparedness as well as other community projects. (Medium, Frontier)
> Becoming a partner and networking; experiencing some nontraditional partnering. (Small, Frontier)
> Legitimacy as a player in the emergency response field—also access to individuals for follow-up. (Medium, Frontier)
> Introduction to all agencies and person's responsible for agencies; knowing resources available from each agency. (Small, Frontier)
> Brainstorming with others and having a local group resource base to work with coalition building. (Small, Frontier)
> Getting to know key contacts in case of an emergency; fostering better communication between LEPC and public health; sharing resources and information; learning from drills and follow-up critiques. (Small, Frontier)
> Our ability to respond seamlessly and well to the community's public health needs in an emergency on all levels (county, tribal, state, and federal). (Rural)
> System for gaining access to resources from other agencies. (Rural)

DISCUSSIONS AND RECOMMENDATIONS

Data collected through the open-ended questions on the Montana Public Health Emergency Preparedness and Response Capacity Assessment provide beginning insight into key challenges and benefits associated with public health agency partnering for preparedness. Gray (1989) characterized collaboration as "a process through which parties who see different aspects of a problem can constructively explore their differences and search for solutions that go beyond their own limited vision of what is possible" (p. 5). Although collaboration is a complex process, survey participants acknowledged the possible synergistic effects of interagency collaboration. Networking opportunities improved public health disaster response infrastructure and contributed to other community-based projects. Although not specifically mentioned, joint training and educational opportunities help professionals develop a common language and an appreciation for the skills, knowledge, contributions, and points of view of others (Butler, Cohen, Friedman, Scripp, & Watz, 2002).

We captured several differences between frontier and rural counties in this investigation. First, the definite test faced by frontier counties to meet a wide range of service area needs, including the complexities of preparedness, may help explain statements' regarding the burden disaster preparedness puts on limited fiscal and human resources. This reality might support sharing resources in a regional approach to preparedness planning and response while maintaining and preserving local identity and unique needs. Secondly, larger rural jurisdictions are more likely to be an established partner in a LEPC. Partnering is a dynamic and transforming process but requires time, skill, commitment, and interest. As more local public health agencies become active contributors in a LEPC, the potential synergistic effects could raise awareness and help identify ways of extending the public health effort toward disaster and other critical issues. Finally, additional qualitative research focusing on public health professionals and their partnership experiences in rural and frontier communities is needed to learn more about successful efforts to strengthen response to disasters and public health essential service number 4, "mobilize community partnerships to identify and solve health problems" (Public Health Functions Steering Committee, 1994, p. 1).

REFERENCES

American Public Health Association. (2002). *One year after the terrorist attacks: Is public health prepared? A report card from the American Public health Association*. Retrieved October 19, 2002, from http://www.apha.org/united

Butler, J., Cohen, M., Friedman, C., Scripp, R., & Watz, C. (2002). Collaboration between public health and law enforcement: New paradigms and partnerships for bioterrorism planning and response. *Emerging Infectious Disease, 8*(10). Retrieved December, 2002, from http://www.cdc.gov/neidod/EID/Vol8no10/02–0400.htm

Centers for Disease Control and Prevention. (2002). *Local public health preparedness and response capacity inventory: A voluntary rapid self-assessment* (Local Version 1.1). Retrieved December, 2002, from http://www.phppo.cdc.gov/od/inventory/

Cowie, F., Elder, M., & Leibowitz, R. (2000). *Realistic approaches to rural and frontier hazardous materials risk management*. Retrieved June 28, 2002, from http://www.state.mt.us/dma/des/Library/Frontier_HazMat.pdf

Denzin, N., & Lincoln, Y. (1998). *Collecting and interpreting qualitative materials*. Thousand Oaks, CA: Sage.

Department of Justice [DOJ]. (2000). *Public health performance assessment: Emergency preparedness*. Rertrieved September 5, 2000, from http://www.phppo.cdc.gov/Homelandsec6rants/Images/Do.15_41May4.pdf

Drexler, M. (2002). *Secret agents: The menace of emerging infections*. Washington, DC: Joseph Henry Press.

Florin, P., Mitchell, R., Stevenson, J., & Klein, I. (2000). Predicting intermediate outcomes for prevention coalitions: A developmental perspective. *Evaluation and Program Planning, 23*, 341–346.

Gebbie, K. (2002, November 12). *Bioterrorism and emergency readiness: Competencies for all public health workers* (Preview Version II). New York: Columbia University School of Nursing

Gray, B. (1989). *Collaborating: Finding common ground for multiparty problems.* San Francisco, CA: Jossey-Bass.

Henderson, D. (1998). Bioterrorism as a public health threat. *Emerging Infectious Disease, 4*(3), 1–6. Retrieved Novermber 20, 2001, from http:www.cdc.gov/ncidod/eid/vol4no31/hendrsn.htm

Koplan, J. (2001, November). *Building infrastructure to protect the public's health.* Paper presented at the National Public Health Training Network [Satellite Downlink from Atlanta, GA].

Kuntz, S. (2004). Association between collaboration and bioterrorism preparedness in Montana: A local rural public health agency perspective. (Publication #: 3126263). Retrieved May 27, 2004, from http://www.hsls.pitt.edu/guides/hist-med/researchresources/dissertations/dissertations.html?topic_id = 12&mmth = 2004/12

Landesman, L., & Leonard, R. (1993). SARA three years later. *Prehospital Disaster Medicine, 8*(1), 39–44.

Lasker, R., Weiss, E., & Miller, R. (2001). Partnership synergy: A practical framework for studying and strengthening the collaborative advantage. *The Milbank Quarterly, 79*(2), 179–205.

Lindell, M., & Perry, R. (2001). Community innovation in hazardous materials management: Progress in implementing SARA Title III in the United States. *Journal of Hazardous Materials, 88,* 169–194.

Mattessich, P., Murray-Close, M., & Monsey, B. (2001). *Collaboration: What makes it work* (2nd ed.). St. Paul, MN: Amherst H. Wilder Foundation.

McHugh, M., Staiti, A., & Felland, L. (2004). How prepared are Americans for public health emergencies: Twelve communities weigh in. *Health Affairs, 23,* 201–209.

Montana County Profiles. (2002). Retrieved January 15, 2003, from http://www.dphhs.state.mt.us/hpsd/pubheal/healplan/profiles/

Montana Department of Public Health and Human Services [MTDPHHS]. (2002). Montana's public health preparedness and response to bioterrorism and other public health threats and emergencies. Cooperative Agreement with the Centers for Disease Control and Prevention (U90/CCU816832–03–1).

Montana Department of Public Health and Human Services. (2003). *An assessment of Montana's capacity to respond to a public health emergency: Statewide report.* Seattle, WA: University of Washington, Northwest Center for Public Health Practice.

Polivka, B., Dresbach, S., Heimlich, J., & Elliott, M. (2001). Interagency relationships among rural early intervention collaboratives. *Public Health Nursing, 18,* 340–349.

Public Health Functions Steering Committee. (1994). *Public health in America.* Retrieved October, 2001, from http://www.health.gov/phfunctions/public.htm

Reynolds, M., & Leahy, E. (2002). Developing a public health training institute through public health improvement efforts: Montana's story. *Journal of Public Health Management Practice, 8*(1), 83–91.

Smilie, J. (2003, May 2). *Using your preparedness capacity assessment results to conduct a gap analysis.* Paper presented at DPHHS Public Health Emergency Preparedness and Response Program, Helena, MT.

U.S. Code. 1986. Title 42, Chapter 116. *Emergency planning and community right-to-know.* Retrieved June 28, 2002, from http://www4.law.cornell.edu/uscode/42/ch116.html

Weiss, E., Miller, R., & Lasker, R. (2001). *Findings from the national study of partnership functioning: Report to the partnerships that participated.* New York: Center for the Advancement of Collaborative Strategies in Health.

Wetter, D., Daniell, W., & Treser, C. (2001). Hospital preparedness for victims of chemical or biological terrorism. *American Journal of Public Health, 91,* 710–716.

CHAPTER TWENTY-ONE

Environmental Risk Reduction for Rural Children

Wade G. Hill and Patricia Butterfield

Rural living is often portrayed as inherently healthy and wholesome, with children enjoying the benefits of fresh air and clean water. The idealized view of rural life is perpetuated by what some have referred to as the "agrarian myth," in which youngsters thrive on living away from the artificiality and materialism of cities (Kelsey, 1994). However, the realities of rural living and their requisite patterns of environmental exposure are complex, dynamic, and multidimensional. Exposure risks to children vary by place, by time, and by age. The risks also vary by parents' occupations, seasonal changes, and jurisdictional policies addressing the use and disposal of local toxicants. Each of these factors, plus many more, creates a complicated web of exposures that influence current and future risks of disease. Exposure patterns in children are so multifaceted that it is not unusual to see very different measures of exposure among three or four children living under the same roof. Such are the challenges in understanding environmental health risks to children living in rural communities.

However, the challenges inherent in assessing complex exposures in children are, in many ways, dwarfed by the ability of the current health care system to document patterns of exposure in groups at risk. Neither exposures to biologic and chemical agents nor their potential health consequences (e.g., asthma, neurodegenerative diseases) are recorded systematically in medical databases. Health providers have a superficial understanding of only the most prevalent exposures (e.g., lead) and are typically at a loss to answer clients' questions about other common exposure risks (e.g., pesticides, solvents, metals).

For more than 200 years, rural areas have been considered the "dumping ground" of a production-based economy. Items (e.g., nuclear waste, antiquated military supplies) and activities (e.g., mining, smelting) considered dangerous, distasteful, or requiring large plots of land have been preferentially located in remote parts of the country. Contaminants from such historic activities have left a legacy of risks for local residents. Because the contamination is not routinely discovered until decades later, the culpable group can no longer be located and the community must rely on federal resources for cleanup and remediation resources. Typically rural municipalities lack both the financial, technical, and scientific expertise (e.g., laboratories, behavioral researchers) to understand local exposures and their commensurate health risks. Small county and regional health departments, which have been understaffed and overmandated since September 11, 2001, often field questions about environmental risks in their area, but lack the time and money to fully pursue investigative efforts. Rural families who live in unincorporated areas may live adjacent to agricultural (e.g., combined animal feeding operations) and industrial facilities, but may be unaware of risks associated with such facilities.

Despite risk patterns that may pose a threat to young children, contaminant patterns in rural communities are understudied and rural citizens are often underrepresented in environmental health research (Malcoe, Lynch, Keger, & Skaggs, 2002). Research in rural communities has focused almost exclusively on the sequelae from a specific agent (e.g., mercury, arsenic) or contaminant site (e.g., Environmental Protection Agency [EPA] Superfund site). Such research has provided an important foundation about the health consequences of living adjacent to a mine, railroad yard, or waste disposal site. However, examining environmental health risks from a single agent perspective provides a myopic view of risks to a family or community, rather than providing families with answers about their overall health risks and what they can do to minimize such risks.

Requirements of rural nursing practice necessarily follow trends in the health status of populations, demographic changes, and the dynamic nature of the determinants of health, illness, and safety. From a population view, perhaps no segment of our society requires more attention in promoting health than young children. It is known that the most rapid mental growth occurs during early childhood and that the early years are critical in the development of intelligence, personality, and social behavior (Bellamy, 2002). Equally important is an understanding that children are particularly susceptible to environmental exposures as the exploratory behaviors of childhood are the principle ways that children learn (Moya, Bearer, & Etzel, 2004).

Rural nurses have a unique opportunity to identify and intervene in cases where environmental exposures to children exist. Despite commonly held notions that rural environments offer isolation from environmental contaminants, many rural areas offer the most potent environmental exposures in the United States. For example, the state of Montana currently has 11 sites of industrial contamination listed on the National Priority List (Superfund), and ranks among the top 20% of states in land releases of toxic contaminants (Scorecard.org, 2004). Although rural childhood environmental exposures may result from effluents of extractive industries or other industrial sites, many chronic environmental exposures occur within the home where caregivers and nurses have significant capacity for intervention. By employing common sense low-cost behaviors, caregivers of young children can prevent environmental exposures that may manifest in negative health outcomes.

ENVIRONMENTAL RISK REDUCTION THROUGH NURSING INTERVENTION AND EDUCATION (ERRNIE)

The Environmental Risk Reduction Through Nursing Intervention and Education study (ERRNIE) is a 5–year project designed primarily to (a) determine the prevalence of multiple environmental exposures among rural children and (b) deliver and evaluate environmental risk reduction education to rural households by public health nurses through a randomized controlled trial. Because nurses generally feel unprepared to manage environmental health issues (Van Dongen, 2002), the ERRNIE project will also evaluate the capacity and needs of public health nurses to integrate environmental health into their practice. The ERRNIE project capitalizes on the existing public health infrastructure that currently accesses at-risk populations through programs such as WIC, immunization clinics, and the Head Start program among others. Childhood exposures of interest in the ERRNIE study are those that occur in or around homes and include ETS, radon, CO, lead, and impurities in well water. In the discussion that follows we focus on the first objective of the ERRNIE study, to determine the prevalence of multiple environmental exposures among rural children.

The conceptual basis for the ERRNIE project is the World Health Organizations Multiple Exposures Multiple Effects (MEME) model first described in the report, "Making a Difference: Indicators to Improve Children's Environmental Health" (Briggs, 2003). This model suggests that neither exposures nor health indicators can be interpreted in simple direct relationships and that health outcomes should be viewed in terms of actions and contexts as well as exposures. The MEME model proposes that the exposure and health outcome dichotomy exists within contextual

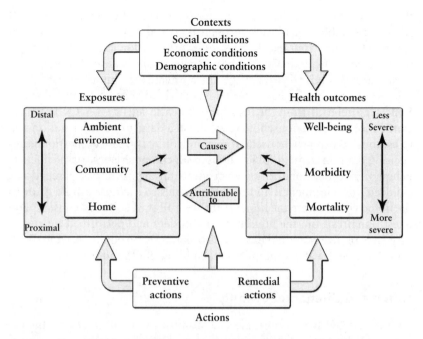

Figure 21.1. The Multiple Exposures Multiple Effects Model

From *Indicators to Improve Children's Environmental Health,* by D. Briggs, 2003, p. 145 Geneva, Switzerland: World Health Organization. Copyright 2003 World Health Organization. Reprinted with permission.

conditions (e.g., social, economic, and demographic conditions) that may influence the nature of the relationship. This idea agrees with the assumption of the ERRNIE project that rural environments offer unique risk factors for environmental exposures, such as lack of municipal water, sewage treatment, and housing regulations. The MEME model also portrays the home environment as the most proximal location for employing preventive actions to limit exposures associated with health outcomes (Fig. 21.1).

METHODS

Design

Because Phase I of the ERRNIE project attempts to understand the prevalence of multiple environmental contaminants among rural children, the project staff used a cross-sectional correlational design. Project staff recruited eligible households through the local public health agency in Gallatin County Montana. To be eligible for the study, each household had to be located in Gallatin County, be receiving public health services, have at least one child under 6 years of age, use a private or community well as the primary source of drinking water, and had to read or speak English fluently. Following referral from the local public health agency, ERRNIE project staff contacted each household to establish a date for home visitation and to establish a primary household respondent. Staff mailed questionnaires eliciting data on demographics, household characteristics, risk reduction behaviors, occupational risks, environmental exposure risk perceptions, children's developmental and health histories to each household prior to the home visit. During the home visit ERRNIE staff collected consents and questionnaires from the household respondent and performed the necessary tests on five potential exposures of interest: carbon monoxide (CO), lead, ETS, well water contaminants, and household radon.

Home and Biomarker Testing

Staff tested CO with a portable CO monitor (Series 450, Dwyer Instruments, Michigan City, IN) following an established protocol that included an assessment of primary and secondary gas heat sources, gas water heaters, gas range tops and ovens, and gas dryers. They tested individual appliances followed by a total system induction which they turned on all gas appliances and tested each appliance. The staff established action level for CO exposures at 9 ppm and referred values at or above this level to the local health department and the client's health care provider. Additionally, staff advised clients not to use the appliance until it had been retested by the local fire department or energy provider (testing is free) and provided health education concerning the cause and health effects of CO exposure.

The project staff also tested each child in the household for exposure to lead and ETS. They accomplished lead testing by using blood lead collection filter paper (Tamarack Medical Lab, Centennial, CO) and a single finger-stick for each child. Action levels for lead exposure were set conservatively at 5 μg/dL; staff retested all values at or above this level for confirmation and trend analysis and referred them to the local public health department and clients health care provider for follow-up. They also collected urine samples (2–3 ml) from household children to assess ETS exposure through cotinine assay (Mayo Medical Laboratories, Rochester, MN). There was no established action level for ETS exposure but staff provided education regarding health effects of passive smoke exposure for all positive findings.

Last, staff assessed possible contaminants from well water and household radon. They collected water samples from each household for a complete well screen (Montana Department of Public Health, Environmental Laboratory) including the assessment of bacteria, nitrates, metals (e.g., lead, arsenic), anions (e.g., sulfate, fluoride), petroleum, and pesticides or herbicides. Because of the complexity of water chemistry and the number of possible contaminants evaluated, a water quality expert evaluated each case independently and performed appropriate follow-up testing and referral for abnormal findings. Staff left a short-term charcoal radon test (DRHOMEAIR, Alpha Energy Laboratories, Carrollton, TX) with each household after reviewing the instructions for performing the test with the primary household respondent. Staff provided any household with a radon level exceeding 4 pCi/L (EPA established action level a long-term radon test as well as referral back to the health department and their usual medical provider for follow-up.

FINDINGS

Sample Description

Thirty-one rural households were referred from the local health department in Gallatin County, Montana, and consented to participate in the ERRNIE project. Each household had an average of 2 adults (range: 1–5) and 2 children (range 1–5) and the primary household respondents were female (100%), aged 21–40 (94%), and Caucasian (97%). Consistent with a population receiving public health services, 58% of the sample either had no source of health insurance or were receiving Medicaid and generally had total household incomes of less than $35,000 (68%).

Children's Exposures

Our findings indicate that rural children in Gallatin County experience preventable environmental exposures within the home and that some experience multiple exposures. Table 21.1 shows the number of households that had exposures exceeding action levels for ETS, radon, CO, lead, and impurities in well water.

About 13% ($n = 4$) of the households and 7% ($n = 4$) of the children in this sample had identifiable exposures to ETS. Urinary cotinine values among these four children ranged from 18 to 41 μg/dL indicating that the children were moderately to heavily exposed to ETS (Pirkle et al., 1996). In total, we found 10 households containing 18 children to have radon levels above the EPA action level of 4 pCi/L. Radon levels within the homes ranged from 4.10 to 24.10 with an average of 10.0

Table 21.1 Children's Environmental Exposures
(*N* = 31 households, 58 children)

	Households		Children	
Type of environmental exposure	*n*	%	*n*	%
Tobacco smoke[a]	4	12.9	4	6.9
Radon[b]	10	32.3	10	31.0
Carbon monoxide[c]	1	3.2	1	1.7
Lead[d]	6	19.4	7	12.1
Impure well water[e]	12	38.7	21	36.2
Multiple	8	25.8	16	27.5

[a]ETS exposure defined as any cotinine value above 5 ng/ml. [b]Radon exposure defined by levels ≥ 4pCi/L. [c]CO exposure defined by ≥ 9 ppm on any appliance. [d]Lead exposure defined by ≥ 5 μg/dL. [e]Impure well water exposure was expert defined as any contaminant that may pose health risk.

pCi/L (SD = 5.85). We found CO levels exceeding 9 ppm in a single house with a single child where a stovetop burner emitted 14 ppm CO with a spot-check.

We found blood lead levels exceeding 5 μg/dL among 7 children (12.1 % of sample) in 6 households and ranged from 5.0 to 7.5 μg/dL with an average of 5.9 μg/dL. We identified well water quality issues as follows: 9 households with total coliform bacteria counts exceeding quality standards, 2 households that had chemical contamination, and 1 household that had naturally occurring fluoride levels exceeding safe levels. In total, almost 39% of the households in this sample experienced some water quality issue that had the potential to effect health.

We found multiple household exposures among 16 children (27.5%) residing in 8 households (25.8%). Combinations of exposures that occurred most frequently included having both radon and water quality problems (3 households), lead exposure and water quality problems (2 households), and ETS exposure and water quality problems (2 households). We found single household containing 3 children to have 3 exposures including lead, ETS, and water quality problems.

DISCUSSION

Data from Phase I of the ERRNIE project support the need for environmental risk reduction interventions among rural populations receiving public health services. These data indicate that many rural children likely experience potent exposures to environmental agents known to have health consequences. Although each exposure carries unique risk of health consequences, exposures that occur in or around the home may be prevented with simple low-cost solutions.

Behaviors aimed at reducing environmental health risks for children focusing in or around the home have been organized into four main categories: (a) environmental modification; (b) caretaker vigilance; (c) food; (d) home, and personal hygiene; (e) and behavioral modification (Schneider & Freeman, 2000). Many of the behaviors within these categories require little to no resources and have the potential to yield significant benefits in risk reduction from exposure to environmental contaminants. Environmental modification includes actions such as placing doormats at home entry areas to collect potential contaminants, designating places isolated from living areas where dirty clothes and shoes are stored, and keeping household chemicals out of reach of children. Caretaker vigilance requires adults who are responsible for children to consider issues such as the hygiene and food preparation practices of day care services and not allowing anyone to smoke in the presence of their children. Food, home, and personal hygiene simply directs adults to wash foods well, maintain safe food cooking and storage practices, and teaching children the importance of hand washing. Last, important aspects of behavioral modification with respect to children's environmental health include enforcing the use of utensils for eating and running tap water for a period of time before drinking.

ETS

Childhood exposures to ETS are known to cause health effects, such as middle ear disease, asthma, bronchitis, pneumonia, and impaired pulmonary function (DiFranza, Aligne, & Weitzman, 2004). Four children in four separate households within Phase 1 of this study were shown to have appreciable and significant exposures to ETS. National averages of serum cotinine for a non-smoking population aged 3–11 years range from 0.109 to 3.37 ng/ml (National Center for Environmental Health, 2003). When adjusting for the differences between urinary and serum concentrations of cotinine (i.e., urinary levels are about 6 times greater; Benowitz, 1999), cotinine values for the children in this study ranged from 3.0 to 6.8 ng/ml placing these children in the top 10% of non smokers in the United States for this age group.

Household Radon

Significant radon exposure occurred in about a third of the sample for both households and children. Although acute effects of radon exposure in children are unlikely, regulatory agencies such as the EPA and International Agency for Research on Cancer have consistently classified radon as carcinogenic to humans (Frumkin & Samet, 2001). The average radon level within our sample was 10.0 pCi/L (SD = 5.85), which translates to a lifetime lung cancer risk of 56 out of 1,000 persons compared with 23 out of 10,000 persons with consistent lifetime exposures to radon at 0.4 pCi/l (U.S. EPA, 2003).

CO Poisoning

Effects of CO poisoning are well-known and include fatigue, headaches, dizziness, impaired vision and coordination, confusion, and possibly death. The U.S. National Ambient Air Quality Standards for indoor air limits CO concentrations to 9 ppm over an 8–hr period (U.S. EPA, 2004) although cumulative measurements over extended periods of time are difficult and costly. Because of this, measurement of CO for this study represents an effort to screen for possible malfunctioning appliances and the potential for harmful levels of CO to be present within the home. Despite finding only a single household with relatively low concentrations of CO (14 ppm) from a single appliance, possible acute health effects from exposure to CO warrant continued attention.

Lead Poisoning

Pediatric lead poisoning has remained a priority environmental health issue since the use of lead-based paints and lead additives to gasoline have brought exposures within close reach of children. Among adults, health effects from lead exposure, such as neurobehavioral abnormalities, tend to be reversible (Baker et al., 1985); however the more centralized nervous system effects occurring in children are not (Needleman, Schell, Bellinger, Leviton, & Allred, 1990). Although a 1991 CDC statement on childhood lead poisoning suggests 10 μg/dL as a screening action guideline, a threshold value below which lead has no apparent adverse developmental effect has not been established (Bellinger, 2004). In fact, some evidence indicates that children with blood lead levels lower than 10 μg/dL experience sustained effects of lower IQ, academic achievement, and cognitive function (Bellinger, Stiles, & Needleman, 1992; Lanphear, Dietrich, Auinger, & Cox, 2000). Blood lead concentrations of 7 (12.1%) children in 6 (19.4%) households ranged from 5.0 to 7.5 μg/dL and indicate that children in this sample were at risk for developmental effects from lead exposure.

Well Water Impurities

Impurities in well water can take many forms each imparting a particular set of health risks. Because of the complexity of well water chemistry, a water quality expert evaluated analysis results from each water sample in this study to determine if health risks were present. Findings indicate that most (75%) well water contamination in this sample occurred as a result of total coliform counts exceeding safety standards. Total coliform is generally thought to be a nonspecific indicator of fecal contamination and may indicate the presence of more pathogenic bacteria, such as Escherichia coli, which is associated with acute gastrointestinal illness (Strauss, King, Ley, & Hoey, 2001). Other contamination findings include two households with chemical contamination thought to be related to solvents leaching from plumbing and one household with naturally occurring fluoride levels exceeding safe standards.

Solutions

Simple low to no-cost solutions exist for each of the five potential exposures of interest in the ERRNIE project. ETS can be easily avoided by designating a place outside of the home to smoke, not smoking in automobiles although children are present, and ventilating the home well. Although full abatement for homes with high radon levels is costly, caretakers can locate sleeping areas for children on upper levels within the home and maximize ventilation. All homes with gas appliances should have CO detectors, which are fairly inexpensive (i.e., $20–30) and malfunctioning appliances should be repaired or replaced. Exposures to lead can be limited or avoided by cleaning floors and walls to minimize dust, using doormats and areas of the home separate from living areas for soiled shoes and clothing, hand washing, and being aware of occupational risk factors where adults may carry lead into the home from work environments. Well water should be tested annually for contaminants, and testing is often subsidized by local health authorities. A number of solutions exist for unsafe well water depending on the type of contaminant involved. Bacterial contamination can usually be addressed cheaply by following a cleaning procedure using a diluted bleach solution within the well, and more complex problems can be addressed by various water cleaning and filtration systems of varying costs. The least costly solution may be to use a municipal source of water for drinking and cooking until more permanent solutions can be found.

CONCLUSIONS AND IMPLICATIONS FOR RURAL NURSING

Although many environmental health problems are necessarily addressed on a population level through policy and regulation, changes toward health protections can be slow and may often be at odds with other forces in the social milieu, such as economics. Although policy may be ideal for broad-based reform to prevent childhood exposures to environmental contaminants, nurses working at the household level have a significant capacity to assist families in understanding and identifying health risks and risk-avoidance strategies.

Families and communities often look to nurses for guidance on health risks, especially those associated with hazards at home or work (National Environmental Education & Training Foundation, 2002). Rural areas provide a context for increased risk of environmental exposures for children that may have both acute and long-term health consequences. Lack of resources, regulatory fragmentation, and the inadequacy of data and data systems contribute to this context (Center for Rural Health Practice, 2004), and rural nurses should become increasingly aware of how they can improve the environmental health of their communities.

REFERENCES

Baker, E. L., White, R. F., Pothier, L. J., Berkey, C. S., Dinse, G. E., Travers, P. H., et al. (1985). Occupational lead neurotoxicity: improvement in behavioural effects after reduction of exposure. *British Journal of Industrial Medicine, 42*(8), 507–516.

Bellamy, C. (2002). Child health. In R. Detels, J. McEwen, R. Beaglehole & H. Tanaka (Eds.), *Oxford textbook of public health* (4th ed., pp. 1603–1622). Oxford: Oxford University Press.

Bellinger, D. C. (2004). Lead. *Pediatrics* (Vol. 113, pp. 1016–1022): Washington, DC: American Academy of Pediatrics.

Bellinger, D. C., Stiles, K. M., & Needleman, H. L. (1992). Low-level lead exposure, intelligence and academic achievement: A long-term follow-up study. *Pediatrics, 90,* 855–861.

Benowitz, N. L. (1999). Biomarkers of ETS exposure. *Environmental Health Perspectives, 107,* Suppl. 2, 349–355.

Briggs, D. (2003). *Indicators to improve children's environmental health.* Geneva, Switzerland: World Health Organization.

Center for Rural Health Practice. (2004). *Bridging the health divide: The rural public health research agenda.* Pittsburgh: University of Pittsburgh.

DiFranza, J. R., Aligne, C. A., & Weitzman, M. (2004). Prenatal and postnatal environmental tobacco smoke exposure and children's health. *Pediatrics* (Vol. 113, pp. 1007–1015): Washington, DC: American Academy of Pediatrics.

Frumkin, H., & Samet, J. M. (2001). Radon. *A Cancer Journal for Clinicians, 51*(6), 337–344, quiz 345–348.

Kelsey, T. W. (1994). The agrarian myth and policy responses to farm safety. *American Journal of Public Health, 84,* 1171–1177.

Lanphear, B. P., Dietrich, K., Auinger, P., & Cox, C. (2000). Cognitive deficits associated with blood lead concentrations < 10 microg/dL in US children and adolescents. *Public Health Reports, 115,* 521–529.

Malcoe, L. H., Lynch, R. A., Keger, M. C., & Skaggs, V. J. (2002). Lead sources, behaviors, and socioeconomic factors in relation to blood lead of Native American and White children: A community-based assessment of a former mining area. *Environmental Health Perspectives, 110* (Suppl. 2), 221–31.

Moya, J., Bearer, C. F., & Etzel, R. A. (2004). Children's behavior and physiology and how it affects exposure to environmental contaminants. *Pediatrics* (Vol. 113, pp. 996–1006). Washington, DC: American Academy of Pediatrics.

National Center for Environmental Health. (2003). *Second National Report on Human Exposure to environmental chemicals.* Retrieved July 28, 2004, from http://www.cdc.gov/exposurereport/2nd/pdf/secondner.pdf

National Environmental Education & Training Foundation. (2002). Nurses and environmental health: Success through action. In *Agency for Toxic Substances and Disease Registry* (Ed.), Washington, DC: Author.

Needleman, H. L., Schell, A., Bellinger, D., Leviton, A., & Allred, E. N. (1990). The long-term effects of exposure to low doses of lead in childhood. An 11–year follow-up report. *New England Journal of Medicine, 322,* 83–88.

Pirkle, J. L., Flegal, K. M., Bernert, J. T., Brody, D. J., Etzel, R. A., & Maurer, K. R. (1996). Exposure of the US population to ETS: The Third National Health and Nutrition Examination Survey, 1988 to 1991. *Journal of the American Medical Association, 275,* 1233–1240.

Schneider, D., & Freeman, N. (2000). *Childrens environmental health: Reducing risk in a dangerous world.* Washington, DC: American Public Health Association.

Scorecard.org. (2004). *Land contamination report: Montana.* Retrieved July 26, 2004, from http://www.scorecard.org/env-releases/land/state.tcl?fips_state_code = 30#ej

Strauss, B., King, W., Ley, A., & Hoey, J. R. (2001). A prospective study of rural drinking water quality and acute gastrointestinal illness. *BMC Public Health, 1*(1), 8.

U. S. Environmental Protection Agency. (2003). *EPA assessment of risks from radon in homes.* Retrieved July 28, 2004, from http://www.epa.gov/radiation/docs/assessment/radon_in_homes.pdf

U. S. Environmental Protection Agency. (2004). *Sources of indoor air pollution— carbon monoxide (CO).* Retrieved July 28, 2004, from http://www.epa.gov/iaq/co.html

Van Dongen, C. J. (2002). Environmental health and nursing practice: A survey of registered nurses. *Applied Nursing Research, 15*(2), 67–73.

CHAPTER TWENTY-TWO

Rural School Health: Who Covers for the Rural School Nurse When There is None?

Laurie Bernhardt Glover

Nearly 150,000 children prekindergarten through 12th grade attend schools in Montana (Montana Office of Public Instruction, 2004). Montana law does not require local districts to provide school nursing services. The school nurse role is as variable as the geographic landscape of this immense rural state. The spectrum ranges from schools with no school nurse to those with full-time nursing services; many school nurses often will divide time between several schools.

Montana's county health departments also frequently include school services as part of their total county health services. Of the total 56 Montana counties, 53 responded to a Montana Department of Public Health and Human Services (MDPHHS) survey detailing school nursing services (Jo Ann Dotson, MDPHHS, personal communication, July 1, 2004). Of the responding counties, 47 (89%) stated their counties did provide at least some school nursing services. However, the number of hours was highly variable, with a range of 0–165 hours (m = 18.9, Mode 2).

My observation during two decades as a Montana public health professional and parent is that in schools with no school nurse, secretaries are incorporating increasingly greater health components into their duties.

It follows that secretaries likely have evolving roles and outlooks on the health status of Montana children. My purpose in this qualitative study was to explore the perceptions of a group of school secretaries in a variety of school settings and identify variables affecting their role comfort.

OVERVIEW OF COMMUNITIES AND METHDOLOGY

Secretaries from six schools participated in the study. Two schools encompassed K–12 populations, whereas the other four were elementary only. Five of the schools were public schools and one was a parochial school. Enrollments ranged from 130–400 for the six schools. Four schools are located in rural towns, and two are located in cities in rural counties. The schools located in cities were blocks away from a hospital and physician offices. Three of the rural towns were 20–30 miles from the nearest professional health care providers. The remaining rural town had local health care provider(s) and a hospital. It was not unusual in the rural towns to have students bused 30 miles one way to school, which could make their homes 60 miles from the nearest health care provider. Five of the schools were located in a county with a population density of 29.3 persons per square mile, and one school was located in a county with a population density of 0.8 persons per square mile (U.S. Bureau of the Census, 1998). This could be considered frontier, although this school was just two blocks away from a hospital and health care provider.

At the time of this study, the leading cause of death for children aged 5–14 and teens and adults aged 15–24 years in Montana was accidents (Montana Department of Public Health and Human Services, 1998). Secretaries in this study uniformly identified injuries as the most common health condition occurring in the children they served.

All secretaries interviewed said health-related duties comprised an average 15%–25% of their total duties. None of the schools involved in the study employed or contracted with a school nurse. Each county in the study had a health department with public health nurses available for school consultation by phone and sometimes by site visit.

I selected school secretaries to include a sampling of rural and urban public and parochial settings. I used semistructured interviews to collect data. I either tape-recorded interviews or recorded them by writing. I open-coded data. I confirmed emerging categories and their properties following consultation with a consultant. I repeated the process of constant data comparison throughout the analysis to allow for the emergence of categories and relationships (Chenitz & Swanson, 1986). I used theoretical coding and memo writing to identify emerging relationships.

FINDINGS

The phenomenon of "knowing" emerged as a process on a continuum with a positive consequence of "role comfort" and a negative consequence of "role ambivalence" or "role discomfort." The conditions in existence for the phenomenon knowing to occur in the study were such factors as age, experience, years of residence in community, and formal and informal education. Knowing, as developed in this study, was more than a set body of acquired knowledge. More broad and abstract in nature, it included knowing the subtleties of the community as well as health content needed for the job.

The following is a paradigm induced from the study by grounded theory. The "Knowing Fosters Role Comfort" paradigm will be the basis for the discussion of the findings (see Figure 22.1).

Conditions of Knowing

I identified conditions from the study as having an effect on the phenomenon of knowing and thus, the hypothetical result of role comfort or discomfort. The age range for the secretaries was 36–69 years (m = 49 years). The years worked at their respective schools ranged from 6–29 (m = 14). All had received a formal education of 12–13 years, and two had obtained a year of vocational health training posthigh school. Years lived in the community ranged from 7–69 (m = 36). Four of the six secretaries had training in first aid, CPR (cardiopulmonary resuscitation), or other health training (not for professional licensure), either obtained on their own or provided by the school.

The Phenomenon of Knowing

Secretaries related knowing their role and responsibilities as pertaining to health services to school children. They identified themselves as being the first and often sole person responsible for injury care, sick child care, calls to parents, referrals, and medications.

> If there's an injury, the staff will send them to me. I am to decide if it's serious enough to call a parent or call paramedics, whatever. Then I will administer the first aid if it's something I can do.

Knowing Fosters Role Comfort

Role ambivalence/Discomfort←——**<KNOWING>**——→**Role comfort**

Conditions of knowing: **age, job and life experience, training, years in community.**
Conditions of role comfort: **proximity to health care, smaller school enrollment.**

Figure 22.1 Study paradigm.

Dealing with a wide range of actual and potential health conditions, the secretaries are aware they need to know what to do for the unexpected. One secretary related, "We have three diabetic students. I know about what happens to them, if they get too high or they get too low, what I need to do to help them. We have severely asthmatic children."

The secretaries were also cognizant of their limitations and freely stated them in the majority of the interviews. They often declared they were asked to "diagnose" conditions by other staff and sometimes parents, yet did not feel qualified to do so: "I don't claim to know what a nurse would know and it's not my place to make any type of decision like that."

All interviewees knew and were able to list the most frequent health problems they saw in the children and also barriers to receiving medical care. Many cited playground injuries and common acute illnesses as those most often needing attention during the school day. However, some were concerned about other less obvious health care needs they observed.

> You know, the one area that I see at my school is during our dental screening ... we do have a lot of kids who need attention that way and just aren't getting it. Insurance these days with the parent's workplace just doesn't cover dental services ... it's just not a priority in some households.

One secretary noted that being in the central office, she had access to information peripheral to basic health, such as which children had emotional problems. She stated, "Not only just medically, emotionally, there are kids that need help too. I'm sure there's ways that people could get help, but whether they choose not to or they don't know how ..."

As secretaries pointed out their limitations, they also listed resources called into play when they have questions. The resource used by all the secretaries interviewed was the local health department. Secretaries were not hesitant to telephone health department nurses for needed information and advice on health matters. One interviewee reported, "I never hesitate to call the county health. We have called the clinic also and talked to the nurses there and they're always very good, but my first choice is always the county health."

Local health care professionals were used by one half of the secretaries. In one case, a local doctor taught the entire school staff about diabetes because two students had the disease. Two rural secretaries turned to local emergency medical responders or teachers with first aid training in their communities with questions. One secretary cited the use of parents who were nurses as resources. Only one secretary listed the use of a medical or health book as a resource.

Two who had prior vocational health training said they used this training in their job performance. One secretary had worked with medical insurance forms in a previous job and used this knowledge to refer parents to financial assistance programs.

Several related they had developed knowledge through years of experience with certain conditions at their school jobs. Others described an inner knowing based on years of personal life experiences or exposure to relatives with medical backgrounds. A secretary related, "The diabetic kids, their parents know that I know enough ... I know how to react to this now ... because we've had them for all the years I've been here. I know what to do with it." Another interviewee reported, "My sister-in-law's a nurse. I have a lot of family in the medical field, so it's not something I don't know a little about. I think more than anything we use our maternal instinct as for what needs to be done."

Finally, the secretaries discussed knowing their communities in varying degrees. Several had lived in their towns their entire lives. One secretary who was a relative newcomer to her community (7 years) described a negative perception of some diversity she observed in her community. "... I don't know, they're a different kind of people with different thoughts of how things should be and that creates a problem too."

Other secretaries who had lived in their communities at least 20 years portrayed an understanding of what mattered to their fellow residents, what worked and didn't work.

> ... You know, I think I am [more trusted because I am a longtime resident]. And only because I have an aide that, the name is not known, so they always ask for me. And she would give the same advice or even better advice than me. This would be the downfall of me living there all my life and knowing people. I can be a little pushy. "Don't you see?" or "Have you done this?"

The parochial school secretary described her church and school community as a small community where everybody knows everybody, even though it is located within a larger Montana town. She went on to state that the school has a fund for those children unable to afford medical care, an example of a community networking to care for its members.

Role Ambivalence or Discomfort vs. Role Comfort

Analysis of demographic and coded qualitative data through comparison and contrasts yielded the following results. The secretaries who reported a higher level of role comfort were those who had vocational health training or first aid and CPR. They also tended to be older, had more years on the job, and had been a community resident longer than the mean time for participants. Two other factors examined in the study appeared to be related to role comfort. Those who perceived themselves as more comfortable in their roles tended to be close in proximity to health care providers and worked in schools with smaller enrollments than those with less perceived role comfort. The assumption is that proximity to health care providers increased the comfort level of the lay provider. Also, the concern of transportation time in serious injuries and illnesses is lessened. My assumption is that smaller school enrollments place fewer demands on the secretary and consequently, increased role comfort.

The secretaries perceived feelings of ambivalence and role discomfort. One secretary, a long-time community resident with no health training, was not in close proximity to health care providers and served a larger school population. She was also younger in age and experience than the average interviewee. "Really none of my duties should have to do with health services, I wouldn't think. There is a lot of responsibility put on me that I'm not always comfortable with."

Secretaries who did not have a higher level of perceived role comfort used words such as "scary," "nerve-wracking," and "luck" when recounting situations they had handled. One secretary was advised that deliberately not getting health training could be in her best interests.

> ... it's always been an issue. Do I want to become certified? Am I more liable if I become certified in CPR? ... Nobody really knows for sure. They seem to think that it's better that I don't become certified in CPR.

Two respondents who had higher perceived role comfort were able to state that and relate it to either formal or informal training or experience. One secretary had vocational and first aid or CPR training as well as many years experience. She was a long-time community resident and in close proximity to health care providers. Her school enrollment was one half of the former secretary's school. "I have a fairly high responsibility level, but am comfortable with it. I think any secretary needs medical training, what to watch for." Another secretary with many years of community residence and experience at her school was able to see her progression in comfort through the years. "It used to be I'd feel stressed about it ... what if I said something wrong? Now, I ask a teacher and/or the principal. I don't worry so much."

RELEVANCE TO SCHOOL NURSING
THEORY AND RESEARCH

Caniparoli (1998) used the defining attributes of age, length of time spent in a community, and establishment of a relationship within the community to describe old-timers. Truly, several of the interviewed secretaries could be viewed as old-timers in their communities. By virtue of their status, they have insight into relevant health and social factors of the school children, as well as the community.

Myers (1998) described an insider as a member of a group, having access to privileged information, an awareness of implicit assumptions and social context, and a longtime resident. Many school secretaries, being both old-timers and insiders, are key contacts for health care and information for school-aged children. School secretaries are important community people with whom nurses should establish contact.

Although this study did not measure community members' perceptions of the secretaries' health role performance, I assumed they are valued because of the care entrusted to them. Also, secretaries reported that they are asked health questions by parents on the job and in the community. Turnbull (1998) called nonprofessional persons who are asked for health care *advice lay consultants*. Interestingly, the four secretaries living in rural towns all said they were asked health questions during off-duty hours. The two secretaries living in the city were not. One rural school secretary said, "There is a role overlap. They might ask me questions in the restaurant after school hours. But I love the parents here; they're all nice."

IMPLICATIONS FOR RURAL NURSING PRACTICE

The findings and implications of this study are limited to the state and communities in which I conducted the interviews. Although similarities exist between Montana and other rural states, more research is recommended before applications to other communities can be made.

Nurses in rural communities should make contact with the school secretary. Nurses could garner valuable information about the community and children in particular and affect the health of the community through health education classes offered to the students and staff. Health information sharing and assistance in establishing health procedure guidelines by nurses could potentially enhance the secretary's role comfort and job performance.

Nurses in their dual roles as professionals and parents can advocate for increased basic health education to school personnel responsible for children's health needs. This advocacy role can be enacted through parent meetings, school board meetings, the media and legislature. School secretaries rarely meet as a group according to the interviewees. Thus public health nurses can use existing telecommunication networks to link with rural schools to provide education on health matters. An example of available technology is Montana's Office of Public Instruction's METNET (Montana Office of Public Instruction, 2004).

Potential problems exist when school secretaries without basic health training provide health care to children. First, school secretaries are vulnerable to liability litigation. Second, the children in their charge are vulnerable to inadequate first aid care. Some secretaries were told by fellow employees that health care training is not in their best interests. School administrators and regulatory agency personnel need to acknowledge potential liabilities and train secretaries just as they train bus drivers. The title secretary is a misnomer as it does not address the scope of duties required of school secretaries. They need to be afforded the training needed for the safe performance of their jobs and informed of the legal boundaries. School administrators must facilitate this training through available or newly funded resources.

As budgets are cut and priorities are set, nurses' voices need to be heard as they argue for continued or reinstated nurse presence in schools. Five of the six interviewed secretaries verbalized a desire for a school nurse who would be an accessible health expert and also could help set guidelines and protocols. Several wished for a nurse employee or nurse volunteer to help with busy periods of medication administration and the occurrence of injuries, such as noon hours.

Nurses with access to school administrators can facilitate enhanced health training to school employees. They can also urge administrators to address liability concerns of school secretaries with factual information.

State and county health agency personnel and their nurse employees should target school secretaries with information on medical insurance programs geared to low-income families. One secretary said she received a Children's Health Insurance Program brochure the first year of its existence in Montana but since then she has had to call for brochures each year. She then mails them to parents and follows up with phone calls encouraging eligible families to apply.

Rural nurses, other health care providers, and school secretaries can be a most effective team when working in coordination to provide health care oversight in the schools. In conclusion, the school secretaries illustrated here have basic health knowledge and awareness of their limitations. They know their school population and community. Nurses have the problem-solving and group process skills to bring together rural community members to discuss and move toward the best health environment for their schools.

REFERENCES

Caniparoli, C. (1998). Old-timer. In H. J. Lee (Ed.), *Conceptual basis for rural nursing* (pp.102–112). New York: Springer Publishing.

Chenitz, W. C., & Swanson, J. A. (1986). *From practice to grounded theory: Qualitative research in nursing*. Menlo Park, CA: Addison-Wesley.

Montana Department of Public and Human Services. (1998). *1997 Montana vital statistics*. Helena, MT: Author.

Montana Office of Public Instruction. (2004). *Enrollment data Fall 2003–04*. Retrieved July 9, 2004, from http://www.opi.state.mt.us

Myers, D. (1998). Insider. In H. J. Lee (Ed.) *Conceptual basis for rural nursing* (pp.125–138). New York: Springer Publishing.

Turnbull, T. (1998). Lay care network. In H. J. Lee (Ed.), *Conceptual basis for rural nursing* (pp. 189–199). New York: Springer Publishing.

U.S. Bureau of the Census. (1998). *1998 estimates of Montana's resident population*. Washington, DC: Author.

CHAPTER TWENTY-THREE

Improving the Health Literacy of Rural Elders: An Interdisciplinary Approach

M. Susan Jones, Marilyn M. Gardner, Janelle A. Peeler,
Serena Merry Britt, and Marilyn Lewis Graves

Almost 25% of the general population of the United States lives in a rural area. In Kentucky, roughly 15% of the rural population is aged 65 or older (U.S. Bureau of Census, 2000). Elders in rural areas are more likely to be poorer than their metropolitan counterparts and are at risk for being underinsured or uninsured. Long traveling distances to obtain services as well as lack of personal transportation are barriers to seniors seeking health care. Rural elders also have poorer perceptions of their health status and are likely to have a higher rate of chronic disease (Bushy, 2000). Research indicates that health literacy is directly related to health outcomes, length and frequency of hospitalizations, and health care expenditures (Davis & Magilvy, 2000; Kovner & Harrington, 2000). The significant dissonance that exists between rural elder's perception of their health and their actual health status can be lessened by improving their health literacy status. Our purpose of this chapter is to describe an interdisciplinary learning experience for health care professionals aimed at improving the health literacy of rural elders and the challenges and rewards of implementing such a program.

PROGRAM DESCRIPTION: AN OVERVIEW

The Health Enhancement of the Rural Elderly (HERE) project is a federally funded program designed to empower rural elders to maximize their use of the health care system by improving health literacy and fostering strong community relationships. The targeted population for this project were people aged 65 and older living in two south central counties in Kentucky identified as rural and poor. The demographics of the counties indicated similarities in population with each county recording approximately 11,000 residents with 20% of the population of each county living below the poverty level. Residents above the age of 65 comprise 14% to 15% of the total population of each county. Both counties are classified as Health Care Professional Shortage Areas (HPSA, Health Resources & Services Administration [HRSA], 2000).

Western Kentucky University faculty members from the disciplines of nursing, social work, and public health collaborated to implement and evaluate this 3-year multicomponent, interdisciplinary project. One component of the project was the use of an interdisciplinary group of students from nursing, social work, and public health to develop educational modules designed for use with the rural elders. These modules addressed the topics of medications, medical terminology, basic anatomy and physiology, and orientation to medical forms. These modules were designed in an effort to enhance the communication among rural elders and their health care providers.

EDUCATIONAL MODELS: A PROCESS OF INTERDISCIPLINARY DEVELOPMENT

The development of the educational modules evolved over the course of this project. Consequently, the process, which entailed four phases of development (see Table 23.1), served to illustrate the collaborative interdisciplinary effort.

Phase 1: Planning

The first 8 months of the 3–year project were spent in planning, networking with community partners, exploring resources in the targeted rural counties, and organizing an advisory panel of community partners with expertise in elder care. Faculty recruited students from within each of their respective programs to enroll in a three-credit hour "independent study" class. The course was team-taught by three faculty members from

Table 23.1 HERE Project: Phases of Education Module Development

Phase I. Planning
Goal: Explore available resources and network to establish community partnerships

Time	Students involved	Process/Content	Format/Length	Strategies Used/Lessons Learned
Year 1 Semester 1	1 UN 1 USW 1GPH	• networking with community • exploring local resources • organizing advisory panel	F: networking & exploring via letters, e-mails, newspaper advertisement, community visits	S: communication skills LL: need to revisit efforts in connecting with community
Year 1 Semester 2	1 GN	• research intervention locations		S: community engagement LL: certain cultural barriers need be addressed

Phase II. Developing Educational Modules
Goal: Develop series of educational modules addressing identified deficiency areas for rural elders

Time	Students involved	Process/Content	Format/Length	Strategies Used/Lessons Learned
Year 1 Semester 2	1 UN 3 USW 2 GN 4 GPH	Educational modules developed: • Basic Anatomy and Physiology • Medical Terms • Advanced Directives and Medical Forms • Pharmacology	F: handouts, learning objectives, lesson plans L: 30 - 60 minutes	S: research, record, and present to faculty and advisory panel LL: need for increased oversight; difficulty in merging U and G students

Table 23.1. (continued)

Phase III: Implementation
Goal: Refine and implement the educational modules within a target community

Year 2 Semester 1	2 USW 2 GN	• each session, each semester covered all four educational modules	F: 2 sessions per location, 4 locations total L: 2 hours each	S: advertising via radio, phone calls, and flyer LL: two 2-hour sessions may be a little much for rural elders
Year 2 Semester 2	1 GN		F: 1 session per location, 4 locations L: 1.5 – 2 hours each	S: shortened sessions to keep rural elders attention
Year 3 Semester 3	3 GN		F and L same as previous semester	LL: each semester, weather can prevent older individuals from attending

Phase IV. Mass Dissemination
Goal: Distribute health literacy information to greater number or rural elders

Year 2 Summer	7 GN	• Created themes and outline	F: video (n=3), brochure, PSA L: 12 minutes per section of video	S: utilize feedback
Year 3 Semester 2	1 GN 1 GSW 1 PGN	• Contact prior to delivering, locations: pharmacies, hospitals, physician offices, senior centers, churches, community groups		LL: few rural physicians offices have TVs

Legend: U = Undergraduate, G = Graduate, PG = Post-graduate, N = Nursing, C = Communications, PH = Public Health, SW = Social Work, F = Format, L = length, S = Strategies, LL = Lessons Learned, PSA = Public Service Announcements the disciplines of nursing, social work, and public health; each academic department issued separate credit for the course.

Phase 2: Developing Educational Modules

The first course was held in the latter part of year one of the grant cycle; undergraduate and graduate students enrolled from the disciplines of nursing, public health, and social work. The primary course objective was to develop a series of educational modules that addressed deficiency areas in rural elders identified in the literature and through consultation with the advisory panel. These deficiency areas included medications, medical terminology, basic anatomy and physiology, and orientation to medical forms including advance directives. Communication skills were woven into each module.

The class was divided into four interdisciplinary teams; each was given the primary responsibility of developing one of the educational modules. Each team was assigned a content expert from the advisory council to use as a consultant. These interdisciplinary student teams, with guidance from faculty members, researched and designed the initial educational modules thought to be appropriate for the targeted audiences. Each educational module had to be theoretically sound and contain learning objectives, lesson plans for teaching the module, written materials to be given to the projected audience, and teaching materials such as audiovisual aids. Students were challenged to make the educational materials interactive, culturally sensitive, and appropriate for rural elders. Throughout the semester, students were required to chronicle their learning experiences through journal entries. Some of the journal process involved answering specific questions related to the project, but students were also encouraged to express their opinions on the process.

At the end of the semester, students made verbal and written presentations of their modules to the interdisciplinary faculty and community advisory board. The advisory committee and the interdisciplinary faculty team gave each interdisciplinary team evaluative feedback. To assist with later refinement of the modules, the presentations were videotaped for use by future students and project staff.

Phase 3: Implementation

A second group of students from within each discipline were recruited the following semester for the third phase of the project. The objective of this phase was to refine and implement the educational modules within a target community. To fulfill the objective of this phase, invitations were extended to rural elders to attend any of four presentations of the modules.

Several strategies were used to implement the educational modules and recruit elderly participants. These strategies included frequent telephone calls, site visits, radio interviews, posting brochures announcing the sessions in church bulletins, newsletters, local newspapers, and using local insiders to gain access.

Again, the class was divided into interdisciplinary teams. Their first task was to incorporate the previous semester's evaluative feedback from the advisory panel and faculty into each module. Next, teams were required to teach the modules to the class and faculty and received substantive critique. Students then implemented the modules at four sites within the target community as part of the project. At each presentation site, the four modules, each lasting approximately 15–20 minutes apiece, were presented.

Based on feedback from students and community members, the project staff decided to share these educational modules with a larger number of rural elders; therefore students began exploring other methods to deliver the educational messages. Because of the short period of time many senior adults are physically able to tolerate sitting through meetings, the modules were condensed and presented in a 2–hour class format and later to a 1–hour class. These modules were presented by invitation at rural churches, rural community centers, community senior citizen centers, and at a statewide leadership conference for women. This change maximized the number of rural elderly receiving the health messages contained in the educational modules. Feedback received from project participants was positive. Participants reported that they considered the information given to be beneficial and indicated that they enjoyed the personal attention given to them in the process of the presentations. It is interesting that as a result of the interactions with the presenters during the group process, the elderly participants were particularly responsive to the discussion of living wills to the point that many immediately requested assistance in completing the forms.

Phase 4: Mass Dissemination

Although the changes in Phase 3 increased the number of rural elders receiving the educational messages, project staff remained concerned about the limited number of elders who participated in the project. Fewer than 10 persons were present at three of the four sessions. The low number of participants was thought to be because rural elder's reluctance to engage in a program offered by someone outside their community. This was further compounded by transportation limitations. Consequently, project staff gave consideration to directing the educational focus to health care providers and disseminating information through other avenues. To address these concerns, graduate students were recruited for directed study to critically study the content and distribution of the educational modules. As a result of their efforts, the modules were redesigned into four 30-second public service announcements, three 12-minute videos, and three educational pamphlets.

CHALLENGES, REWARDS, AND LESSONS LEARNED

Although the benefits of an integrated interdisciplinary model are both great and evident, challenges arose. Anticipating these challenges and recognizing the rewards was central to successfully meeting the educational goals of such a model. Learning from these challenges contributed to the rich, rewarding outcomes experienced by students and faculty alike.

Student Recruitment

Because students were expected to function within self-managing teams, the search for independent learners and self-starters who were open to working in a multidisciplinary setting was crucial to a successful educational experience. Willingness to work outside their primary area of study and motivation and acceptance of different theoretical models was necessary for success. For the educator, having the time and tools to effectively screen students for these characteristics resulted in a greater number of faculty and student expectations being met.

Many students involved reported that their primary motivation in deciding to participate in the class included an interest in rural health and elders. However, those students who foresaw the advantages of interdisciplinary experiences were open and better prepared for the variety of student interests and expertise encountered. In recording experiences in journals a student wrote, "It will be a good opportunity to work with students from other departments, and I look forward to seeing how the differing disciplines can all contribute to a comprehensive final product."

During the first three phases, primarily recruiting students from the departments of nursing, social work, and public health was sufficient. However, completing the educational pamphlets, public service announcements, and educational videos entailed collaboration with experts outside of these disciplines. Although there were opportunities to effectively use students from areas outside the health professions, efforts to recruit from other disciplines such as communications, speech, and education were met with limited success. If faculty had the time and opportunity to informally engage faculty from other departments, while at the same time educating them on the goals of the HERE project, perhaps the recruitment would have resulted in a better response from students in other areas of study.

Student Preparation

Interdisciplinary learning is very student directed. Within a multidisciplinary system, there is often a lack of common language between professions. The variations in the educational experiences and socialization between professionals contribute to differing perspectives and values, professionally and personally. The existing hierarchy, as well as role competition and turf issues at the university, further exacerbated the current system's inability to function in interdisciplinary teams, instead "causing defined roles to predominate over meeting patients' needs" (Greiner & Knebel, 2003). These obstacles were often present among the faculty and students unless structure was implemented. Providing students with the opportunity to establish objectives and plans to reach them must be balanced with enough direction and guidance to foster student comfort. As experienced in the first year of this project, providing students with only the long-term goals of the project and letting the teams establish specific objectives, resulted in some student confusion, as reflected in this journal entry: "... in the beginning it was very confusing about what was expected for us to do and how we were to work together to develop modules." Such frustration made evident the need for additional faculty support and guidance, especially during the initial stages of the class when there was confusion or incongruity in student-professor expectations.

In subsequent semesters, faculty offered students a detailed syllabus that outlined the specific level of expectations and described assignments and grading criteria with more clarity. As a result, students generally reported a more positive experience and worked independently and more efficiently from the very start.

Group Process

Interdisciplinary learning requires an ability to work effectively in groups. With the HERE project, problems that developed with group activities were not entirely different from those one would find in most group processes. The project team experienced difficulty in scheduling meeting times so that all could attend and participate often.

Initially faculty members were limited in their opportunities to assist students in the resolution of most of these problems because of time constraints. In later semesters, limiting group size as well as developing assignments that were appropriate for the schedules, interests, and living locations of students proved advantageous.

Part of the value of interdisciplinary learning is found in students learning to compromise, assign tasks, be responsible to peers, and problem solve to overcome the challenges of working in a group. Faculty attempting to intervene and resolve all these problems for the students subtracts from the benefits and experience of group process. During this experience the faculty discovered that lending time, encouragement, and support to the students, as well as assisting them in the exploration of various avenues of resolution, is crucial. Journaling provided an effective means for the students to communicate concerns and reactions as well as to reflect and process thoughts and feelings. Ultimately, this assignment allowed faculty to more easily support, assist, and respond through written feedback.

To best prepare students, reduce frustrations, and limit difficulties, it was imperative for the faculty to initially inform students of the common pitfalls and anticipated problems of group work. This aided in developing strategies to respond to problems as well as enhance student learning. By learning to effectively respond to these particular group challenges, students are likely to be more successful in working with interdisciplinary groups in a professional practice setting. Developing student skills in adaptability is essential for practitioners to effectively work with other practitioners to ultimately maximize patient care in a rural setting.

During various phases of the project's planning, implementation, and evaluation, the faculty members also experienced many challenges experienced by students. As with the students, each HERE faculty member brought to the project specific areas of expertise, interests, and theoretical frameworks. Discussing differences and negotiating solutions capitalized on these individual strengths creating a collaborative and productive work environment. Consequently, the faculty also benefited.

CONCLUSIONS

Engaging students in an interdisciplinary educational model for learning enabled students to understand and respond to such work, while effectively using differing health care theories and orientations. Ultimately, students became aware of the importance of engaging expertise from differing areas while at the same time recognizing their own professional and educational expertise and limits.

Interdisciplinary learning can be a highly effective and greatly beneficial model for education as well as professional practice, but it has its own set of challenges. Working with others within one's primary discipline can be challenging in and of itself; adding group members from other areas of practice and study calls for even greater patience and increased understanding of group dynamics. On the other hand, the rewards can be greater. A student identified the value of the interdisciplinary process as illustrated in this journal excerpt:

I thought it was a great idea by the faculty committee to split all of the students into groups to focus on different aspects of the module so that each student could assist and build on each others thoughts, views and conclusions on key issues pertaining to important issues about our module.

Despite this particular 3-year service-based, interdisciplinary project's onset of challenges, the project reached the overall goal of conducting multiple interventions within the two-targeted counties. Over the 2-year intervention period, the students encountered many elders who were interested in the topics of the modules. To reach elders who were unable to attend the educational modules, students created public service announcements, informational videos, and brochures. The venue of communication for the public service announcements will involve local radio stations, while the videos and brochures will be distributed to pharmacies, the offices of health care providers, and public libraries. Because of the amount of interest indicated by local elders, funding is being sought so that the project may continue and expand to other rural counties in southern Kentucky.

Although all the students participating in the HERE project shared a common interest of elderly rural health care, their philosophical and theoretical orientations were often different and related to those orientations found within their primary area of study. Facilitating student opportunities to learn and work in a collaborative environment with others from differing backgrounds, experiences, and theoretical bases provided both faculty and students with a rich, comprehensive learning experience reflective of the interdisciplinary nature of today's health care settings.

REFERENCES

Bushy, A. (2000). Community and public health nursing in rural environments. In M. Stanhope, & B.J. Lancaster (Eds), *Community and public health nursing* (4th ed., pp. 315–333). St. Louis, MO: Mosby.

Davis, R., & Magilvy, J. K. (2000). Quiet pride: The experience of chronic illness by rural older adults. *Journal of Nursing Scholarship, 32,* 385–390.

Greiner, A., & Knebel, E. (2003). *Health professions education: Bridge to quality.* Washington, DC: National Academy Press.

Health Resources and Services Administration. (2000). Health Professionals Shortage Areas (HRSAs). Retrieved November 21, 2004, from http://belize.hrsa.gov/newhpsa/newhpsa.cfm

Kovner, C. T., & Harrigngton, C. (2000). Counting nurses. *American Journal of Nursing, 100* (5), 33.

U.S. Bureau of the Census. (2000). Urban and rural classification census 2000: Urban and rural criteria. Retrieved October 18, 2003, from www.census.gov/prod/2001

The Culture of Rural Communities: An Examination of Rural Nursing Concepts at the Community Level

Nancy Findholt

In the late 1970s, faculty members and graduate students at Montana State University-Bozeman College of Nursing initiated a 6-year ethnographic study to explore the health beliefs and practices of rural Montana residents (Long & Weinert, 1989; Weinert & Long, 1987). Several of the concepts that emerged from this research were later validated by a quantitative survey and became the foundation for a theory of rural nursing. These concepts included work beliefs and health beliefs, isolation and distance, self-reliance, lack of anonymity, outsider or insider, and old-timer or newcomer. My purpose in this chapter is to describe how these concepts were manifested over two decades later and at the community-level in three rural communities in Oregon.

The findings that I present here represent a portion of the results I obtained from a study (Findholt, 2004) examining the influence of rurality on community participation in a community health development initiative. Although many researchers have sought to identify the factors that influence community participation, most previous studies have focused on the characteristics of people who participate and those that do not, the reasons people choose to participate, or the characteristics of organizations that facilitate or hinder participation (Wandersman & Florin, 2000). Very few investigators have explored how community characteristics affect participation, yet these characteristics may have a significant effect on the forms or levels of participation that are possible, as well as on the outcomes of participation that can be achieved. This study of rural community participation was guided by a conceptual framework that posited that the ability of a rural community to participate in health development is both facilitated and hindered by factors in the culture, physical setting, and social structure of the community. Among the cultural factors included in the conceptual framework were three that were derived from the MSU research. These were (a) the priority given to health, (b) perceived efficacy of collective action, and (c) insider or outsider differentiation.

Priority given to health was defined as the priority assigned to health programs as compared to economic programs at the community level. It corresponded to the concept of "work beliefs and health beliefs." The Montana State University study found that rural residents assessed their health needs in relation to work roles and work activities (Weinert & Long, 1987). Being productive in their role was of primary importance to these individuals, and health problems were often ignored unless they interfered with the ability to work. On the basis of these findings, I proposed in the current study that rural communities would place a higher value on economic development than on health development.

Perceived efficacy of collective action referred to the belief of community members in their ability to work together to solve problems. This cultural variable corresponded to the concept of "self-reliance." The Montana State University findings revealed that rural people were self-reliant in coping with personal and family health problems and preferred self-care, or care provided by family and friends, over professional care (Weinert & Long, 1987). Thus, in the current study I proposed that rural residents, as a whole, would have confidence in their collective ability to solve problems, including problems related to health.

Finally, *insider or outsider differentiation* was a phrase chosen to refer to the degree to which community members, as a group, accepted and trusted individuals based upon their tenure in the community. It was derived from the concepts of "insider or outsider" and "old-timer or newcomer." The ethnographic data collected in Montana suggested that rural people organized their social environment around these concepts and determined who to accept and who to trust based upon variables such as length of residence, family history, and type of occupation (Weinert & Long, 1987). Therefore, I anticipated that, in a rural community, a health development leader who was well-known to residents and perceived as an insider would be more likely accepted than a leader who was viewed as an outsider.

I did not include the concepts of "isolation and distance" and "lack of anonymity" in the conceptual framework for this study and, therefore, they were not among the cultural factors that I intentionally explored. However, as described in this chapter, some of the qualitative findings did provide insight into the presence of these characteristics in the rural communities.

METHODS

This research employed a multiple-case study design featuring three communities that were engaged in the Community Health Improvement Partnership, a health development initiative offered by the Office of Rural Health (2002) in Oregon. Besides being selected for their involvement in the health development effort, the communities chosen as cases were required to meet specific criteria for rurality that were established using the Rural-Urban Commuting Area (RUCA) scale. The RUCA scale classifies census tracts based upon size and daily commuting patterns (Rural Health Research Center, 2002). Communities participating in this study were required to have a main town of no more than 9,999 people, no primary or secondary commuting flow greater than 5% to an urban area, and no secondary flow greater than 30% to a large town. I used these criteria to restrict the sample to communities with small populations that were unlikely to be influenced by urban culture. I labeled the three communities chosen for the sample as Community A, B, and C.

I collected data reported in this chapter through key informant interviews and focus groups with community members. The key informants were health professionals or members of local health boards. The focus group participants included school administrators, small business owners, retirees, employees of social service organizations, and others from the nonhealth sectors of the community. All of the respondents were participants in the health development planning team. I conducted twenty-one key informant interviews and six focus groups.

I designed the interview questions to solicit the respondents' perceptions of their community and of community members' views, rather than their personal opinions. To assess the priority given to health, I asked the respondents how their community ranked health in comparison with other concerns, such as the economy, environment, or infrastructure. I assessed perceived efficacy of collective action by asking the respondents whether most residents believed that, by working together, they could bring about general improvements in the community, and whether residents believed they had the collective ability to improve the community's health. I assessed insider or outsider differentiation by asking whether the leader of the health development initiative was perceived by residents as an insider and whether this perception had an effect on their acceptance of the leader.

I used semistructured interviews to facilitate comparability of the data across communities; however, I also encouraged the respondents to describe other community characteristics they believed had influenced participation in the health development initiative. It was through these opportunities that the comments concerning isolation and lack of anonymity emerged.

Data analysis occurred concurrently with data collection and consisted of three interwoven processes described by Miles and Huberman (1994). These were data reduction, data display, and conclusion drawing and verification. Data reduction involved simplifying and abstracting the raw data through a process of writing summaries, coding, and writing memos. Data display occurred as I compressed the data and organized it into matrices. I developed within-case displays first and later "stacked" these to create cross-case displays. I accomplished conclusion drawing and verification by making contrasts and comparisons across different communities and different data sources, looking for evidence of patterns and examining exceptions to patterns, following up on surprises, and looking for negative evidence.

DESCRIPTION OF THE COMMUNITIES

The communities that participated in this study were not towns, but were regions with boundaries that corresponded to the service area of the local hospital. The service area boundaries were delineated by the Office of Rural Health (2003) when the communities were chosen to participate in the health development initiative. Table 24.1 shows demographics of communities A, B, and C

Community A was, in many respects, the neediest and most rural of the three communities. It was a sparsely populated and isolated coastal region, 72 miles by winding roads from the county seat, with the oldest and poorest residents, and an economy that was floundering. The traditional industries of forestry and fishing had declined significantly in recent years, forcing many families to leave the area. An effort was being made to attract tourists and to recruit new businesses, but at the time of this study, the economy remained depressed.

Community B encompassed a large portion of a county located in the ranch and farm lands of eastern Oregon. Of the three communities included in the study, Community B was the farthest from a metropolitan area of 50,000 or more residents. However, its main town was over twice as large as Community A's and a major interstate highway traversed the community. Besides agriculture, which was a large component of the economy, many people were employed in human services (health care, education, and social services) or in wood products manufacturing, an industry that had been developed to replace the loss of jobs in forestry. Demographic statistics for

Table 24.1. Selected Demographic Characteristics of Study Communities
as Compared with Oregon

Community characteristic	Community A	Community B	Community C	Oregon
Size	7,641 residents with one main town, population 4,230	14,266 residents with one main town, population 9,840	44,479 residents with two main towns, population 9,532 & 5,903	N/A
Median age	47.3	45	44	40
% White race	91.7	94.3	90.6	82.7
% below poverty	15.8	14.4	13.9	11.6
% Population age 25+ without high school diploma	19.6	20	15.1	14.9

Note. From *Demographic-Socioeconomic, and Health Status Report,* by Office of Rural Health, 2003, Oregon Health Sciences University, Portland, and from *Oregon Population Report,* by Portland State University, Population Research Center, 2002, Portland State University, Oregon.

this region revealed a community that was older and poorer than the state as a whole, yet was younger and less poor than Community A.

Community C was the largest, least rural, and least needy of the study communities. This community was an entire county located on the coast in western Oregon. There were two main towns in the county, both of which were less than 60 miles from a major metropolitan corridor. The region was popular as a weekend and vacation retreat and as a retirement destination, and had an economy based on tourism. Residents described the community as having two populations: (a) the retirees, who were generally well educated and financially comfortable, and (b) the people who struggled to make ends meet by working in the tourist industry. Both groups were quite transient; the community had few long-term residents. Overall, the population was poorer, older and less educated than the state as a whole, but was closer to the state demographic averages than either Communities A or B.

RESULTS

Priority Given to Health

The case study data revealed that the priority given to health matters, in comparison with the economy, was relatively high in these communities. Although some of the respondents believed that economic development or issues, such as infrastructure improvement and education, were more important to their community than health development, approximately half of the people from each study site said that health was one of their community's top concerns.

One reason that was cited for the high priority given to health was the change in the communities' demographics. Respondents explained that, as the percentage of residents who were poor or old had increased, there had been a corresponding increase in the need for health care services, which in turn had placed a burden on the community, resulting in greater attention being given to health issues. In Communities A and C, the influx of retirees was also cited as a reason for the high priority given to health. It was noted that the retirees expected adequate health care services. Furthermore, respondents in all of the study sites observed that health had become a higher priority in their communities as local leaders learned that to recruit business and to attract newcomers, they needed to have a strong health care system.

Perceived Efficacy of Collective Action

The degree to which residents had confidence in their collective ability to improve the community varied across the study sites. Most of the respondents in Community A reported that residents believed that, by working together, they could achieve positive change. Similarly, in Community B, it was noted that some, and possibly most, of the residents had confidence in collective action. However, in Community C, over half of the people I interviewed stated that a large segment of the population was pessimistic or negative about community efforts.

In contrast to the varying degrees of confidence concerning general community improvement, the findings show that residents in all of the communities were quite skeptical about their ability to resolve community health problems. A primary reason given for the skepticism was that the complexity and magnitude of the rural health care crisis made the problems seem overwhelming. However, lack of experience in making health improvements and the failure of other social programs were also cited as factors that contributed to residents' skepticism.

Insider or outsider Differentiation

In Communities A and C, two people were identified as being the leader of the health development initiative. One of these was viewed as a community insider and the other as an outsider. In Community B, only one person was identified as the leader. She was well-known among members of the agricultural sector, but was unknown to other residents.

Whether leaders were perceived as an insider or an outsider appeared to have little effect on how they were accepted by residents in any of the study sites. Although a few respondents said that familiarity was essential in establishing credibility and trust, most thought that the leader's skills and personality were more important. It is interesting that one theme that emerged across the communities was that having a leader who was unknown was beneficial to the health development effort in that it allowed the process to be perceived as an unbiased and impartial. Respondents explained that, in a small community, where residents know the leaders' opinions on issues, they are apt to assume that planning projects led by a known leader will be slanted in favor of that leader's agenda.

Although the concepts of insider versus outsider and old-timer versus newcomer had little relevance in terms of the communities' acceptance of the health development leader, these concepts did emerge as factors that defined, and in some cases divided, the residents in two of the study sites. In Communities A and B, individuals who had resided in these communities for as long as 24 years were described by themselves or by others as newcomers, a finding which suggests that they were not fully integrated into the community. In addition, many of the respondents in Community A reported that tension existed among the newcomers who were interested in changing the community, and the old-timers who wanted things to remain the same. On the other hand, in Community C, several respondents commented that the concepts of old-timer and newcomer had little meaning because there were so many newcomers. As one person stated, "We're so used to different people.... It's not something that divides the community at all."

Lack of Anonymity

Lack of anonymity was mentioned only in Community A. Respondents there noted that one of the challenges of serving on a health planning team in a small community was that team members knew each other well and interacted often, thus they were reluctant to be confrontational or to express opinions that conflicted with others in the group. This had the effect of reducing openness during discussions. One person observed, "That's the thing that I think is the hardest part about this process in a small community, is the inability to ... be frank about things."

Isolation and Distance

The comments concerning isolation and distance emerged during discussions of collective efficacy. Because of the distances that separated the study communities from larger communities, respondents perceived that they were isolated. For example, one individual from Community A observed that the next largest community was 70 miles away and "may as well be on the moon."

Some of the respondents believed that their community's isolation was a positive factor in that residents realized they needed to work together to solve problems. As one person explained: "We're just not sitting there, looking for someone else to solve the problems because, you know, we're out here in all this ground and there ain't no cavalry. There's no cavalry. We've just got to figure out what to do." However, it was also noted that isolation and distance contributed to a sense of collective depression, a sense of skepticism about whether positive change was possible, and a feeling of being disenfranchised. Furthermore, isolation made it difficult for rural communities to solve problems because their access to resources was very limited.

DISCUSSION

The discovery that health development was a rather high priority in these communities was unexpected in light of the earlier findings from Montana. One explanation for the inconsistency between this study's findings and those reported by Montana State University researchers might be that many of the Montana subjects were people who were still working, whereas the participants in the current study were from aging communities with many residents who were no longer working. Just as it is logical to assume that an individual's interest in health would increase with age, so too might a community's interest in health increase as its population ages. It is important to note, however, that one of the reasons cited for the high priority given to health in the Oregon communities was that health services were necessary for economic development. This perspective of health as a means to an economic end was very similar to the Montana observations.

The high level of skepticism among residents concerning their collective ability to resolve community health problems was also unexpected given that Weinert and Long (1987) had found that rural people had confidence in their ability to manage personal and family health problems. It is possible that Oregon residents had less confidence in their ability to address health concerns than Montana residents. However, it is also likely that solving community health problems was perceived by rural people as different, and perhaps more complex, than solving problems pertaining to their own health or the health of family members.

Another finding that was unanticipated was that the communities' acceptance of the health development leader was, for the most part, not influenced by residents' perception of the leader as an insider or an outsider. I had assumed that, if the concepts of insider and outsider divided the community, which was clearly the case in Community A, then insider status would be a critical element in assuring that the leader was accepted. However, the respondents' comments suggested that, in a small community where people know the local leaders and are aware of their opinions, familiarity might actually hinder residents' acceptance of the leader. This finding relates to lack of anonymity, which is discussed next.

The case study data pertaining to lack of anonymity were consistent with those obtained by Weinert and Long (1987). The comments made by respondents in Community A concerning the difficulties of serving on a planning team with people they knew well were very similar to remarks made by rural nurses who were part of the Montana sample. These nurses had reported that, because their patients were often also their neighbors, friends, or family members, it was difficult for them to separate their professional and personal roles (Long & Weinert, 1989).

The findings pertaining to the residents' perception of their isolation were inconsistent with Weinert and Long's (1987) results. Although the Oregon respondents described their communities as isolated, Montana residents who lived outside of town and traveled more than 50 miles to receive routine health care did not view themselves as isolated (Long & Weinert, 1989).

In summary, only one of the concepts that were identified in the early Montana research was evident in the community-level data collected in Oregon. This concept was lack of anonymity, a characteristic pertaining more to the small size of a community than to rurality per se.

CONCLUSION

These findings, drawn from a study of rural community participation in a health development initiative, provide insight into the culture of rural communities and serve to extend rural nursing theory by revealing how the concepts identified in the initial theory work were manifested at the community-level in Oregon. The many inconsistencies between this study's findings and those of the early Montana research may be due to several factors, but one likely cause is that the culture of rural communities has changed in the 20-plus years since the initial data were collected. Given the loss of jobs in traditional rural industries, advances in telecommunications and transportation, relocation of retirees to rural areas, and other major social changes that have impacted rural communities, it follows that rural culture has been altered.

The results of this study have relevance to all nurses who have an interest in improving rural health, and especially to those who practice in a rural setting. The health of rural Americans is closely linked to factors in the culture, economy, demography, and geography of rural places (Ricketts, 1999). Thus, to successfully impact the health of rural people, nurses need to have an understanding of rural communities. Furthermore, for nurses interested in community-based practice in a rural setting, it is important to understand community-level perspectives of health as well as community-level influences on health decision making.

The findings from this study were limited by several factors, including the small size and limited diversity of the sample, the potential for bias in the use of health development committee members as representatives of their community, and by the lack of an urban comparison group. Further research is needed to explore whether the characteristics identified in this research are unique to rural communities, and to confirm their applicability in other rural settings.

REFERENCES

Findholt, N.E. (2004). *The influence of rurality on community participation in a community health development initiative.* Unpublished doctoral dissertation, Oregon Health and Science University, Portland.

Long, K. A., & Weinert, C. (1989). Rural nursing: Developing the theory base. *Scholarly Inquiry for Nursing Practice, 3*(2), 113–127.

Miles, M. B., & Huberman, A. M. (1994). *Qualitative data analysis* (2nd ed.). Thousand Oaks, CA: Sage.

Office of Rural Health (ORH). (2003). *Demographic, socioeconomic, and health status report.* Portland: Oregon Health and Science University.

Portland State University (PSU), Population Research Center. (2002). *Oregon population report.* Retrieved February 19, 2003, from http://www.upa.pdx.edu/CPRC/

Ricketts, T. C. (1999). Introduction. In T. C. Ricketts, III (Ed.), *Rural health in the United States* (pp. 1–6). New York: Oxford University Press.

Rural Health Research Center. (2002). *Rural–urban commuting area codes (RUCAs).* Retrieved February 3, 2003, from http://wwww.fammed.washington.edu/wwamirhrc/rucas/rucas.html

Wandersman, A., & Florin, P. (2000). Citizen participation and community organizations. In J. Rappaport & E. Seidman (Eds.), *Handbook of community psychology* (pp. 247–272). New York: Kluwer Academic/Plenum.

Weinert, C., & Long, K. A. (1987). Understanding the health care needs of rural families. *Family Relations, 36,* 450–455.

PART VI

Looking Ahead

The last part contains two chapters that present potential direction for future rural nursing theory development. The first is written by Lee and McDonagh and provides suggestions for furthering the rural nursing theory base from the core group of nurse scientists from Montana State University-Bozeman in the United States and the University of Calgary in Alberta, Canada. The last chapter by Shreffler-Grant and Reimer contains content that looks at education, practice, and policy issues as they relate to the changing rural nursing theory base.

CHAPTER TWENTY-FIVE

Further Development of the Rural Nursing Theory Base

Helen J. Lee and Meg K. McDonagh

Our purpose in this chapter was to synthesize the information gleaned from the rural nursing theory base literature review found in chapter 2 of this book and the comparison study, "Exploring Rural Nursing Theory Across Borders" found in chapter 3 of this book. Recommendations for structural change in the descriptive middle range theory published by Long and Weinert (1989) are made and a plan for making those changes is proposed.

FINDINGS OF THE LITERATURE REVIEW AND COMPARISON STUDY

We state the three theoretical statements from the 1989 rural nursing theory base below and followed them with suggestions for changes in the first and second theoretical statements of the 1989 theory base.

Theoretical Statement #1

... rural dwellers define health primarily as the ability to work, to be productive, to do usual tasks (Long & Weinert, 1989, p. 120)

313

Knowledge of the health perceptions of individuals, families, and communities is essential to understanding their motivation for illness treatment, health maintenance, and health promotion (Long, 1993). Participants in the early rural nursing theory base studies perceived their health as being able to function. However, the findings of the literature review (Chapter 2) and the comparison study (Chapter 3) suggest a changing view, a more holistic perception of health. Although the earlier emphasis on role performance still may be peculiar to certain age and occupational groups within rural communities, the theoretical descriptive statement regarding health perception needs expansion to incorporate additional definitions and perceptions of health. An example of a differing perception of health includes the views of those who consider themselves healthy in spite of having one or more chronic health conditions such as heart disease and diabetes.

Because rural residents define health in a variety of ways, we suggest these revised descriptive statements:

1. Rural residents define health as being able to do what they want to do; it is a way of life and a state of mind; there is a goal of maintaining balance in all aspects of their lives.
2. Older rural residents and those with ties to extractive industries are more likely to define health in a functional manner—to work, to be productive, and to do usual tasks.

Theoretical Statement #2

... rural dwellers are self-reliant and resist accepting help or services from those seen as 'outsiders' or from agencies seen as national or regional 'welfare programs.' (Long & Weinert, 1989, p. 120)

Corollary to statement #2: ... help, including needed health care, is usually sought through an informal rather than a formal system (Long & Weinert, 1989, p. 120).

The second theoretical statement refers to rural persons' health-seeking behaviors. Key concepts from the 1989 model include self-reliance, seeking care from insiders, and use of the informal system. Within the review of literature (Chapter 2), self-reliance continues to be the foremost characteristic identified in rural persons. However, changes were seen in the seeking of care from insiders and the use of the informal system. Participants in the comparison study (Chapter 3) indicated they were seeking care from insiders and outsiders and using both the informal and formal systems of care. Insiders, defined as long-time accepted members of the community (Myers, 1998), and outsiders, who are unconnected with the local population (Bailey, 1998), can be involved in providing formal care delivered by private or government agencies. Decision making regarding which type of care was sought was dependent upon what sickness (short duration & curable), illness (chronic, serious, & potentially life-threatening), or injury was present at the time (Chapter 3).

We propose these two statements as revisions of Theoretical Statement #2:

1. *Rural residents are self-reliant and make decisions to seek care for illness, sickness, or injury depending on their self assessment of the severity of their present health condition and of the resources needed and available.*
2. *Rural residents with infants and children who experience illness, sickness, or injury will seek care more quickly than for themselves.*

Theoretical Statement #3

"... health care providers in rural areas must deal with a lack of anonymity and much greater role diffusion than providers in urban or suburban" (Long & Weinert, 1989, p. 120)

The above statement focuses on concepts pertaining to the health care providers' professional practice environment; it indicates health care provider experience a lack of anonymity and role diffusion. Because this statement is well supported in the literature review, no changes are recommended.

The lack of anonymity that health care providers experience in rural communities is in itself a paradox. On the one hand, it is often the familiarity and knowing of community members and the lack of anonymity or being known by them that draws health care professionals to rural areas. Yet, it is often this same attribute of rural practice that can later drive them away.

THE CONCEPT OF DISTANCE

Although not a part of the three theoretical statements in the 1989 rural nursing theory paper, the concept of distance held a prominent place in the rural health care literature review (Chapter 2). Also, the comparison study authors (Chapter 3) acknowledged the importance of distance in their findings and indicated that increasing distances to services for Canadian residents determines the difference between rural and northern locations in the provinces. Other expressions referring to very sparsely populated areas include frontier and remote. Frontier is a term that appears in U.S. literature (Eliason, 1986). Remote is a term found in the Australian (Brown, Young, & Byles, 1999; Fitzgerald, Pearson, & McCutcheon, 2001; Jiro-jwong & MacLennan, 2002) and Canadian (Hanson, 2004; Racher & Vollman, 2002) rural health and nursing literature.

EMERGING CONCEPTS FROM THE COMPARISON STUDY

New concepts emerging from the comparison study included health-seeking behavior and choices (Chapter 3). Themes of distance and resources also emerged from the findings of the comparison study and from the literature review examining the rural nursing theory base (Chapter 2).

Health-Seeking Behaviors

Health-seeking behaviors were defined as "conscious behaviors designed to promote healthy relationships among physical, mental, social and spiritual aspects of one's life so that life balance is maintained" (Chapter 3, p. 34). Three subthemes, symptom-action-time-line (SATL) process, resources, and self-reliance, are a part of health-seeking behaviors. The SATL process (Buehler, Malone, & Majerus, 1998) is used to identify symptoms of sickness, illness or injury and then seek the appropriate level of requisite care. The level of care sought may be self, lay, or professional depending upon the perceived seriousness and type of symptom. Accessing resources is a part of the SATL process. Self-reliance, defined as behaviors to promote or maintain health without seeking assistance from others, was prevalent in the data from Montana and the Canadian provinces of Alberta and Manitoba. It is considered a subtheme of health-seeking behavior because of its paramount influence in seeking health care in sparsely populated rural areas.

Choices

Choices, the making of decisions to live in a rural environment and accessing health care resources, was a new theme that emerged from the comparison study. Explicitly evident in the Montana data and implicitly identified in the Canadian study through the participants' expressions of the benefits of living in rural environments, the theme is associated with the concept of place. Although we think of place in a geographical context, it is a broader entity that shapes one's political, economic, spatial, geographic, and cultural experiences and views of the world (Kelly, 2003). De la Rue and Coulson (2003) found that rural participants' well-being and health were very influenced by the "geographical location of living on the land" (p. 5). Place provided these rural residents with a kind of emotional or spiritual connectedness that affected the outcomes of their health care experiences.

Distance and Resources.

As indicated in multiple studies in the literature review (Chapter 2) and in the comparison study (Chapter 3), distance and resources are concepts that directly impact access to health care services. Authors Gulzar (1999) and Racher and Vollman (2002) discuss the complexity of processes in accessing health services. The rurality or remoteness of a given place affects access to health services. Within the rural environment, such factors as geographical, political, and economical, as well as the acceptability and educational preparation of health care providers, all influence the residents' access *to* and choice *of* health resources. Studying patterns of health care use and feedback loops among residents may add to the understanding of the complexity of accessing health care services in rural and remote areas (Racher & Vollman). Delivery of health services across sparsely populated areas presents unique challenges because of the vast distances involved and the scarcity of health professionals. For example, the greater the nurse-to-patient or physician-to-patient ratios and the more rural or remote the community is from large urban centers, the more limited the health resources are for rural and remote community members.

FUTURE DIRECTION

Theories are developed with the purposes of describing, explaining, and predicting phenomena (Fawcett, 2000). The intent of the earlier theory development work at the College of Nursing at Montana State University-Bozeman was to use the descriptive research conducted in the naturally occurring sparsely populated rural areas to develop a middle range theory, one that would provide a framework for nurses providing care for individuals living in that environmental setting (Shannon, 1982). What evolved was a descriptive theory, the most basic type of middle range theory (Fawcett, 1999). Middle range theory focuses "on a limited dimension of the reality of nursing" and grows at the "intersection of practice and research to provide guidance for everyday practice and scholarly research rooted in the discipline of nursing" (Smith & Liehr, 2003, p. xi).

Although controversy exists about the placement and abstraction level of middle range theories within the hierarchical structure of nursing theories (Peterson & Bredow, 2004), the basic structure of theories, regardless of level, is similar—concepts and relational statements that describe or link those concepts (Fawcett, 1999). The interweaving of those concepts and statements provide a pattern of ideas, a coherent way of viewing phenomena (Smith & Liehr, 2003). The pattern, once published and subjected to testing, should be open to change and the incorporation of new ideas.

Subjecting the middle range rural nursing theory to testing in several studies (Lee & Winters, 2004; Bales, 2000a, 2000b; Thomlinson et al., 2002). Chapter 3 (pp. 27–39) demonstrates the need for change in the published rural nursing theory base. This change is evident because of the newly emerging concepts and above proposed theoretical statements revisions.

Vision for the Future

Because of the descriptive nature of the middle range rural nursing theory, additional descriptive research is needed (Fawcett, 1999). Analysis of the concepts that emerged from the testing of the theory is needed. The analysis methods can take several approaches, including the Wilson method (Walker & Avant, 1995), the evolutionary method (Rodgers, 1993), and the empirical or inductive approach (Morse, 1995), or a combination thereof. Testing of the proposed changes in the rural nursing theory relational statements through qualitative studies (ethnography, grounded theory, phenomenology, historical inquiry) needs to take place in other sparsely populated areas. Development and testing of instruments to measure the concepts is needed. Conducting surveys to measure attributes, attitudes, knowledge, and opinions using open-ended and structured interview schedules and questionnaires is needed (Fawcett, 1999). With a compilation of these focused research efforts can emerge a model, a schema, or a list of logically ordered statements that, when presented, provides guidance for the care of persons in a variety of sparsely populated areas (Smith & Liehr, 2003).

Moving the Work Forward

A core group of nurse researchers from Montana and Alberta hold monthly teleconferences and periodic face-to-face meetings to review and critique theoretical material and models. Members of this North American Study group discuss and plan projects to further rural nursing theory development while offering research and educational opportunities to graduate students within their course work or independent studies. A rural nursing research and theory development listserv, developed at the Third International Congress of Rural Nurses in Binghamton, New York provides a mechanism for online discussion for furthering rural nursing research and theory development.

The NAS and listserv members already identified these following questions for exploration: (a) Are these health-seeking behaviors unique to rural residents? (b) Will health-seeking behavior activities of the SATL process fit under the same middle range theory framework as those for health promotion? (c) How do illness variables affect rural persons' health-seeking behaviors? (d) How do illness variables affect rural persons' choices of health care providers? (e) Are rural dwellers more accepting of "outside" services if they are provided by health care professionals working in partnerships with the rural community and local health professionals?

CONCLUSION

As we have argued in this chapter, the middle range rural nursing theory as published by Long and Weinert (1989) is in need of revision. Advances in health service technologies and care along with changes in the perceptions and behaviors of rural residents over the past 20 years, may account for some of the emerging concepts that we identified. Continued research and theoretical development efforts will increase the potential for a middle range theory that can provide acceptable and appropriate nursing care to rural persons.

REFERENCES

Bailey, M. C. (1998). Outsider. In H. J. Lee (Ed.), *Conceptual basis for rural nursing* (pp. 139–148). New York: Springer Publishing.

Bales, R. L. (2002a, April). *Health needs and perceptions: A study of six persons in Cooke City, MT.* Paper presented at the Proceedings of the 35th Annual Communicating Nursing Research Conference, Palm Springs, CA.

Bales, R. L. (2002b). *Health perceptions, needs, and behaviors of remote rural women of childbearing and childrearing age.* Unpublished master's thesis, Montana State University–Bozeman, Bozeman, MT.

Brown, W. J., Young, A. F., & Byles, J. E. (1999). Tyranny of distance? The health of mid–age women living in five geographical areas of Australia. *Australian Journal of Rural health, 7,* 148–154.

Buehler, J. A., Malone, M., & Majerus, J. M. (1998). Patterns of responses to symptoms in rural residents: The Symptom-action-time-line process. In H. J. Lee (Ed.), *Conceptual basis for rural nursing* (pp. 318–328). New York: Springer Publishing.

de la Rue, M., & Coulson, I. (2003). The meaning of health and well–being: Voices from older rural women. *The International Electronic Journal of Rural and*

Remote Health Research, Education, Practice, and Policy, 3(192), 1–10. Retrieved September, 5, 2004, from http://rrh.deakin.edu.au

Eliason, G. (1986). Frontier areas: Problems for delivery of health services. *Rural Health Care, 8*(5), 1, 3.

Fawcett, J. (1999). *The relationship of theory and research* (3rd ed.). Phildelphia: Davis.

Fawcett, J. (2000). *Analysis and evaluation of contemporary nursing knowledge: Nursing models and theories.* Philadelphia: Davis.

Fitzgerald, M., Pearson, A., & McCutcheon, H. (2001). Impact of rural living on the experience of chronic illness. *Australian Journal of Rural Health, 9,* 235–240.

Gulzar, L. (1999). Access to health care. *Journal of Nursing Scholarship, 31,* 13–19.

Hanson, P. G. (2004). Canadian perspectives: Aboriginal perspectives in rural health promotion practice. In J.M. Wiegmann, Health promotion of families in rural settings (pp. 593–594), In P. J. Bomar (Ed.), *Promoting health in families.* CPH 20, pp. 581–604. Philadelphia: Elsevier.

Jirojwong, S., & MacLennan, R. (2002). Management of episodes of incapacity by families in rural and remote Queensland. *Australian Journal of Rural Health, 10,* 249–255.

Kelly, S. E. (2003). Bioethics and rural health: Theorizing place, space, and subjects. *Social Science & Medicine, 56,* 2277–2288.

Lee, H. J., & McDonagh, M. K. (2004, April). *The rural nursing theory base.* Paper presented at the 37th Communicating Nursing Research Conference, Portland OR.

Lee, H. J., & Winters, C. A. (2004). Testing rural nursing theory: Perceptions and needs of service providers. *Online Journal of Rural Nursing and Health Care, 4*(1). Retrieved June 3, 2004, from http://www.rno.org/journal/issues/v.1.4/is-sues-1/Lee_article.htm.

Long, K. A. (1993). The concept of health: Rural perspectives. *Nursing Clinics of North America, 28,* 123–130.

Long, K. A., & Weinert, C. (1989). Rural nursing: Developing the theory base. *Scholarly Inquiry for Nursing Practice: An International Journal, 3,* 113–127.

Morse, M.J. (1995). Exploring the theoretical basis of nursing using advanced techniques of concept analysis. *Advances in Nursing Science, 17*(3), 31–46.

Myers, D. D. (1998). Insider. In H. J. Lee (Ed.), *Conceptual basis for rural nursing* (pp. 125–138). New York: Springer Publishing.

Peterson, S. J., & Bredow, T. S. (2004). *Middle range theories: Application to nursing research.* Philadelphia: Lippincott Williams & Wilkins.

Racher, F. E., & Vollman, A. R. (2002). Exploring the dimensions of access to health services: Implications for nursing research and practice. *Research and Theory for Nursing Practice: An International Journal, 16*(2), 77–90.

Rodgers, B. L. (1993) Concept analysis: An evolutionary view. In B. L. Rogers & K. A Knaft, *Concept development in nursing: Foundations, techniques and applications* (pp. 73–92). Philadelphia: Saunders.

Shannon, A. M. (1982). Introduction: Nursing in sparsely populated areas. *Western Journal of Nursing Research, 4* (3)suppl, 70–71.

Smith, M. J., & Liehr, P. R. (2003). *Middle range theory for nursing.* New York: Springer Publishing.

Thomlinson, E., McDonagh, M. K., Reimer, M., Crooks, K., & Lees, M. (2002, October). *Health beliefs of rural Canadians: Implications for practice.* Poster presented at the 3rd International Congress of Rural Nurses, Binghamton, NY.

Walker, L., & Avant, K. (1995). *Strategies for theory construction nursing* (3rd ed.). Norwalk, CT: Appleton-Century-Crafts.

CHAPTER TWENTY-SIX

Implications for Education, Practice, and Policy

Jean Shreffler-Grant and Marlene A. Reimer

As an applied discipline, nursing has traditionally measured the relevance of theory by the extent to which it can inform practice, education, and health care policy. Our purpose in this chapter was to make more explicit the relevance of key elements of the rural theory base. We discuss selected educational, practice, and health care policy implications of the key concepts and theoretical statements as reported by Long and Weinert (1989) and Lee and McDonagh in Chapter 2 of this book. We explore how these implications may need to change as rural nursing theory is revised and extended. We also present exemplars from the United States, Canada, and Australia to illustrate how the key concepts and theoretical statements can inform education, practice, and health care policy that address rural populations and their health across international borders.

IMPLICATIONS OF THE FIRST THEORETICAL STATEMENT

How a group of citizens perceive health, manage their health, and seek health care has broad implications for education, practice, and policy that transcend national borders. The first theoretical statement is: "rural dwellers define health primarily as the ability to work, to be productive, to do usual tasks" (Long & Weinert, 1989, p.120). The interrelated concepts associated with this statement are work beliefs and health beliefs; health is defined in relation to work and health needs are secondary to work needs.

Education

On the basis of the original rural nursing theory work, the first theoretical statement suggests that nursing programs should include the concept of role performance as health in curricula so that nurses include actual or potential effects of a health problem on the ability to work and to do usual tasks in their assessments and plans of care. Nursing educators should also offer opportunities for students to learn how clients' definitions of health influence their health and illness management behaviors.

Practice

In the practice arena, the first theoretical statement suggests that rural health services should be oriented, structured, and timed to fit with the rhythm of work and role performance. In addition, the benefits of preventive care may be better communicated by framing them according to what will assist the person to continue to work and do their usual tasks. Recent statistics from both Canada and the United States demonstrate the need to find new ways to approach preventive care among rural dwellers based on trends in health indicators such as obesity, hypertension, smoking, and having regular health care visits (Fried, Prager, MacKay, & Xia, 2003; Mitura & Bollman, 2003).

Policy

Policy implications of the original work include establishing funding mechanisms whereby health services can be offered near where people work and scheduled around the cycle of rural work. Rural residents may not seek timely health services if work must be delayed or disrupted to seek care (Sellers, Poduska, Propp, & White, 1999).

The original theory development work on definitions of health, as well as beliefs about work and health was conducted in the United States. Research participants were principally Caucasian rural dwellers, the majority population in the Rocky Mountain and High Plains area in which this work was conducted (90.6% of Montana population, U.S. Bureau of the Census, 2004). It was not intended to characterize these concepts for American Indians, the primary minority population in the same rural areas (6.2% of the Montana population, U.S. Census, 2004). Canadian research on health beliefs of rural dwellers, as reported in Chapter 3 by Winters, et al., was also drawn primarily from Caucasians living in the western part of the country. Further research is warranted to explore how Native American and Aboriginal people living in rural areas define health and how their conception of health is the same or different from the dominant population. In any case, it is unlikely that one definition of health or one set of health beliefs would emerge that would characterize health beliefs among different Aboriginal communities or tribes, any more than it is likely among Caucasian groups of different cultures.

As discussed by Lee and McDonagh in Chapter 2, rural dwellers' views of health may now be more diverse across different geographic areas, age and ethnic groups, and occupations than when the original theory development work began and may require a reconceptualization of definitions of health, work beliefs, and health beliefs. Of particular note are the subpopulations among rural dwellers.

Discussion

Martin (1997) pointed out that farming and ranching are now experienced more as a lifestyle than as an occupation, thus calling for different approaches to affect behavior change. Another example can be found within rural subpopulations where unemployment has now persisted for multiple generations. Defining health based on ability to work may not be relevant for those who have never had regular work (Long, 1993). Some rural areas are now more racially and ethnically diverse than in the past. Culturally based beliefs about what it means to be healthy are likely to result in different definitions of health among racial and ethnic groups. Migration of urban residents to rural areas has resulted in a subpopulation of exurban rural dwellers who bring their urban values and expectations about health and health care with them (Troughton, 1999). The "graying" of rural areas is well documented in the literature, as people age in place and younger people migrate out for employment and other opportunities (McLaughlin & Jensen, 1998; Ricketts, Johnson-Webb, & Randolph, 1999). With improved health care and healthier lifestyles, people are living many more years postretirement than they once did. How health is defined among this rural population may well have nothing to do with what we traditionally think of as work, but instead may be more consistent with the concept of health as role performance or ability to do usual tasks. Healthy elders may define health as the ability to actively participate in leisure, voluntary activities, and travel. Elders in poor health may define health as nothing more than the ability to complete their activities of daily living. Further research and exploration is warranted to refine the definitions of health for these multiple rural subpopulations.

IMPLICATIONS OF THE SECOND
THEORETICAL STATEMENT

The second theoretical statement is: "rural dwellers are self-reliant and resist accepting help or services from those seen as 'outsiders' or from agencies seen as national or regional 'welfare' programs" (Long & Weinert, 1989, p. 120). Related key concepts are self-reliance, outsider, insider, old-timer, and newcomer.

Education

The second theoretical statement underlines the importance of a participative, community development approach in which rural dwellers identify and design health initiatives to fit with their own needs and resources. This approach is consistent with the second theoretical statement as originally conceptualized, as well as the proposed newer subtheme of symptom-action-time-line and the new theme involving choices discussed by Lee and McDonagh in Chapter 25. The importance of working in partnership with rural dwellers and communities is essential content for nursing curricula so that graduates can and will apply the principles of community development and participatory action in rural practice. Skills essential for partnership development and maintenance should also be included in nursing curricula. As a middle-range theory of rural health-seeking behavior evolves, this theory should be derived and validated in partnership with rural residents themselves so that it is consistent with their local needs and beliefs.

Practice

Goeppinger (1993) advocated partnership as a core intervention strategy in health promotion with rural populations at both individual and aggregate levels. Considering the rural tendency to "make do" and what Weissert, Knott, and Stieber (1994) referred to as the "asymmetry of information between citizens and health professionals ... about what constitutes good care" (p. 366) in traditional care models, empirical testing of the partnership model in promoting the health of rural residents is needed. A Canadian example of a new tool to support participative community development for rural citizens is a workbook currently being tested in Manitoba, Canada (Ryan-Nicholls, 2004). The workbook is designed to help rural citizens assess the health of their communities, and identify goals and strategies to improve the sustainability of rural communities. In the United States, Findholt (2004) studied how rurality influenced community participation in health development initiatives. She found that having a structured process for the initiative appeared to compensate for some of the resource and experiential limitations in rural communities. Communities, for example, that had limited experience and success with previous planning efforts were not hindered in their current efforts because they had structured support and resources from a state level Office of Rural Health.

Policy

The question of what health care resources are necessary and sufficient in rural and remote areas, given the distance to other sources of care, continues as a focus of debate and policy shifts for which evidence for decision making is scarce. The major constraint is the lack of sufficient population to justify a full mix of acute care, long-term care, and supported residential and home care services (Keyzer, 1995). In a study of home care resources for rural families with cancer, Buehler and Lee (1992) found that the more rural the family, the more limited and inadequate the formal resources available to assist them. These investigators also found that the longer the dying trajectory and the greater the deterioration of the person with cancer, the more resources became inadequate and the greater the caregiver burden. These findings illustrate one of many policy questions that has emerged: the relationship between length of illness and sustainability of resources through the trajectory of illness in rural versus urban environments. It would seem that a mix of formal and informal resources and the resiliency of each to prolonged illness vary but few studies have systematically addressed this phenomenon.

The Australian Rural Health Strategy adopted in 1994 (Keyzer, 1995) called for "relocation of resources away from services based on existing facilities towards services based on expressed demand" (p. 28). They advocated changes that would shift power bases from traditional rural primary and hospital care delivery to a system that relied much more on nurse practitioners and interdisciplinary collaboration. However, 10 years later tension still exists in Australia and elsewhere between the economic arguments for downsizing and closure of rural facilities versus advocacy for aging in place, new life-saving treatments that require pretransfer interventions at local health care facilities, and other new technologies such as telehealth that minimize the need for travel to urban locations for health care (Ricketts, 2000).

In the US, the Critical Access Hospital (CAH) has gained broad support as an alternative to closure of local rural hospitals and is being implemented in rural areas across the nation. CAHs must be located in remote areas and are limited to short-stay lower-intensity services in exchange for more flexibility in staffing and other licensure requirements and more favorable Medicare reimbursement as compared with traditional rural hospitals. The underlying goal is to shift the facility's emphasis from inpatient and surgical services to emergency, out-patient, primary, and long-term care, which are services that may be more sustainable in remote rural areas because they better match the needs of area residents (Alpha Center, 1990). One of the prototypes for this national model of care was a grassroots effort initiated by a partnership of rural citizens and legislators in a remote rural area in Montana. There are currently 35 CAHs in Montana (Montana Hospital Association, 2004) and over 600 across rural areas nationwide (Hagopian, Johnson, Fordyce, Blades, & Hart, 2003).

IMPLICATIONS OF THE THIRD
THEORETICAL STATEMENT

Education

Finally, the third theoretical statement regarding health care providers' lack of anonymity, role diffusion, and professional isolation (Long & Weinert, 1989) suggest that students planning for rural practice should be given opportunities to develop skills to function in a generalist role or what McLeod, Browne, and Leipert (1998) refer to as a multispecialist role that is characteristic of rural nursing practice. Offering undergraduate students a rural elective experience is one such strategy, particularly when it not only involves placement in a rural site but also seminars on rural health and practice issues. Students with an interest in rural practice should have opportunities to develop strategies to cope with or overcome practice isolation, such as skill development in the use of mentors, consultants, and telehealth applications. Through full engagement with their communities, nurses who are newcomers in rural areas may begin to appreciate the familiarity of life in a rural community and gradually be seen as insiders rather than outsiders which may mediate the negative aspects of lack of anonymity and practice isolation. Some nurses, of course, are already insiders having come from the particular community. The sense of practice isolation may be less acute for them but the practical issues of limited access to educational opportunities and ready consultation are nevertheless present to varying degrees.

Practice and Policy

Dealing with lack of anonymity, role diffusion, and practice isolation may contribute to recruitment difficulties and high turnover of rural health care professionals that contribute to shortages of providers in rural practice settings. Here too, policy makers can look to innovative approaches and exchange of best practices. For example, the Rural Physician Action Plan in Alberta recognized that (a) medical students from rural areas were more likely to go into rural practice but (b) rural applicants were often disadvantaged in the interview and selection processes for medical school because of lack of sophistication in interviewing and preparation of materials (I. Pfeiffer, personal communication, March 4, 2004). An experienced recruiter was hired to help rural applicants prepare for admission interviews. Thus, they went to a root cause with what appear to be positive results.

Another innovative strategy for addressing shortages of nurses and other health care providers in rural areas can be seen in the growth of educational outreach efforts via distance technology to rural areas. Rural residents or insiders who are more likely to select rural practice upon graduation can access all or part of educational programs without leaving their rural communities for significant periods of time. Another successful approach for recruitment of health professionals in rural areas has been educational scholarships for rural residents or "grow your own" programs (Hagopian et al., 2003).

CONCLUSIONS

The radical changes necessary to shift education, practice, and policy for rural health require a strong theory base and depth of understanding of rural health and practice that can emanate only through experience and research. Those who focus on rural health are used to thinking in terms of local contextual factors and the unique nature of a single rural area, region, or nation. Through engagement in across-border collaborative research and scholarly work on rural nursing theory, we and our respective teams have deepened our understanding of the extent to which larger issues of health care reform are also shifting. At the end of the day, the relevance of rural nursing theory and concepts as described in this book will likely be measured by its ability to evolve and change as new knowledge shapes it and to positively influence education, practice, and health care policy—and thereby improve the health of rural citizens on both sides of the border.

REFERENCES

Alpha Center. (1990). *Alternative models for delivering essential health care services in rural areas*. Washington, DC: Author.

Buehler, J. A., & Lee, H. J. (1992). Exploration of home care resources for rural families with cancer. *Cancer Nursing, 15*, 299–308.

Fried, V. M., Prager, K., MacKay, A. P., & Xia, H. (2003). *Chartbook on trends in the health of Americans. Health, United States, 2003.* Hyattsville, MD: National Center for Health Statistics.

Findholt, N. (2004). *The influence of rurality on community participation in a community health development initiative.* (Unpublished doctoral dissertation, Oregon Health & Sciences University, Portland).

Goeppinger, J. (1993). Health promotion for rural populations: Partnership interventions. *Family and Community Health, 16*(1), 1–10.

Hagopian, A., Johnson, K, Fordyce, M., Blades, S., & Hart, L. G. (2003). Health workforce recruitment and retention in critical access hospitals. *CAH/FLEX National Tracking Project, 3*(5). Retrieved April 9, 2004, from http://rupri.org/rhfp–track/results/vol3num5.pdf

Keyzer, D. M. (1995). Health policy and rural nurses: A time for reflection. *Collegian, 2*(1), 28–35.

Long, K. A. (1993). The concept of health: Rural perspectives. *Nursing Clinics of North America, 28* (1), 123–130.

Long, K. A., & Weinert, C. (1989). Rural nursing: Developing the theory base. *Scholarly Inquiry for Nursing Practice: An International Journal, 3,* 113–127.

Martin, S. R. (1997). Agricultural safety and health: Principles and possibilities for nursing education. *Journal of Nursing Education, 36*(2), 74–78.

McLaughlin, D. K., & Jensen, L. (1998). The rural elderly: A demographic portrait. In R. T. Coward & J. A. Krout (Eds.), *Aging in rural settings: Life circumstances & distinctive features* (pp. 15–43). New York: Springer Publishing.

McLeod, M., Browne, A. J., & Leipert, B. (1998). Issues for nurses in rural and remote Canada. *Australian Journal of Rural Health 6,* 72–78.

Mitura, V., & Bollman, R. D. (2003). The health of rural Canadians: A rural–urban comparison of health indicators. *Rural and Small Town Canada Analysis Bulletin, 4*(6), 1–21. (Available from the Agriculture Division, Statistics Canada, Ottawa)

Montana Hospital Association. (2004). *Critical Access Hospital List.* Retrieved June 23, 2004, from http://www.mtha.org/mhref4.htm

Ricketts, T. C. (2000). The changing nature of rural health care. *Annual Review of Public Health, 21,* 639–657.

Ricketts, T. C., Johnson–Webb, K. D., & Randolph, R. K. (1999). Populations and places in rural America. In T. C. Ricketts (Ed.), *Rural health in the United States* (pp. 7–24). New York: Oxford University Press.

Ryan–Nicholls, K. (2004). Rural Canadian community health and quality of life: Testing of a workbook to determine priorities and move to action. (Preliminary Report). *The International Electronic Journal of Rural and Remote Health Research, Education, Practice and Policy, 4*(278), 1–10. Retrieved June 23, 2004, from http://rrh.deakin.edu.au

Sellers, S. C., Poduska, M. D., Propp, L. H., & White, S. I. (1999). The health care meanings, values, and practices of Anglo–American males in the rural Midwest. *Journal of Transcultural Nursing, 10,* 320–330.

Trouhton, M. J. (1999). Redefining "rural" for the twenty-first century. In W. Rampy, J. Kulig, I. Townshend, & V. McGowan (Eds.), *Health in rural settings: Contexts for action* (pp 21–38). Lethbridge, AB, Canada: University of Lethbridge.

U.S. Bureau of the Census. Retrieved June 23, 2004, from http://quickfacts.census. gov/qfd/states/30000.html

Weissert, C. S., Knott, J. H., & Stieber, B. E. (1994). Education and the health professions: Explaining policy choices among the States. *Journal of Health Politics, Policy and Law,* 19, 361–392.

APPENDIX

An Analysis of Key
Concepts for Rural Nursing

Helen J. Lee and Charlene A. Winters

Long and Weinert (1998) noted that during the initial "process of data organization ... some concepts appeared repeatedly in the ethnographic data collected in several different areas of the state" (p. 9). Following the initial publication of their article in 1989, faculty in the Rural Nursing Theory Special Committee within the Montana State University-Bozeman College of Nursing embarked on a plan to analyze identified concepts. Their efforts were enhanced through course work involvement of graduate nursing students enrolled in Montana State University's College of Nursing rural generalist program. The purpose of this appendix is to summarize the analyzed concepts contained in the first edition of Conceptual Basis of Rural Nursing. The summary provides a quick reference of the analyzed concepts and allows for easy identification of areas needing further work.

The concepts are organized according to the framework provided in the rural nursing theory base. Following each theoretical statement are concept summaries pertinent to that particular statement. Each concept summary is presented using the analysis framework selected by the chapter authors. Elements of the framework, whether explicit and implicit, contained in the chapters are presented; elements not evident are indicated by statements such as "none given" or "not identified."

FIRST STATEMENT: HOW RURAL
DWELLERS DEFINE HEALTH

The first statement indicates that "... rural dwellers define health primarily as the ability to work, to be productive, to do usual tasks (p. 10)." Work beliefs and health beliefs were key concepts while isolation and distance were identified as related concepts. Health, isolation, and distance were three of the four concepts analyzed.

Health beliefs (Long, 1998)

Analysis framework: Smith's (1983) four models of health—clinical, role
    performance, adaptive, eudemonistic
Definition: Rural dwellers often conceptualize health within the role
    performance model
Defining attributes (p. 213):

1. "ability to work ...[and] perform one's daily activities" (Long, p. 213)
2. "determine health needs primarily in relation to work activities" (Long, p. 213)
3. "as a result of their environment, rural dwellers are more frequently called upon to be independent and self-reliant" (Long, p. 212)

Antecedents: Beliefs held will affect "health-promotion behaviors, health
    care seeking, and acceptance of preventive and treatment interven-
    tions" (Long, p. 211).
Consequences: Knowledge of client's concept of health is important for
    development of relevant and acceptable assessment approaches and
    intervention strategies (Long, p. 213–214).
Empirical referents: none identified

Isolation (Lee, Hollis, & McClain, 1998)

Analysis framework: Walker & Avant, 1995
Definition: none given
Essential attributes:

1. separation—"being divided from the rest" (Lee et al., p. 69)
2. relativeness—"something dependent on external conditions for its specific nature ... existing or having its specific nature only by relation to something else; not absolute or independent" (Lee et al., p. 69)
3. perception—"consciousness or awareness" (Lee et al., p. 69)

Antecedents: "presence of an indicator directing attention to the condition of isolation (geographical terrain, distance, changes imposed by weather, economic costs, time or personal preference) (Lee et al., p. 69)

Consequences: "decreased communication or interaction with other individuals that results in social or professional isolation" (Lee et al., p. 70)

Empirical referents: None identified

Distance (Henson, Sadler, & Walton, 1998)

Method of analysis: Walker & Avant, 1988

Definition: "implies a degree of separation between two or more entities.... The nature of separation may be in space, time or behavior." (Henson et al., 1998, p. 51)

Essential attributes:

1. mileage—"total number of miles traveled" (Henson et al., p. 56)
2. time—"measurement in minutes it takes to travel from one place to another" (Henson et al., p. 56)
3. perception—"variation in awareness of data that is different from others' awareness" (Henson et al., p. 56)

Antecedent: "access to health care" (Henson et al., p. 58)

Consequence: "potential for compromised health care" (Henson et al., p. 58)

Empirical referents

Objective:

1. "distance" (miles, kilometers) (Henson et al., p. 58)
2. "travel time" (Henson et al., p. 58)
3. MSU Rurality Index (county of residence population, distance to emergency care); (Weinert & Boik, 1995)

Subjective: "perception" (Henson et al., p. 58)

SECOND STATEMENT: SELF-RELIANCE

The second statement is "... rural dwellers are self-reliant and resist accepting help or services from those seen as 'outsiders' or from agencies seen as national or regional 'welfare' programs. A corollary to this statement is that help, including needed health care, is usually sought through an informal rather than a formal system (p. 11)." Key concepts analyzed were self-reliance, outsider, insider, old-timer, newcomer, resources, informal networks, and lay care network.

Self-Reliance (Chafey, Sullivan, & Shannon, 1998)

Method of analysis: Qualitative research inquiry (Morse, 1995)
Definition:

1. "the capacity to provide for one's own needs" (Agich, 1993, as cited in Chafey et al., p. 158)
2. "the desire to do for one self and care for oneself" (Long & Weinert, 1989, as cited in Chafey et al., p. 158)

Sample: Cohort of nine women between 70–85 years of age living in small rural towns
Interview: Structured guide developed to elicit participants' perceptions of self-reliance (p. 160).
Characteristics:
    Primary

1. learned— a skill emanating from previous learning events that started in their youth (family chores & assumption of responsibilities), continued into adulthood and was reinforced by later life events (retirement, death of a parent or spouse). (Chafey et al., p. 162)
2. decisional choice—"making one's own decisions and choices" (Chafey et al., p. 164)
3. independence— independence or dependence on self, dependence of others, self-assertion or freedom of action, and self-identity" (Chafey et al., p. 166)

    Secondary— embodied an aspect of their self-reliance experience

1. self-confidence (Chafey et al., p. 170)
2. self-competence (Chafey et al., p. 170–171)

Outsider (Bailey, 1998)

Method of analysis: Walker and Avant (1988)
Definition: "being exterior to the group, matter, or boundary in question" (Bailey, p. 140)

Defining attributes:

1. differentness— "in terms of cultural orientation, standards, lifestyle, education, religion, occupation, social status, worldview, interests, or experience": "the quality or state of being different" (Bailey, p. 143–144)
2. unfamiliarity— with the matter in question (Bailey, p. 144)
3. unconnectedness—"having no family of personal ties" (Bailey, p. 144)

Antecedents: "... lacking understanding or knowledge of the social context, beliefs, rituals, customs and history of the community" (Bailey, p.144)
Consequences: "... one may be excluded from access to knowledge and information, not be accepted, not be recognized, be isolated, and be distrusted" (Bailey, p. 144)
Empirical referents: none identified

Insider (Myers, 1998)

Method of analysis: Walker and Avant (1995)
Definition: "... someone who is a member of a group and has access to special or privileged information" (Myers, p. 127)
Defining attributes:

1. "member of a group" (Myers, p. 132)
2. "having access to privileged information" (Myers, p. 132)
3. "an awareness of implicit assumptions and social context" (Myers, p. 132)
4. "a long-time occupant" (Myers, p. 132)

Antecedents: "acceptance by the group" (Myers, p. 135)
Consequences (Myers, p. 135):

1. "power ... because of having information that others lack" (Myers, p. 135)
2. "reserved social position ... that is unavailable to others" (Myers, p. 135)
3. "lack of objectivity" (Myers, p. 135)
4. "committed to the group" (Myers, p. 135)

Empirical referents: none identified

Old-Timer (Caniparoli, 1998)

Method of analysis: Walker and Avant (1995)
Definition:

1. "one who is long established in a place or position" (Caniparoli, p. 103)
2. "a man who has lived in the county a long time" (American slang; p. 103)

Defining attributes:

1. "age" (Caniparoli, p. 108)
2. "length of time spent in a community" (Caniparoli, p. 108)
3. "establishment of a relationship within the community" (Caniparoli, p. 108)

Antecedents: "identification as an old-timer" (Caniparoli, p. 110)
Consequences: "establishes a relationship within the community ... [that] can be viewed as positive or negative depending on the role of the viewer" (Caniparoli, p. 110)
Empirical referents: none identified

Newcomer (Sutermaster, 1998)

Method of analysis: Walker and Avant (1995)
Definition: "one than has recently arrived" (Sutermaster, p. 113)
Defining attributes:

1. "newly arrived" (Sutermaster, p. 120)
2. "unaware of the history of the area/institution" (Sutermaster, p. 120)
3. "their existence may result in change" (Sutermaster, p. 120)

Antecedents: Individuals or families would have had a need or desire to move" (Sutermaster, p. 121).
Consequences: "There is a new individual or family living in the community" (Sutermaster, p. 121).
Empirical referents: none identified

Resources (Ballantyne, 1998)

Method of analysis: Walker and Avant (1995)

Definition: "Resources are properties, resorts, or assets that are finite by nature and are made available for use by populations through an allocation process. Resources are accessed and used in response to a population's or individual's motivation for need satisfaction.... . Furthermore, these three elements can be visualized in a circle with the flow of energy between the allocated resource, accessibility of the resource, and use of the resource." (Ballantyne, p. 181)
Defining attributes:

1. property—"resource is a property or an asset that has value for consumption by populations in need of that property" (Ballantyne, p. 181)
2. expedient—"continuance or plan for solution of a particular problem" (Ballantyne, p. 181)
3. resort—"turning inward to one's resources" (Ballantyne, p. 181)

Antecedents: knowledge of availability (Ballantyne, p. 187)
Consequences: access to health care
Empirical referents: none identified

Informal Networks (Grossman & McNerney, 1998)

Method of analysis: Walker and Avant (1995)
Definition: "'networks are interconnected relationships, durable patterns of interactions, and interpersonal threads that comprise a social fabric'" (Grossman & McNerney, pp. 201–202)
Defining attributes:

1. volunteer; includes family members, coworkers, and neighbors who offers assistance free of charge (Grossman & McNerney, p. 204)
2. information exchange (Grossman & McNerney, p. 204)
3. support— has two components: emotional component (being a friend, listening) and physical (assistance with daily living, health promotion and maintenance activities) (Grossman & McNerney, p. 204)
4. guidance; "may be given as advice, consultation (availability of resources, referral to health care providers, sources of alternative treatments), and information" (Grossman & McNerney, p. 204)

Antecedents:

1. "a bond ... the tie that exists among ... the core of the informal network (family, friends, neighbors, and coworkers)" (Grossman & McNerney, p. 206):

2. "are generated in response to a perceived need" (Grossman & Mc-Nerney, p. 206):

Consequences: "the perceived need is met or not met" (Grossman & McNerney, p. 206)
Empirical referents: none identified

Lay Care Network (Turnbull, 1998)

Method of analysis: Walker and Avant (1988)
Definition: none given
Defining attributes:

1. interconnection or net— "An interconnection is the means by which one thing connects with another, whereas a net consists of fibers woven together for catching something" (Turnbull, p. 195),
2. of the people— "belonging to, concerned with, or performed by the 'people' in a nonprofessional capacity" (Turnbull, p. 195)
3. sense of concern — "the idea that one develops or maintains an interest in the well-being of a person or object, to oversee with the intent to protect" (Oxford , 1989 as cited in Turnbull, p. 195).

Antecedents: none identified
Consequences: none identified
Empirical referents: none identified
Conclusion: Turnbull (1998) recommends "further refinement of the concept, 'lay care provider,' and suggests a change in the wording of the concept itself" (p. 198). The literature review clearly delineates between "lay providers" and "informal care providers" whereas the wording, lay care providers, combines two different concepts.

THIRD STATEMENT: LACK OF ANONYMITY AND ROLE DIFFUSION

The third statement is "… health care providers in rural areas must deal with a lack of anonymity and much greater role diffusion than providers in urban or suburban settings (p. 11)." The key concepts are lack of anonymity and role diffusion. Related concepts are familiarity and professional isolation. Analyzed were anonymity, familiarity, and professional isolation.

Lack of anonymity (Lee, 1998)

Method of analysis: Walker & Avant (1995)
Definition: "a condition in which one cannot remain nameless or unknown" (Lee, p. 77)
Defining attributes:

1. visible— "that which can be seen, is apparent or obvious" (Lee, p. 83)
2. identifiable— being able to recognize or establish; the condition or character of a person" (Lee, p. 83)
3. diminished personal/professional boundaries: borders or perimeters through which one functions are smaller, more circumscribed" (Lee, p. 83)

Antecedents: "Lack of anonymity occurs in an environmental context characterized by a low level of stimulation. It contains fewer number of individuals and/or objects (e.g., automobiles, buildings) needing to be considered in the normal deliberation of one's activities." (Lee, pp. 83–84)
Consequences: "... a relationship [in which] one's actions are visible and readily observed" (Lee, p. 84). Greater difficulty in maintaining personal and professional privacy exists because of the relationship.
Empirical referents: none identified

Familiarity (McNeely & Shreffler, 1998)

Method of analysis: Walker and Avant (1995)
Definition: "an antithetical concept that includes the positive ideas of thorough knowledge of or an acquaintance with and closeness and intimacy, such as one would find in a family or deep friendship, and the contrasting perspective of offensive, unwarranted, intimate conduct that might include behaviors such as flirting, sexual harassment, domestic violence, abusive relationships, or incest" (McNeely & Shreffler, p. 91).
Defining attributes:

1. "friendly relationship or close acquaintance" (McNeely & Shreffler, p. 98)
2. "intimacy" (McNeely & Shreffler, p. 98)
3. "informality" (McNeely & Shreffler, p. 98)
4. "the exhibited familiarity is welcome or unwelcome depending on the perceptions of the receiver" (McNeely & Shreffler, p. 98)

Antecedents: none identified
Consequences: none identified
Empirical referents: none identified

Professional Isolation (Shreffler, 1998)

Method of analysis: Walker & Avant, 1988
Definition: none given
Defining attributes:

> "... an actual separation from or a deficiency in a resource needed to fulfill one's professional responsibilities or needs (objective component)" (Shreffler, p. 426)
> "professional need is perceived as partially or wholly unmet (subjective component)" (Shreffler, p. 426)
> "the actual separation or deficiency is on a continuum" (Shreffler, p. 426)
> "the individual is not voluntarily separating her/himself from an available professional resource" (Shreffler, p. 426)
> "the objective component is more likely to be present in rural areas" (Shreffler, p. 426)

Antecedents:

> The individuals experience "... separation from or deficiency in resources needed to fulfill professional responsibilities," and have "needs for resources to fulfill their professional responsibilities," "can make choices about the use of available resources" and "are able to perceive whether professional needs are met" (Shreffler, p. 429).

Consequences: "are specific to the need that is unmet and the vulnerabilities of the individual in the occupation or job position" (Shreffler, p. 429)
Empirical referents:

1. "... the availability of the needed resource is measured and found deficient" (Shreffler, p. 429)
2. "individuals ... express awareness of an unmet need or exhibit signs of the consequence of the unmet need" (Shreffler, pp. 429–430).

CONCLUSION

In this appendix, we summarize the concepts found in the first edition of *Conceptual Basis of Rural Nursing*. Most of the analyses were conducted using the Wilson method (Walker & Avant, 1995). However, some of the elements (e.g., definition, antecedents, consequences, empirical referents) were not addressed. Furthermore, some key concepts were not analyzed (e.g., work beliefs, role diffusion). Further development of the concepts is needed. Paramount is the need for validation of concepts with rural dwellers.

REFERENCES

Bailey, M. C. (1998). Outsider. In H. J. Lee (Ed.), *Conceptual basis for rural nursing* (1st ed., pp. 139–148). New York: Springer Publishing.

Ballantyne, J. (1998). Health resources and the rural client. In H. J. Lee (Ed.), *Conceptual basis for rural nursing* (1st ed., pp. 178–198). New York: Springer Publishing.

Caniparoli, C. D. (1998). Old–timer. In H. J. Lee (Ed.), *Conceptual basis for rural nursing* (1st ed., pp. 102–112). New York: Springer Publishing.

Chafey, K., Sullivan, T., & Shannon, A. (1998). Self reliance: Characteristics of their own autonomy by elderly rural women. In H. J. Lee (Ed.), *Conceptual basis for rural nursing* (1st ed., pp. 156–177). New York: Springer Publishing.

Grossman, L. L, & McNerney, S. (1998). Informal networks. In H. J. Lee (Ed.), *Conceptual basis for rural nursing* (1st ed., pp. 200–208). New York: Springer Publishing.

Henson, D., Sadler, T., & Walton, S. (1998). Distance. In H. J. Lee (Ed.), *Conceptual basis for rural nursing* (1st ed., pp. 51–60). New York: Springer Publishing.

Lee, H. J. (1998). Lack of anonymity. In H. J. Lee (Ed.), *Conceptual basis for rural nursing* (1st ed., pp. 76–88). New York: Springer Publishing.

Lee, H. J., Hollis, B. R., & McClain, K. A. (1998). Isolation. In H. J. Lee (Ed.), *Conceptual basis for rural nursing* (1st ed., pp. 139–148). New York: Springer Publishing.

Long, K. A. (1998). The concept of health: Rural perspectives. In H. J. Lee (Ed.), *Conceptual basis for rural nursing* (1st ed., pp. 139–148). New York: Springer Publishing.

Long, K A., & Weinert, C. Rural nursing: Developing the theory base. In H. J. Lee (Ed.),*Conceptual basis for rural nursing* (1st ed., pp. 3–18). New York: Springer Publishing.

McNeely, A. G., & Shreffler, M. J. (1998). Familiarity. In H. J. Lee (Ed.), *Conceptual basis for rural nursing* (1st ed., pp. 89–101). New York: Springer Publishing.

Morse, M. J. (1995). Exploring the theoretical basis of nursing using advanced techniques of concept analysis. *Advances in Nursing Science, 17* (3), 31–46.

Myers, D. D. (1998). Insider. In H. J. Lee (Ed.), *Conceptual basis for rural nursing* (1st ed., pp. 125–138). New York: Springer Publishing.

Shreffler, M. J. (1998). Professional isolation: A concept analysis. In H. J. Lee (Ed.), *Conceptual basis for rural nursing* (1st ed., pp. 420–432). New York: Springer Publishing.

Smith, J. A. (1983). *The idea of health: Implications for the nursing profession.* New York: Teachers College Press.

Sutermaster, D. J. (1998). Newcomer. In H. J. Lee (Ed.), *Conceptual basis for rural nursing* (1st ed., pp. 113–124). New York: Springer Publishing.

Turnbull, T. S. (1998) Lay care network. In H. J. Lee (Ed.), *Conceptual basis for rural nursing* (1st ed., pp. 189–199). New York: Springer Publishing.

Walker, L., & Avant, K. (1988). *Strategies for theory construction in nursing.* Norwalk, CT: Appleton-Century-Crafts

Walker, L., & Avant, K. (1995). *Strategies for theory construction in nursing* (3rd ed.). Norwalk, CT: Appleton-Century-Crofts.

Weinert, C., & Bork, R. (1995). MSU ruality index: Development and evaluation. *Research in Nursing and Health, 18,* 453–464.

INDEX

Aboriginal people, need for more
    research on health beliefs, 324
Acceptability
    component of choice of health care,
        166–176
    definition, 96
Acceptability Scale. See Scale,
        Appendix A, 175–176
    description, 169–170
    results of testing, 170–172
Access to health care services
    conceptual framework for
        acceptability study, 167–168
    distance and resources, 317
    literature support for, rural nursing
        theory, 24
Access within reason. See Themes,
        Health perceptions, needs, and
        behaviors
Accountability, related to
        interpersonal knowing, 188
'Aces,' 190, 195.
    See also Pinch Hitter Theory of
        Rural Nursing
Acts of balancing. See Enduring acts
    of balancing
Advice lay consultants, rural school
    secretaries, 288
Affirming affirmations, lack of
    anonymity
    Personally. See Perceptions, lack of
        anonymity
    Professionally. See Perceptions, lack
        of anonymity

American Association of Critical Care
        Nurses (AACN).
    See Professional nurse
        organizations
    Telemedicine, 251–252
American Indian. See Native
        American
American Nurses' Association (ANA).
    See Professional nursing
        organizations
    Social Policy Statement, rural
        nursing study framework, 182,
        207
        Core, 183, 210
        Boundary, 183, 210–211
        Dimensions, 182–183, 208–210
        Intersections, 182, 207–208
        Nature and scope, 182–183
    Telenursing, 252
Anonymity. See Lack of anonymity
Antecedents
    distance, 333
    health beliefs, 332
    informal networks, 337–338
    insider, 335
    isolation, 333
    lack of anonymity, 339
    newcomer, 336
    old-timer, 336
    outsider, 335
    professional isolation, 340
    resources, 337
Attributes, defining/essential
    distance, 333

Attributes, defining/essential
    (*continued*)
  familiarity, 339
  health beliefs, 332
  informal networks, 337
  insider, 335
  isolation, 332
  lack of anonymity, 339
  lay care network, 338
  newcomer, 336
  old-timer, 336
  outsider, 335
  professional isolation, 340
  resources, 337
  self-reliance, 334
Autonomy
  Continuum with job variety and
    satisfaction, community health,
    212–214
  See Opportunities, men in nursing

Balancing, enduring acts of. *See* Rural
    family health
Barriers in continuing education. *See*
    Deterrents
Becoming hardy. *See* Resilience,
    developing
Benefits, public health emergency
    preparedness, 265–266
Boundary of rural nursing. *See* ANA,
    Social Policy statement

Cancer, isolated rural women living
    with. *See* Chronic illness
    experience
Carbon monoxide (CO) exposure
  Testing procedures, 274
  Exposure of rural children, 276,
    278
Challenge
  educational, using interdisciplinary
    approach, 297–299
  public health emergency
    preparedness, 263–265
  See Opportunities, men in nursing
Characteristics
  old-timers. *See* Themes, old-timers
  self-reliance, 334
Children, rural,
  environmental risk reduction,
    270–281

Children first. *See* Themes, health
    perceptions, needs, and
    behaviors
Choice (s)
  characteristic of self-reliance, 334
  component of acceptability of
    health care, 166–176
  in strategizing safety, 108
  newly emerging theme, 316–317
  sub-themes
    residence, 35, 36–37
    health care provider, 35, 36–37
  theme, exploring nursing theory
    across borders, 35, 36–37
Choosing. *See* Safety, strategizing,
    perinatal experiences of rural
    women
Chronic illness experience, isolated
    rural women, 153–165
Community functions of old-timers.
    See Themes, old-timers
Community support. *See* Themes,
    health needs and perceptions
Comparison study, exploring rural
    nursing theory across borders,
    27–39
Computer education
  academic education, obtaining,
    252–254
  continuing education, obtaining,
    251–252
  Consequences
    distance, 333
    health beliefs, 332
    informal networks, 338
    insider, 335
    isolation, 333
    lack of anonymity, 339
    newcomer, 336
    old-timer, 336
    outsider, 335
    professional isolation, 340
    resilience, 92–93
    resources, 337
Consumer, conscientious. *See* Themes,
    health needs and perceptions of
    rural persons
Context, northern. *See* Resilience,
    developing
Continuing education. *See also*
    computer education

deterrents, 249–250
professional nursing organizations, 254
rural nurses, 187–188, 248–256
telenursing, 252
telemedicine, 251–252
Conscientious consumer. *See* Themes, health needs and perceptions
Core of rural nursing. *See* ANA Social Policy statement
Critical Access Hospitals (CAH), 166–167, 235–236, 326–327
results of accessibility study, 170–172

Data ordering scheme, rural nursing theory development, 7–8
Declining (deterioration). *See* Consequence of resilience
Definition
autonomy, 212
distance, 333
familiarity, 339
frontier, 130, 198
health beliefs, 332
job satisfaction, 212
job variety, 212
informal networks, 337
insider, 335
lack of anonymity, 9, 339
old-timer, 336
outsider, 334
newcomer, 336
remote isolated, 81
remote rural/rural remote, 54–55, 68, 81
resources, 337
rural, 81, 111, 130, 206
rural nursing, 4, 195–196
self-reliance, 9, 334
Definition(s) of health
part of first theoretical statement, 9–10, 11, 313
proposed revision of first statement, 314
sub-themes of definition of health
illness, 34
sickness, 34
theme, exploring nursing theory across borders, 34
Definition, rural. *See* Definition, rural

Delay in seeking health care, rural persons, 193, 195, 210
Deterrents to continuing education, 249–250
Dimensions of rural nursing. *See* ANA, Social Policy statement
Distance
concept analysis summary, 333
identified as key concept, rural nursing theory base, 8–9
literature support for, rural nursing theory, 23–24
need for further research, 315–316
place in further theory development, 317–318
sub-themes. *See* Themes, exploring rural nursing theory across borders
rural, 35, 37
northern, 35, 37
theme, exploring nursing theory across borders, 35, 37
Distance as a way of life. *See* Themes, health perceptions, needs, and behaviors
Distance disadvantage in an emergency. *See* Themes, health perceptions, needs, and behaviors

Education and professional development, rural nurses, 187
Education, computer. *See* Computer education
Education, continuing. *See* Continuing education
Educational modules
Phases of development, HERE project, 292–297
Educational outreach
addressing nursing shortage, 328, 248–256
Efficacy, perceived, of collective community action. *See* perceived efficacy
Elders. *See* 'graying' of rural areas
Empirical referents
distance, 333
professional isolation, 340
Emerging themes for theory development
choices, 316–317
health-seeking behaviors, 316

Enduring acts of balancing, rural families creating health, 110–126
  family caring 120–121
  family identity, 117–118
  family relationships 119
  family work 121
  times of transition, 117
Environmental risk patterns, rural areas, 271
Environmental Risk Reduction through Nursing Intervention and Education study (ERRNIE), 272–281
Environmental tobacco smoke (ETS) exposure of rural children, 275
  testing procedures, 274
Episodic evaluation. See Themes, health perceptions, needs, and behaviors
Essential attributes. See Attributes, defining/essential
Expanded practice. See Opportunities, men in nursing

Familiarity, concept analysis summary, 339–340
Fine tuning. See Safety, strategizing, perinatal experiences of rural women
Fish Out of Water: Novice to Expert. See Themes, rural nursing generalist
Flowing Like a River, metatheme. See Themes, rural nursing generalist
Following through. See Safety, strategizing, perinatal experiences of rural women
Formal health systems, component of second theoretical statement, 10, 21–22, 314–315
Frontier, definition. See Definition, frontier
Frontier areas, preparedness. See Preparedness, public health emergency
Future direction for rural nursing theory, 317–318

Generalist, rural nurse
  acute care setting, 218–231
  community health setting, 205–217

and continuing education, 248
hospital, 186
and rural nursing theory, 10, 12, 14
Going with the Flow: Fluid Role. See Themes, rural nursing generalist
Golden hour of emergency medicine, 219
'Graying' of rural areas, 324

Hardiness. See Themes, health needs and perceptions
Hardy, becoming. See Resilience, developing
Health Care Professional Shortage Areas (HPSA), 292
Health literacy, improving elders, 291–300
Health beliefs
  changing, 324
  concept analysis summary, 332
  identified as key concept, rural nursing theory base, 8–9
Health promotion, 21, 314, 319, 325
Health-seeking behaviors,
  Emerging concept, comparison study, 34–35, 316
  Sub-themes of emerging concept, comparison study
  Symptom-action-time-line, 34, 36
  Resources, 34, 36
  Self-reliance, 35, 36
Health Enhancement of the Rural Elderly project (HERE), 291–300
Historical perspectives, rural nursing theory base, 17–18
Holistic health. See Themes, health perceptions, needs, and behaviors
Hospitals, rural, 219
  See Critical access hospitals (CAH)

Illness, sub-theme of Definition of health. See Definition of health, sub-themes
Implications, education
  based on first rural nursing theory statement, 323
  based on second rural nursing theory statement, 325
  based on third rural nursing theory statement, 327

from study, rural nursing generalist, 229–230

Implications, nursing administration from study, rural nursing generalist, 228–229

Implications, nursing practice
based on first rural nursing theory statement, 323
based on second rural nursing statement, 325–326
based on third rural nursing statement, 327–328
based on rural nursing, developing the theory base 13–14
from study, health needs and perceptions of rural persons, 53–65
from study, exploring rural nursing theory across borders, 37–38
from study, lack of anonymity, 203
from study, old-timers 50–51
from study, rural nursing generalist, 227–228
from study, rural school health, 288–289
from study, women of childbearing and childrearing age, 76–77

Implications, nursing research
from study, men working as rural nurses, 245
from study, rural nursing generalist, 230
from study, women of childbearing and childrearing age, 77

Implications, policy
based on first rural nursing theory statement, 323–324
based on second rural nursing theory statement, 326–327
based on third rural nursing theory statement, 327–328

Implications, rural nursing theory
from study, exploring rural nursing theory across borders, 37–38
from study, lack of anonymity, 202–203
from study, rural school health, 287–288

Improving health literacy for rural elders, 291–300

Inadequate insurance. See Themes, health needs and perceptions

Independence, identified as key concept, rural nursing theory base, 9

Influence on community. See Themes, old-timers

Informal health system
part of second theoretical statement, 10, 21–22, 314–315314

Informal networks, concept analysis summary, 337

Informed risk. See Themes, health needs and perceptions

Insider
concept analysis summary, 335
differentiation at community level, 306–307
identified as key concept, rural nursing theory base, 8–9
rural nursing practice, 179
rural school secretaries, 288

Instruments
Acceptability Scale, 175–176

Interdisciplinary approach
challenges, rewards, lessons learned, 297–299
improving health literacy of rural elders, 291–300
phases, I—IV, 292–297

Interpersonal knowing, rural nursing practice, 188, 194

Interpersonal relationships. See Interpersonal knowing

Intersections of rural nursing. See ANA, Social Policy statement

Interventions, environmental risk, 279

Isolation
concept analysis summary, 332–333
identified as key concept, rural nursing theory base, 8–9
examination at community level, 307–308

Isolation, professional concept analysis summary, 340

Job responsibilities
community based nurses, 207–210
percentage of time spent 207

Job satisfaction. See Autonomy, continuum of

Job variety. See Autonomy, continuum of

Joint Commission on Accreditation of Hospitals, 184

Knowing fosters role comfort rural school secretaries, 284–288

Lack of anonymity
  concept analysis summary, 339
  examination at community level, 307
  identified as key concept, rural nursing theory base, 8–9
  part of third theoretical statement, 10, 12, 315
  perceptions of lack, 197–204
  and rural nursing, 196
Lay care network
  concept analysis summary, 338
Lay care resources, use of, 144
Lead poisoning
  exposure of rural children, 276, 278
  testing procedures, 274
Lessons learned
  educational, using interdisciplinary approach, 297–299
Life in a Fish Bowl: Contextual Knowledge of Patients. See Themes, rural nursing generalist
Listserv, rural nursing and theory development, 318–319
Literacy, health, improving rural elders, 291–300

Maintaining balance. See Themes, online support group intervention
Making the best of the North. See Resilience, developing
Meaningful relationships. See Opportunities, men in nursing
Medicine, practicing, as related to rural nursing, 189–190, 238
Metatheme: Flowing Like a River. See Themes, rural nurse generalist
Middle range theory, 18, 317–318
Models
  Multiple Exposures Multiple Effects, 272–272
  Smith's four models of health, 332

MSU Rurality Index, empirical referent for concept of distance, 333
Moving the theory development work forward, 318–319
Multiple sclerosis (MS), isolated rural women living with. See Chronic illness experience

Name descriptors of older residents. See Themes, old-timers
Native American
  need for more research on health beliefs, 324
  women, sample for SATL process, 130–131
Nature and scope of nursing, 182–183, 190–195
Newcomer
  concept analysis summary, 336
  identified as key concept, rural nursing theory base, 8–9
  and rural nurses, 186, 195
North American Study group (NAS), moving the work forward, 318–319
Northern, sub-theme of distance. See Distance, sub-themes
Northern context. See Resilience, developing
Novice to Expert. See Themes, Rural nursing generalist, Fish Out of Water
Nurse generalist. See Generalist, rural nurse
Nursing. See Definition, rural nursing
Nursing shortages. See Shortages, nursing

Old-timer
  characteristics. See Themes, old-timers
  community functions. See Themes, old-timers
  concept analysis summary, 336
  exploration of concept, 43–52
  identified as key concept, rural nursing theory base, 8–9
  name descriptors. See Themes, old-timers
  perceptions of their influence in the community. See Themes, old-timers

and rural nurses, 186, 192
rural nursing practice, 179
rural school secretaries, 287–288
Online support group intervention.
  See Chronic illness experience
Opportunities, men in nursing
  autonomy, 239–240
  challenge, 242
  expanded practice, 237–239
  meaningful relationships, 240–242
  recruitment, 243
  rural rewards, 242–243
Others first. *See* Themes, online
  support group intervention
Outsider
  concept analysis summary, 334–335
  differentiation at community level,
    306–307
  identified as key concept, rural
    nursing theory base, 8–9

Patterns of responses. *See* Symptom-
  action-time-line process
  (SATL)
Perinatal experiences of rural women.
  See Safety, strategizing
Perceived efficacy of collective
  community action, 302, 306
Perceptions, lack of anonymity
  personally affirming, 199
  personally threatening, 201–202
  professionally affirming, 199–200
  professionally threatening,
    200–201
Philosophical bases, rural nursing
  practice, 179–196
Physical and emotional isolation. *See*
  Themes, online support group
  intervention
'Pinch Hitter Theory of Rural
  Nursing,' 190–191
Preparedness, public health
  emergencies, 259–269
  benefits, 265–266
  challenges, 263–265
Prevention for life. *See* Themes,
  health perceptions, needs, and
  behaviors
Process stages/phases. *See* Symptom-
  action-time-line process
  (SATL)

Professional nursing organizations
  and continuing education. *See
  also* Computer education
  American Association of Critical
    Care Nurses (AACN), 254
  American Nurses' Association
    (ANA), 254
  Rural Nurse Organization (RNO),
    254
  Sigma Theta Tau International
    (STTI), 254
Professional isolation. *See* Isolation,
  professional
Professional resources, use of, 144
Public Health Emergency
  Preparedness and Response
  Capacity Assessment
  (PHEPRCA),
  Montana, 261–262
  qualitative portion report, 259–
    269

Qualitative research designs
  descriptive, 55–56
  ethnographic, 4–5, 29–33, 183
  exploratory descriptive, narrative,
    218–219
  feminist grounded theory, 80–82
  grounded theory, 45–46, 68–69,
    111–114, 130–131, 198, 283
  hermeneutic phenomenology,
    234–237
  multiple case study, 303–304
  secondary analysis, 155
  symbolic interactionism, 98–100
  textual discourse analysis, 262
Quantitative research designs
  cross sectional correlational,
    273–274
  survey, 6–7, 168–169

Radon, household
  exposure of rural children, 275–
    276, 277–278
  testing procedures, 275
Recruitment. *See* Opportunities, men
  in nursing
Resilience, developing, to manage
  vulnerability, 79–95
  becoming hardy, 88
  consequences, 92–94

making the best of the north, 89–90
northern context, 83–86
supplementing the north, 90–92
Relational statements. *See* Rural
nursing theory development,
theoretical statements
Resources
concept analysis summary, 336–337
place in further theory development,
317
sub-theme. *See* Health-seeking
behaviors, sub-themes
Retroductive theory generation, 6, 18
Rewards
educational, using interdisciplinary
approach, 297–299
Rheumatoid diseases, isolated rural
women living with. *See*
Chronic illness, experience
Risk, informed. *See* Themes, health
needs and perceptions
Role comfort, rural school secretaries,
286–287
Role diffusion, third theoretical
statement, 10, 12, 315
Role discomfort/ambivalence, rural
school secretaries, 286–287
Rural
being 180–181
definition. *See* Definition, rural
sub-theme of distance. *See* Distance,
sub-themes
Rural areas
preparedness. *See* Preparedness,
public health emergency
Rural communities, description, 185–
186
Rural children. *See* Children, rural
Rural elders
improving health literacy, 291–300
Rural families creating health. *See*
Enduring acts of balancing
Rural family health. *See* Enduring acts
of balancing
Rural health, priority, on community
level, 302, 305–306
Rural, knowing, 181–182
Rural nurse, description of
home health nurses (HHN),
206–217
hospital nurses, 186

public health nurses (PHN),
206–217
tribal, 206–217
Rural nurse generalist. *See*
Generalists, rural nurse
Rural nursing, defining. *See*
Definitions, rural nursing
Rural nursing theory development
suggested revision for first
theoretical statement, 314
suggested revision for second
theoretical statement, 315
theoretical statement, first, 9–10, 313
literature support for, 20–21
theoretical statement, second, 10,
314
literature support for, 21–22
theoretical statement, third, 10, 315
literature support for, 22–23
Rural Physician Action Plan in
Alberta, 328
Rural rewards. *See* Opportunities,
men in nursing
Rural school health. *See* School
health, rural
Rurality index. *See* MSU Rurality
Index

Safety, strategizing, perinatal
experiences of rural women,
96–109
choosing phase, 102–103
fine tuning phase, 104–106
following through phase, 103–104
seeking information phase, 102
Satisfaction, job. *See* Autonomy,
continuum of
Seeking information. *See* Safety,
strategizing, perinatal
experiences of rural women
School health, rural, 282–290
Scope of rural nursing, 182–183,
194–195
Self care, strategies to treat symptoms,
143
See Symptom-action-time-line
Self-reliance
Concept analysis summary, 334
identified as key concept, rural
nursing theory base, 8–9,
11–12

revised second theoretical
statement, 314–315
sub-theme, health-seeking
behaviors. See Health-Seeking
behaviors, sub-theme
theme, rural nursing generalist. See
Rural nursing generalist, Still
Waters Run Deep
theme, health needs and perceptions
of rural persons. See Themes,
Health needs and perceptions
Shortage, nursing
and male nurses, 232–233
See Educational outreach
Sickness, sub-theme of definition of
health. See Definition of health,
sub-themes
Sigma Theta Tau International.
See Professional nursing
organizations
Still Waters Run Deep: Self Reliance.
See Themes, rural nursing
generalist
Story, Western Slant, 224–227
Strategizing safety. See Safety,
strategizing
Superfund Amendments and Reauthorization Act (SARA), 260
Supplementing the North. See
Resilience, developing
Surviving (stability). See Consequences
of resilience
Symptom-action-time-line process
(SATL)
lay resources stage, 133–134, 139
patterns of responses, 129–137
professional resources stage,
134–135, 139
recommendations for revision,
147–149
self-care stage, 132–133, 139
symptom identification stage, 132, 139
sub-theme. See Health seeking
behaviors
theme. See Themes, exploring rural
nursing theory across borders
time line variations, 135, 144
updating, 138–152

Telemedicine. See Continuing
education

Telenursing. See Continuing education
Themes, exploring nursing theory
across borders
choices, 35
definitions of health, 34
distance, 35
health-seeking behaviors, 34–35
Themes, health needs and perceptions,
57–64
community support, 61
conscientious consumer, 59
hardiness, 58–59
inadequate insurance, 61–62
informed risk, 59–61
self-reliance, 57–58
Themes, health perceptions, needs,
and behaviors of remote rural
women of childbearing and
childrearing age, 69–79
access within reason, 75–76
children first, 74–75
distance as a way of life, 69–71
distance as a disadvantage in an
emergency, 69–73
episodic evaluation, 73–74
holistic health, 76
prevention for life, 75–76
Themes, men in nursing. See
Opportunities, men in nursing
Themes, old-timers
name descriptors of older residents,
47
characteristics of old-timers, 47–48
community functions of old-timers
48–50
old-timers perceptions of their
influence in the community, 50
Themes, online support group
intervention
maintaining balance, 158–159
others first, 159
physical and emotional isolation,
158
uncertainty/searching for answers,
158
vigilance: Finance, physical,
emotional, 159–160
ways of coping, 160–161
Themes, rural nursing generalist
Fish Out of Water: Novice to
Expert, 222

Themes, rural nursing generalist
    (continued)
  Going with the Flow: Fluid Role,
    221–222
  Life in a Fish Bowl: Contextual
    Knowledge of Patients,
    222–223
  Metatheme: Flowing Like a River,
    223
  Still Waters Run Deep: Self
    Reliance, 222
Themes. See Emerging themes for
    theory development
Threatening affirmations, lack of
    anonymity
  personally. See Perceptions, lack of
    anonymity
  professionally. See Perceptions, lack
    of anonymity
Thriving (growth). See Consequences,
    resilience
Time line variations. See Symptom-
    action-time-line process (SATL)
Tobacco smoke. See Environmental
    tobacco smoke
Trial by Fire, 222

Uncertainty. See Themes, online
    support group intervention

Variety, job. See Autonomy,
    continuum
Vigilance. See Themes, online support
    group intervention
Vision for the future, 318

Vulnerability to health risks
  inadequate health care, 87–88
  physical health and safety, 86
  psychosocial health, 87
  See Resilience, developing to
    manage vulnerability

Ways of coping. See Themes, online
    support group intervention
Well water contaminants,
  exposure of rural children, 276,
    278–279
  testing procedures, 275
Western Slant. See Story, Western
    Slant
Women's health research
  chronic illness experience of rural
    women, 153–165
  health perceptions, needs, and
    behaviors of remote rural
    women of childbearing and
    childrearing age, 66–78
  rural and remote women
    developing resilience to manage
    vulnerability, 79–95
  strategizing safety, perinatal
    experiences of rural women,
    96–109
Women to Women (WTW). See
    Chronic illness experience
Work beliefs
  enduring acts of balancing, 123
  identified as key concept, rural
    nursing theory base, 8–9